Air Fryer, Electric and Woo  er

Cookbook [6 I

Thousands of Flaming Recipes with Advanced Tricks to Smoke Just

Everything

By

Chef Carlo Leone

The trademarks that are used are without any consent, and the publication of the trademark is without permission or backing by the trademark owner. All trademarks and brands within this book are for clarifying purposes only and are the owned by the owners themselves, not affiliated with this document.

Author: Chef Carlo Leone

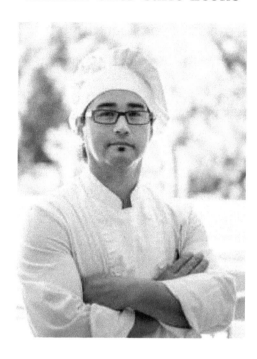

Chef Carlo Leone is the leading authority on the science and application of the carnivore diet. He used his best years of experience to build the perfect diet recipes to reverse self-immunity, chronic inflammation and mental health problems helping hundreds of people. Chef Carlo Leone went viral after showing some of his best recipes through social networks in the late 2018. The great reviews spurred him to find the perfect medium to teach him about his delicious masterpieces. Here we can officially celebrate the 7 new releases of Chef Carlo Leone taken from the brand-new series: "The Butcher Boot Camp". A real collection of kitchen manuals that will leave a mark on the palate of all your friends and family.

Table of Contents

Air Fryer Cookbook for Two

Vegan Air Fryer Cookbook

The Complete Air Fryer Cookbook with Pictures

The Healthy Air Fryer Cookbook with Pictures

Wood Pellet Smoker Grill Cookbook

The Ultimate Electric Smoker Cookbook

Air Fryer Cookbook for Two

Cook and Taste Tens of Healthy Fried Recipes with Your Sweetheart. Burn Fat, Kill Hunger, and Improve Your Mood

By

Chef Carlo Leone

Table of Contents

Introduction:

You have got the set of important knives, toaster oven, coffee machine, and quick pot along with the cutter you want to good care of. There may be a variety of things inside your kitchen, but maybe you wish to make more space for an air fryer. It's easy to crowd and load with the new cooking equipment even though you've a lot of them. However, an air fryer is something you will want to make space for.

The air fryer is identical to the oven in the way that it roasts and bakes, but the distinction is that elements of hating are placed over the top& are supported by a big, strong fan, producing food that is extremely crispy and, most importantly with little oil in comparison to the counterparts which are deeply fried. Usually, air fryers heat up pretty fast and, because of the centralized heat source & the fan size and placement, they prepare meals quickly & uniformly. The cleanup is another huge component of the air frying. Many baskets & racks for air fryers are dishwasher protected. We recommend a decent dish brush for those who are not dishwasher secure. It will go through all the crannies and nooks that facilitate the movement of air without making you crazy.

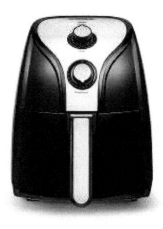

We have seen many rave reviews of this new trend, air frying. Since air frying, they argue, calls for fast and nutritious foods. But is the hype worth it? How do the air fryers work? Does it really fry food?

How do air fryers work?

First, let's consider how air fryer really works before we go to which type of air fryer is decent or any simple recipes. Just think of it; cooking stuff without oil is such a miracle. Then, how could this even be possible? Let's try to find out how to pick the best air fryer for your use now when you understand how the air fryer works.

How to pick the best air fryer

It is common to get lost when purchasing gadgets & electrical equipment, given that there're a wide range of choices available on the market. So, before investing in one, it is really ideal to have in mind the specifications and budget.

Before purchasing the air fryer, you can see the things you should consider:

Capacity/size: Air fryers are of various sizes, from one liter to sixteen liters. A three-liter capacity is fine enough for bachelors. Choose an air fryer that has a range of 4–6 liters for a family having two children. There is a restricted size of the basket which is used to put the food. You will have to prepare the meals in batches if you probably wind up using a tiny air fryer.

Timer: Standard air fryers arrive with a range timer of 30 minutes. For house cooking, it is satisfactory. Thought, if you are trying complex recipes which take a longer cooking time, pick the air fryer with a 1-hour timer.

Temperature: The optimum temperature for most common air fryers is 200 degrees C (400 f). You can quickly prepare meat dishes such as fried chicken, tandoori, kebabs etc.

The design, durability, brand value and controls are other considerations you might consider.

Now that you know which air fryer is best for you let's see the advantages of having an air fryer at your place.

What are the benefits of air fryers?

The benefits of air fryers are as follows:

Cooking with lower fat & will promote weight loss

Air fryers work with no oils and contain up to 80 percent lower fat than most fryers relative to a traditional deep fryer. Shifting to an air fryer may encourage loss of weight by decreasing fat & caloric intake for anyone who consumes fried food regularly and also has a problem with leaving the fast foods.

Faster time for cooking

Air frying is easier comparing with other cooking techniques, such as grilling or baking. Few air fryers need a preheat of 60 seconds, but others do not need a preheat any longer than a grill or an oven. So if there is a greater capacity or multiple compartments for the air fryer basket, you may make various dishes in one go.

Quick to clean

It's extremely easy to clean an air fryer. And after each use, air frying usually does not create enough of a mess except you cook fatty food such as steak or chicken wings. Take the air fryer out and clean it with soap & water in order to disinfect the air fryer.

Safer to be used

The air fryer is having no drawbacks, unlike hot plates or deep frying. Air fryers get hot, but splashing or spilling is not a risk.

Minimum use of electricity and environment friendly

Air fryers consume far less electricity than various electric ovens, saving your money & reducing carbon output.

Flexibility

Some of the air fryers are multi-functional. It's possible to heat, roast, steam, broil, fry or grill food.

Less waste and mess

Pan-fries or deep fryer strategies leave one with excess cooking oil, which is difficult to rid of and usually unsustainable. You can cook fully oil-less food with an air fryer. All the pieces have a coating of nonstick, dishwasher safe and nonstick coating.

Cooking without the use of hands

The air fryer includes a timer, & when it is full, it'll stop by itself so that you may feel secure while multitasking.

Feasible to use

It is very much convenient; you can use an air fryer whenever you want to. Few air fryers involve preheating, which is less than 5 minutes; with the air fryer, one may begin cooking immediately.

Reducing the possibility of the development of toxic acrylamide

Compared to making food in oil, air frying will decrease the potential of producing acrylamides. Acrylamide is a compound that, under elevated temperature cooking, appears in certain food and may have health impacts.

Chapter 1: Air fryer breakfast recipes

1. Air fryer breakfast frittata

Cook time: 20 minutes

Servings: 2 people

Difficulty: Easy

Ingredients:

- 1 pinch of cayenne pepper (not necessary)

- 1 chopped green onion

- Cooking spray

- 2 tbsp. diced red bell pepper

- ¼ pound fully cooked and crumbled breakfast sausages

- 4 lightly beaten eggs

- ½ cup shredded cheddar-Monterey jack cheese blend

Instructions:

1. Combine eggs, bell pepper, cheddar Monterey Jack cheese, sausages, cayenne and onion inside a bowl & blend to combine.

2. The air fryer should be preheated to 360 ° f (180° c). Spray a 6 by 2-inch non-stick cake pan along with a spray used in cooking.

3. Place the mixture of egg in the ready-made cake tray.

4. Cook for 18 - 20 minutes in your air fryer before the frittata is ready.

2. Air fryer banana bread

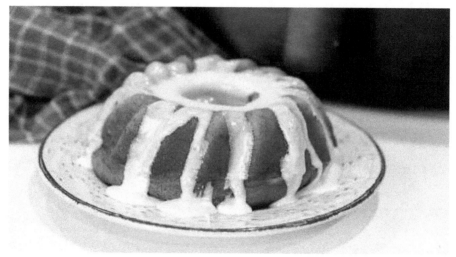

Cook time: 28 minutes

Serving: 8 people

Difficulty: Easy

Ingredients:

- 3/4 cup flour for all purposes

- 1/4 tbsp. salt

- 1 egg

- 2 mashed bananas overripe

- 1/4 cup sour cream

- 1/2 cup sugar

- 1/4 tbsp. baking soda

- 7-inch bundt pan

- 1/4 cup vegetable oil

- 1/2 tbsp. vanilla

Instructions:

1. In one tub, combine the dry ingredients and the wet ones in another. Mix the two slowly till flour is fully integrated, don't over mix.

2. With an anti-stick spray, spray and on a 7-inch bundt pan & then pour in the bowl.

3. Put it inside the air fryer basket & close. Placed it for 28 mins to 310 degrees

4. Remove when completed & permit to rest in the pan for about 5 mins.

5. When completed, detach and allow 5 minutes to sit in the pan. Then flip on a plate gently. Sprinkle melted icing on top, serve after slicing.

3. Easy air fryer omelet

Cook time: 8 minutes

Serving: 2 people

Difficulty: Easy

Ingredients:

- 1/4 cup shredded cheese

- 2 eggs

- Pinch of salt

- 1 teaspoon of McCormick morning breakfast seasoning – garden herb

- Fresh meat & veggies, diced

- 1/4 cup milk

Instructions:

1. In a tiny tub, mix the milk and eggs till all of them are well mixed.

2. Add a little salt in the mixture of an egg.

3. Then, in the mixture of egg, add the veggies.

4. Pour the mixture of egg in a greased pan of 6 by 3 inches.

5. Place your pan inside the air fryer container.

6. Cook for about 8 to 10 mins and at 350 f.

7. While you are cooking, slather the breakfast seasoning over the eggs & slather the cheese on the top.

8. With a thin spoon, loose the omelet from the pan and pass it to a tray.

9. Loosen the omelet from the sides of the pan with a thin spatula and pass it to a tray.

10. Its options to garnish it with additional green onions.

4. Air-fried breakfast bombs

Cook time: 20 mins

Serving: 2

Difficulty: easy

Ingredients:

- Cooking spray

- 1 tbsp. fresh chives chopped

- 3 lightly beaten, large eggs

- 4 ounces whole-wheat pizza dough freshly prepared

- 3 bacon slices center-cut

- 1 ounce 1/3-less-fat softened cream cheese

Instructions:

1. Cook the bacon in a standard size skillet for around 10 minutes, medium to very crisp. Take the bacon out of the pan; scatter. Add the eggs to the bacon drippings inside the pan; then cook, stirring constantly, around 1 minute, until almost firm and yet loose. Place the eggs in a bowl; add the cream cheese, the chives, and the crumbled bacon.

2. Divide the dough into four identical sections. Roll each bit into a five-inch circle on a thinly floured surface. Place a quarter of the egg mixture in the middle of each circle of dough. Clean the underside of the dough with the help of water; wrap the dough all around the mixture of an egg to form a purse and pinch the dough.

3. Put dough purses inside the air fryer basket in one layer; coat really well with the help of cooking spray. Cook for 5 to 6 minutes at 350 degrees f till it turns to a golden brown; check after 4 mins.

5. Air fryer French toast

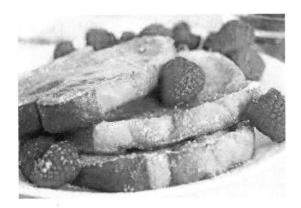

Cook time: 15 mins

Serving: 2 people

Difficulty: easy

Ingredients:

- 4 beaten eggs

- 4 slices of bread

- Cooking spray (non-stick)

Instructions:

1. Put the eggs inside a container or a bowl which is sufficient and big, so the pieces of bread will fit inside.

2. With a fork, mix the eggs and after that, place each bread slice over the mixture of an egg.

3. Turn the bread for one time so that every side is filled with a mixture of an egg.

4. After that, fold a big sheet of aluminum foil; this will keep the bread together. Switch the foil's side; this will ensure that the mixture of an egg may not get dry. Now put the foil basket in the air fryer basket. Make sure to allow space around the edges; this will let the circulation of hot air.

5. With the help of cooking spray, spray the surface of the foil basket and then put the bread over it. On top, you may add the excess mixture of an egg.

6. For 5 mins, place the time to 365 degrees f.

7. Turn the bread & cook it again for about 3 to 5 mins, until it's golden brown over the top of the French toast & the egg isn't runny.

8. Serve it hot, with toppings of your choice.

6. Breakfast potatoes in the air fryer

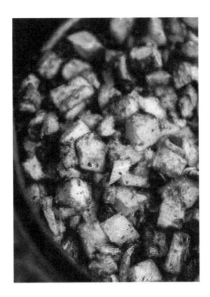

Cook time: 15 mins

Servings: 2

Difficulty: easy

Ingredients:

- 1/2 tbsp. kosher salt

- 1/2 tbsp. garlic powder

- Breakfast potato seasoning

- 1/2 tbsp. smoked paprika

- 1 tbsp. oil

- 5 potatoes medium-sized. Peeled & cut to one-inch cubes (Yukon gold works best)

- 1/4 tbsp. black ground pepper

Instructions:

1. At 400 degrees f, preheat the air fryer for around 2 to 3 minutes. Doing this will provide you the potatoes that are crispiest.

2. Besides that, brush your potatoes with oil and breakfast potato seasoning till it is fully coated.

3. Using a spray that's non-stick, spray on the air fryer. Add potatoes & cook for about 15 mins, shaking and stopping the basket for 2 to 3 times so that you can have better cooking.

4. Place it on a plate & serve it immediately.

7. Air fryer breakfast pockets

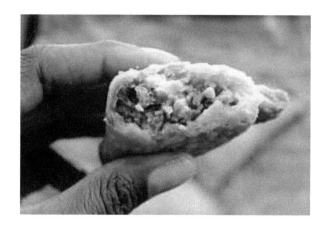

Cook time: 15 mins

Serving: 5 people

Difficulty: easy

Ingredients:

- 2-gallon zip lock bags

- Salt & pepper to taste

- 1/3 + 1/4 cup of whole milk

- 1 whole egg for egg wash

- Cooking spray

- 1-2 ounces of Velveeta cheese

- Parchment paper

- 1 lb. of ground pork

- 2 packages of Pillsbury pie crust

  - 2 crusts to a package

- 4 whole eggs

Instructions:

1. Let the pie crusts out of the freezer.

2. Brown the pig and rinse it.

3. In a tiny pot, heat 1/4 cup of cheese and milk until it is melted.

4. Whisk four eggs, season with pepper and salt & add the rest of the milk.

5. Fumble the eggs in the pan until they are nearly fully cooked.

6. Mix the eggs, cheese and meat together.

7. Roll out the pie crust & cut it into a circle of about 3 to 4 inches (cereal bowl size).

8. Whisk 1 egg for making an egg wash.

9. Put around 2 tbsp. of the blend in the center of every circle.

10. Now, eggs wash the sides of the circle.

11. Create a moon shape by folding the circle.

12. With the help of a fork, folded edges must be crimped

13. Place the pockets inside parchment paper & put it inside a ziplock plastic bag overnight.

14. Preheat the air fryer for 360 degrees until it is ready to serve.

15. With a cooking spray, each pocket side must be sprayed.

16. Put pockets inside the preheated air fryer for around 15 mins or till they are golden brown.

17. Take it out from the air fryer & make sure it's cool before you serve it.

8. Air fryer sausage breakfast casserole

Cook time: 20 mins

Serving: 6 people

Difficulty: easy

Ingredients:

- 1 diced red bell pepper

- 1 lb. ground breakfast sausage

- 4 eggs

- 1 diced green bell pepper

- 1/4 cup diced sweet onion

- 1 diced yellow bell pepper

- 1 lb. hash browns

Instructions:

1. Foil line your air fryer's basket.

2. At the bottom, put some hash browns.

3. Cover it with the raw sausage.

4. Place the onions & peppers uniformly on top.

5. Cook for 10 mins at 355 degrees.

6. Open your air fryer & blend the casserole a little if necessary.

7. Break every egg inside the bowl and spill it directly over the casserole.

8. Cook for the next 10 minutes for 355 degrees.

9. Serve with pepper and salt for taste.

9. Breakfast egg rolls

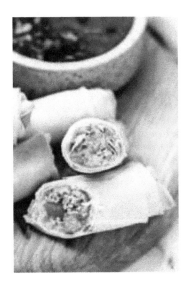

Cook time: 15 mins

Servings: 6 people

Difficulty: easy

Ingredients:

- Black pepper, to taste

- 6 large eggs

- Olive oil spray

- 2 tbsp. chopped green onions

- 1 tablespoon water

- 1/4 teaspoon kosher salt

- 2 tablespoons diced red bell pepper

- 1/2 pound turkey or chicken sausage

- 12 egg roll wrappers

- The salsa that is optional for dipping

Instructions:

1. Combine the water, salt and black pepper with the eggs.

2. Cook sausage in a non-stick skillet of medium size, make sure to let it cook in medium heat till there's no pink color left for 4 minutes, splitting into crumbles, then drain.

3. Stir in peppers and scallions & cook it for 2 minutes. Put it on a plate.

4. Over moderate flame, heat your skillet & spray it with oil.

5. Pour the egg mixture & cook stirring till the eggs are cooked and fluffy. Mix the sausage mixture.

6. Put one wrapped egg roll on a dry, clean work surface having corners aligned like it's a diamond.

7. Include an egg mixture of 1/4 cup on the lower third of your wrapper.

8. Gently raise the lower point closest to you & tie it around your filling.

9. Fold the right & left corners towards the middle & continue rolling into the compact cylinder.

10. Do this again with the leftover wrappers and fillings.

11. Spray oil on every side of your egg roll & rub it with hands to cover them evenly.

12. The air fryer must be preheated to 370 degrees f.

13. Cook the egg rolls for about 10 minutes in batches till it's crispy and golden brown.

14. Serve instantly with salsa, if required.

10. Air fryer breakfast casserole

Cook time: 45 mins

Servings: 6 people

Difficulty: medium

Ingredients:

• 1 tbsp. extra virgin olive oil

• Salt and pepper

• 4 bacon rashers

• 1 tbsp. oregano

• 1 tbsp. garlic powder

- 2 bread rolls stale

- 1 tbsp. parsley

- 320 grams grated cheese

- 4 sweet potatoes of medium size

- 3 spring onions

- 8 pork sausages of medium size

- 11 large eggs

- 1 bell pepper

Instructions:

1. Dice and peel the sweet potato in cubes. Mix the garlic, salt, oregano and pepper in a bowl with olive oil of extra virgin.

2. In an air fryer, put your sweet potatoes. Dice the mixed peppers, cut the sausages in quarters & dice the bacon.

3. Add the peppers, bacon and sausages over the sweet potatoes. Air fry it at 160c or 320 f for 15 mins.

4. Cube and slice the bread when your air fryer is heating & pound your eggs in a blending jug with the eggs, including some extra parsley along with pepper and salt. Dice the spring onion.

5. Check the potatoes when you hear a beep from the air fryer. A fork is needed to check on the potatoes. If you are unable to, then cook for a further 2 to 3 minutes. Mix the basket of the air fryer, include the spring onions & then cook it for an additional five minutes with the same temperature and cooking time.

6. Using the projected baking pans, place the components of your air fryer on 2 of them. Mix it while adding bread and cheese. Add your mixture of egg on them & they are primed for the actual air fry.

7. Put the baking pan inside your air fryer & cook for 25 minutes for 160 c or 320 f. If you planned to cook 2, cook 1 first and then the other one. Place a cocktail stick into the middle & then it's done if it comes out clear and clean.

11. Air fryer breakfast sausage ingredients

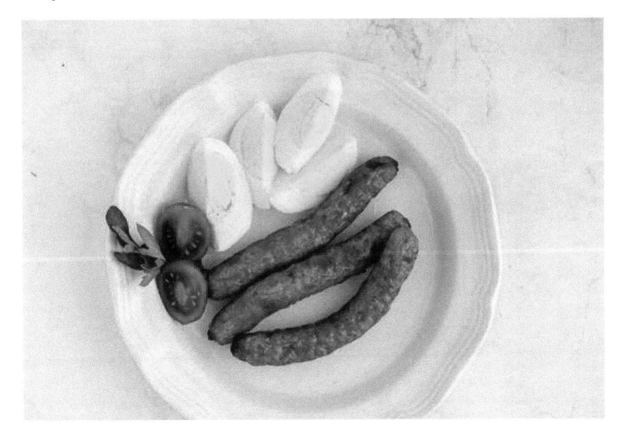

Cook time: 10 mins

Serving: 2 people

Difficulty: easy

Ingredients:

- 1 pound breakfast sausage

- Air fryer breakfast sausage ingredients

Instructions:

1. Insert your sausage links in the basket of an air fryer.

2. Cook your sausages or the sausage links for around 8 to 10 minutes at 360°.

12. Wake up air fryer avocado boats

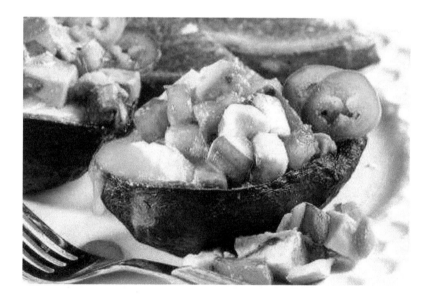

Cook time: 5 mins

Servings: 2

Difficulty: easy

Ingredients:

- 1/2 teaspoon salt

- 2 plum tomatoes, seeded & diced

- 1/4 teaspoon black pepper

- 1 tablespoon finely diced jalapeno (optional)

- 4 eggs (medium or large recommended)

- 1/4 cup diced red onion

- 2 avocados, halved & pitted

- 1 tablespoon lime juice

- 2 tablespoons chopped fresh cilantro

Instructions:

1. Squeeze the avocado fruit out from the skin with a spoon, leaving the shell preserved. Dice the avocado and put it in a bowl of medium-sized. Combine it with onion, jalapeno (if there is a need), tomato, pepper and cilantro. Refrigerate and cover the mixture of avocado until ready for usage.

2. Preheat the air-fryer for 350° f

3. Place the avocado shells on a ring made up of failing to make sure they don't rock when cooking. Just roll 2 three-inch-wide strips of aluminum foil into rope shapes to create them, and turn each one into a three-inch circle. In an air fryer basket, put every avocado shell over a foil frame. Break an egg in every avocado shell & air fry for 5 - 7 minutes or when needed.

4. Take it out from the basket; fill including avocado salsa & serve.

12. Air fryer cinnamon rolls

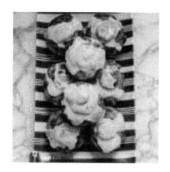

Cook time: 15 mins

Serving: 2 people

Difficulty: easy

Ingredients:

- 1 spray must non-stick cooking spray

- 1 can cinnamon rolls we used Pillsbury

Instructions:

1. put your cinnamon rolls inside your air fryer's basket, with the help of the rounds of 2. Parchment paper or by the cooking spray that is non-stick.

2. Cook at around 340 degrees f, 171 degrees for about 12 to 15 minutes, for one time.

3. Drizzle it with icing, place it on a plate and then serve.

13. Air-fryer all-American breakfast dumplings

Cook: 10 minutes

Servings: 1 person

Difficulty: easy

Ingredients:

• Dash salt

• 1/2 cup (about four large) egg whites or liquid egg fat-free substitute

• 1 tbsp. Pre-cooked real crumbled bacon

• 1 wedge the laughing cow light creamy Swiss cheese (or 1 tbsp. reduced-fat cream cheese)

• 8 wonton wrappers or gyoza

Instructions:

1. By using a non-stick spray, spray your microwave-safe bowl or mug. Include egg whites or any substitute, salt and cheese wedge. Microwave it for around 1.5 minutes, mixing in between until cheese gets well mixed and melted and the egg is set.

2. Mix the bacon in. Let it cool completely for about 5 minutes.

3. Cover a wrapper of gyoza with the mixture of an egg (1 tablespoon). Moist the corners with water & fold it in half, having the filling. Tightly push the corners to seal. Repeat this step to make seven more dumplings. Make sure to use a non-stick spray for spraying.

4. Insert the dumplings inside your air fryer in one single layer. (Save the leftover for another round if they all can't fit). Adjust the temperature to 375 or the closest degree. Cook it for around 5 mins or till it's crispy and golden brown.

Chapter 2: Air fryer seafood recipe

1. Air fryer 'shrimp boil'

Cook time: 15 mins

Servings: 2 people

Difficulty: easy

Ingredients:

- 2 tbsp. vegetable oil

- 1 lb. easy-peel defrosted shrimp

- 3 small red potatoes cut 1/2 inch rounds

- 1 tbsp. old bay seasoning

- 2 ears of corn cut into thirds

- 14 oz. smoked sausage, cut into three-inch pieces

Instructions:

1. Mix all the items altogether inside a huge tub & drizzle it with old bay seasoning, peppers, oil and salt. Switch to the air fryer basket attachment & place the basket over the pot.

2. Put inside your air fryer & adjust the setting of fish; make sure to flip after seven minutes.

3. Cautiously remove & then serve.

2. Air fryer fish & chips

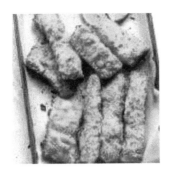

Cook time: 10 mins

Serving: 6 people

Difficulty: easy

Ingredients:

- Tartar sauce for serving

- ½ tbsp. garlic powder

- 1 pound cod fillet cut into strips

- Black pepper

- 2 cups panko breadcrumbs

- ½ cup all-purpose flour

- ¼ tbsp. salt

- Large egg beaten

- Lemon wedges for serving

- 2 teaspoons paprika

Instructions:

1. In a tiny tub, combine the flour, adding salt, paprika and garlic powder. Put your beaten egg in one bowl & your panko breadcrumbs in another bowl.

2. Wipe your fish dry with a towel. Dredge your fish with the mixture of flour, now the egg & gradually your panko breadcrumbs, pushing down gently till your crumbs stick. Spray both ends with oil.

3. Fry at 400 degrees f. Now turn halfway for around 10 to 12 mins until it's lightly brown and crispy.

4. Open your basket & search for preferred crispiness with the help of a fork to know if it easily flakes off. You may hold fish for an extra 1 to 2 mins as required.

5. Serve instantly with tartar sauce and fries, if required.

3. Air-fryer scallops

Cook time: 20 mins

Servings: 2 people

Difficulty: easy

Ingredients:

- ¼ cup extra-virgin olive oil

- ½ tbsp. garlic finely chopped

- Cooking spray

- ½ teaspoons finely chopped garlic

- 8 large (1-oz.) Sea scallops, cleaned & patted very dry

- 1 tbsp. finely grated lemon zest

- ⅛ tbsp. salt

- 2 tbsps. Very finely chopped flat-leaf parsley

- 2 tbsp. capers, very finely chopped

- ¼ tbsp. ground pepper

Instructions:

1. Sprinkle the scallops with salt and pepper. Cover the air fryer basket by the cooking spray. Put your scallops inside the basket & cover them by the cooking spray. Put your basket inside the air fryer. Cook your scallops at a degree of 400 f till they attain the temperature of about 120 degrees f, which is an international temperature for 6 mins.

2. Mix capers, oil, garlic, lemon zest and parsley inside a tiny tub. Sprinkle over your scallops.

4. Air fryer tilapia

Cook time: 6 mins

Servings: 4 people

Difficulty: easy

Ingredients:

- 1/2 tbsp. paprika

- 1 tbsp. salt

- 2 eggs

- 4 fillets of tilapia

- 1 tbsp. garlic powder

- 1/2 teaspoon black pepper

- 1/2 cup flour

- 2 tbsp. lemon zest

- 1 tbsp. garlic powder

- 4 ounces parmesan cheese, grated

Instructions:

1. Cover your tilapia fillets:

Arrange three deep dishes. Out of these, put flour in one. Blend egg in second and make sure that the eggs are whisked in the last dish mix lemon zest, cheese, pepper, paprika and salt. Ensure that the tilapia fillets are dry, and after that dip, every fillet inside the flour & covers every side. Dip into your egg wash & pass them for coating every side of the fillet to your cheese mixture.

2. Cook your tilapia:

Put a tiny sheet of parchment paper in your bask of air fryer and put 1 - 2 fillets inside the baskets. Cook at 400°f for around 4 - 5 minutes till the crust seems golden brown, and the cheese completely melts.

5. Air fryer salmon

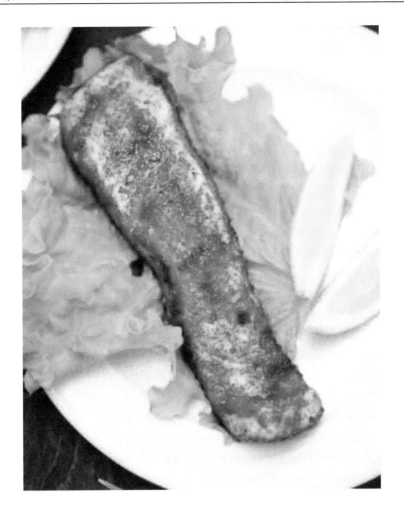

Cook time: 7 mins

Serving: 2 people

Difficulty: easy

Ingredients:

- 1/2 tbsp. salt

- 2 tbsp. olive oil

- 1/4 teaspoon ground black pepper

- 2 salmon fillets (about 1 1/2-inches thick)

- 1/2 teaspoon ginger powder

- 2 teaspoons smoked paprika

- 1 teaspoon onion powder

- 1/4 teaspoon red pepper flakes

- 1 tbsp. garlic powder

- 1 tablespoon brown sugar (optional)

Instructions:

1. Take the fish out of the refrigerator, check if there are any bones, & let it rest for 1 hour on the table.

2. Combine all the ingredients in a tub.

3. Apply olive oil in every fillet & then the dry rub solution.

4. Put the fillets in the Air Fryer basket.

5. set the air fryer for 7 minutes at the degree of 390 if your fillets have a thickness of 1-1/2-inches.

6. As soon as the timer stops, test fillets with a fork's help to ensure that they are ready to the perfect density. If you see that there is any need, then you cook it for a further few minutes. Your cooking time may vary with the temperature & size of the fish. It is best to set your air fryer for a minimum time, and then you may increase the time if there is a need. This will prevent the fish from being overcooked.

6. Blackened fish tacos in the air fryer

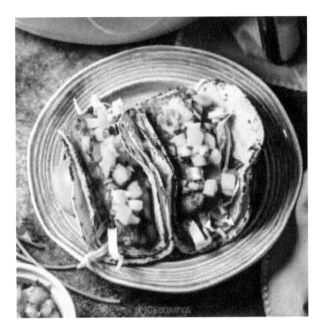

Cook time: 9 mins

Serving: 4 people

Difficulty: easy

Ingredients:

- 1 lb. Mahi mahi fillets (can use cod, catfish, tilapia or salmon)

- Cajun spices blend (or use 2-2.5 tbsp. store-bought Cajun spice blend)

- ¾ teaspoon salt

- 1 tbsp. paprika (regular, not smoked)

- 1 teaspoon oregano

- ½-¾ teaspoon cayenne (reduces or skips to preference)

- ½ teaspoon garlic powder

- ½ teaspoon onion powder

- ½ teaspoon black pepper

- 1 teaspoon brown sugar (skip for low-carb)

Additional ingredients for tacos:

- Mango salsa

- Shredded cabbage (optional)

- 8 corn tortillas

Instructions:

1. Get the fish ready

2. Mix cayenne, onion powder, brown sugar, salt, oregano, garlic powder, paprika and black pepper in a deep mixing tub.

3. Make sure to get the fish dry by using paper towels. Drizzle or brush the fish with a little amount of any cooking oil or olive oil. This allows the spices to stick to the fish.

4. Sprinkle your spice mix graciously on a single edge of your fish fillets. Rub the fish softly, so the ingredients stay on the fish.

5. Flip and brush the fish with oil on the other side & sprinkle with the leftover spices. Press the ingredients inside the fish softly.

6. Turn the air fryer on. Inside the basket put your fish fillets. Do not overlap the pan or overfill it. Close your basket.

7. Air fry the fish

8. Set your air fryer for 9 mins at 360°f. If you are using fillets which are thicker than an inch, then you must increase the cooking time to ten minutes. When the air fryer timer stops, with the help of a fish spatula or long tongs, remove your fish fillets.

9. Assembling the tacos

10. Heat the corn tortillas according to your preference. Conversely, roll them inside the towel made up of wet paper & heat them in the microwave for around 20 to 30 seconds.

11. Stack 2 small fillets or insert your fish fillet. Add a few tablespoons of your favorite mango salsa or condiment & cherish the scorched fish tacos.

12. Alternatively, one can include a few cabbages shredded inside the tacos & now add fish fillets on the top.

7. Air fryer cod

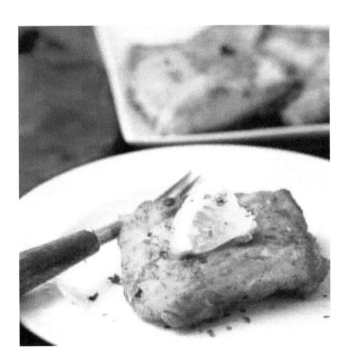

Cook time: 16 mins

Servings: 2 people

Difficulty: easy

Ingredients:

- 2 teaspoon of light oil for spraying

- 1 cup of plantain flour

- 0.25 teaspoon of salt

- 12 pieces of cod about 1 ½ pound

- 1 teaspoon of garlic powder

- 0.5 cup gluten-free flour blend

- 2 teaspoon of smoked paprika

- 4 teaspoons of Cajun seasoning or old bay

- Pepper to taste

Instructions:

1. Spray some oil on your air fryer basket & heat it up to 360° f.

2. Combine the ingredients in a tub & whisk them to blend. From your package, take the cod out and, with the help of a paper towel, pat dry.

3. Dunk every fish piece in the mixture of flour spice and flip it over & push down so that your fish can be coated.

4. Get the fish inside the basket of your air fryer. Ensure that there is room around every fish piece so that the air can flow round the fish.

5. Cook for around 8 minutes & open your air fryer so that you can flip your fish. Now cook another end for around 8 mins.

6. Now cherish the hot serving with lemon.

8. Air fryer miso-glazed Chilean sea bass

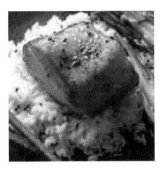

Cook time: 20 mins

Serving: 2 people

Difficulty: easy

Ingredients:

- 1/2 teaspoon ginger paste

- Fresh cracked pepper

- 1 tbsp. unsalted butter

- Olive oil for cooking

- 1 tbsp. rice wine vinegar

- 2 tbsp. miring

- 1/4 cup white miso paste

- 2 6 ounce Chilean sea bass fillets

- 4 tbsp. Maple syrup, honey works too.

Instructions:

1. Heat your air fryer to 375 degrees f. Apply olive oil onto every fish fillet and complete it with fresh pepper. Sprat olive oil on the pan of the air fryer and put the skin of the fish. Cook for about 12 to 15 minutes till you see the upper part

change into golden brown color & the inner temperature now reached 135-degree f.

2. When the fish is getting cooked, you must have the butter melted inside a tiny saucepan in medium heat. When you notice that the butter melts, add maple syrup, ginger paste, miso paste, miring and rice wine vinegar, mix all of them till they are completely combined, boil them in a light flame and take the pan out instantly from the heat.

3. When your fish is completely done, brush the glaze and fish sides with the help of silicone pastry. Put it back inside your air fryer for around 1 to 2 extra minutes at 375 degrees f, till the glaze is caramelized. Complete it with green onion (sliced) & sesame seeds.

Instructions for oven

1. Heat the oven around 425 degrees f and put your baking sheet and foil sprayed with light olive oil. Bake it for about 20 to 25 minutes; this depends on how thick the fish is. The inner temperature must be around 130 degrees f when your fish is completely cooked.

2. Take out your fish, placed it in the oven & heat the broiler on a high flame. Now the fish must be brushed with miso glaze from the sides and the top & then put the fish inside the oven in the above rack. If the rack is very much near with your broiler, then place it a bit down, you might not want the fish to touch the broiler. Cook your fish for around 1 to 2 minutes above the broiler till you see it's getting caramelize. Make sure to keep a check on it as it happens very quickly. Complete it with the help of green onions (sliced) and sesame seeds.

9. Air fryer fish tacos

Cook time: 35 mins

Serving: 6 people

Difficulty: Medium

Ingredients:

• ¼ teaspoon salt

• ¼ cup thinly sliced red onion

• 1 tbsp. water

• 2 tbsp. sour cream

• Sliced avocado, thinly sliced radishes, chopped fresh cilantro leaves and lime wedges

• 1 teaspoon lime juice

• ½ lb. skinless white fish fillets (such as halibut or mahi-mahi), cut into 1-inch strips

• 1 tbsp. mayonnaise

• 1 egg

• 1 package (12 bowls) old el Paso mini flour tortilla taco bowls, heated as directed on package

• 1 clove garlic, finely chopped

- ½ cup Progresso plain panko crispy bread crumbs

- 1 ½ cups shredded green cabbage

- 2 tbsp. old el Paso original taco seasoning mix (from 1-oz package)

Instructions:

1. Combine the sour cream, garlic, salt, mayonnaise and lime juice together in a medium pot. Add red onion and cabbage; flip to coat. Refrigerate and cover the mixture of cabbage until fit for serving.

2. Cut an 8-inch circle of parchment paper for frying. Place the basket at the bottom of the air fryer.

3. Place the taco-seasoning mix in a deep bowl. Beat the egg & water in another small bowl. Place the bread crumbs in another shallow dish. Coat the fish with your taco seasoning mix; dip inside the beaten egg, then cover with the mixture of bread crumbs, pressing to hold to it.

10. Air fryer southern fried catfish

Cook time: 13 mins

Servings: 4 people

Difficulty: easy

Ingredients:

- 1 lemon

- 1/4 teaspoon cayenne pepper

- Cornmeal seasoning mix

- 1/4 teaspoon granulated onion powder

- 1/2 cup cornmeal

- 1/2 teaspoon kosher salt

- 1/4 teaspoon chili powder

- 2 pounds catfish fillets

- 1/4 teaspoon garlic powder

- 1 cup milk

- 1/4 cup all-purpose flour

- 1/4 teaspoon freshly ground black pepper

- 2 tbsp. dried parsley flakes

- 1/2 cup yellow mustard

Instructions:

1. Add milk and put the catfish in a flat dish.

2. Slice the lemon in two & squeeze around two tbsp. of juice added into milk so that the buttermilk can be made.

3. Place the dish in the refrigerator & leave it for 15 minutes to soak the fillets.

4. Combine the cornmeal-seasoning mixture in a small bowl.

5. Take the fillets out from the buttermilk & pat them dry with the help of paper towels.

6. Spread the mustard evenly on both sides of the fillets.

7. Dip every fillet into a mixture of cornmeal & coat well to create a dense coating.

8. Place the fillets in the greased basket of the air fryer. Spray gently with olive oil.

9. Cook for around 10 minutes at 390 to 400 degrees. Turn over the fillets & spray them with oil & cook for another 3 to 5 mins.

11. Air fryer lobster tails with lemon butter

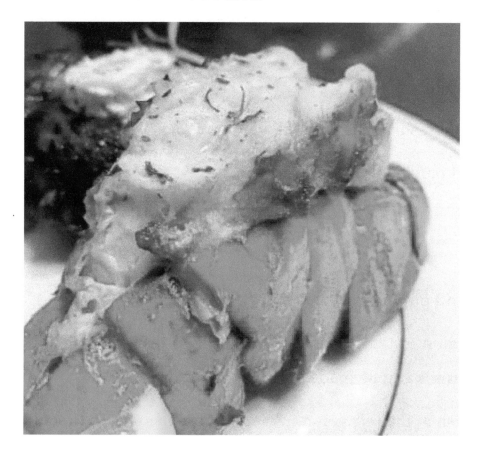

Cook time: 8 mins

Serving: 2 people

Difficulty: easy

Ingredients:

- 1 tbsp. fresh lemon juice

- 2 till 6 oz. Lobster tails, thawed

- Fresh chopped parsley for garnish (optional)

- 4 tbsp. melted salted butter

Instructions:

1. Make lemon butter combining lemon and melted butter. Mix properly & set aside.

2. Wash lobster tails & absorb the water with a paper towel. Butter your lobster tails by breaking the shell, take out the meat & place it over the shell.

3. Preheat the air fryer for around 5 minutes to 380 degrees. Place the ready lobster tails inside the basket of air fryer, drizzle with single tbsp. melted lemon butter on the meat of lobster. Cover the basket of the air fryer and cook for around 8 minutes at 380 degrees f, or when the lobster meat is not translucent. Open the air fryer halfway into the baking time, and then drizzle with extra lemon butter. Continue to bake until finished.

4. Remove the lobster tails carefully, garnish with crushed parsley if you want to, & plate. For dipping, serve with additional lemon butter.

12. Air fryer crab cakes with spicy aioli + lemon vinaigrette

Cook time: 20 mins

Servings: 2 people

Difficulty: easy

Ingredients:

For the crab cakes:

- 1. Avocado oil spray

- 16-ounce lump crab meat

- 1 egg, lightly beaten

- 2 tbsp. finely chopped red or orange pepper

- 1 tbsp. Dijon mustard

- 2 tbsp. finely chopped green onion

- 1/4 teaspoon ground pepper

- 1/4 cup panko breadcrumbs

- 2 tbsp. olive oil mayonnaise

For the aioli:

- 1/4 teaspoon cayenne pepper

- 1/4 cup olive oil mayonnaise

- 1 teaspoon white wine vinegar

- 1 teaspoon minced shallots

- 1 teaspoon Dijon mustard

For the vinaigrette:

- 2 tbsp. extra virgin olive oil

- 1 tbsp. white wine vinegar

- 4 tbsp. fresh lemon juice, about 1 ½ lemon

- 1 teaspoon honey

- 1 teaspoon lemon zest

To serve:

- Balsamic glaze, to taste

- 2 cups of baby arugula

Instructions:

1. Make your crab cake. Mix red pepper, mayonnaise, ground pepper, crab meat, onion, panko and Dijon in a huge bowl. Make sure to mix the ingredients well. Then add eggs & mix the mixture again till it's mixed well. Take around 1/4 cup of the mixture of crab into cakes which are around 1 inch thick. Spray with avocado oil gently.

2. Cook your crab cakes. Organize crab cakes in one layer in the air fryer. It depends on the air fryer how many batches will be required to cook them. Cook for 10 minutes at 375 degrees f. Take it out from your air fryer & keep it warm. Do this again if required.

3. Make aioli. Combine shallots, Dijon, vinegar, cayenne pepper and mayo. Put aside for serving until ready.

4. Make the vinaigrette. Combine honey, white vinegar, and lemon zest and lemon juice in a ting jar. Include olive oil & mix it well until mixed together.

5. Now serve. Split your arugula into 2 plates. Garnish with crab cakes. Drizzle it with vinaigrette & aioli. Include few drizzles of balsamic glaze if desired.

Chapter 3: Air Fryer Meat and Beef recipe

1. Air fryer steak

Cook time: 35 mins

Servings: 2

Difficulty: Medium

Ingredients:

- Freshly ground black pepper

- 1 tsp. freshly chopped chives

- 2 cloves garlic, minced

- 1(2 lb.) Bone-in rib eye

- 4 tbsp. Butter softened

- 1 tsp. Rosemary freshly chopped

- 2 tsp. Parsley freshly chopped

- 1 tsp. Thyme freshly chopped

- Kosher salt

Instructions:

1. In a tiny bowl, mix herbs and butter. Put a small layer of the wrap made up of plastic & roll in a log. Twist the ends altogether to make it refrigerate and tight till it gets hardened for around 20 minutes.

2. Season the steak with pepper and salt on every side.

3. Put the steak in the air-fryer basket & cook it around 400 degrees for 12 - 14 minutes, in medium temperature, depending on the thickness of the steak, tossing half-way through.

4. Cover your steak with the herb butter slice to serve.

2. Air-fryer ground beef wellington

Cook time: 20 mins

Serving: 2 people

Difficulty: easy

Ingredients:

- 1 large egg yolk

- 1 tsp. dried parsley flakes

- 2 tsp. flour for all-purpose

- 1/2 cup fresh mushrooms chopped

- 1 tbsp. butter

- 1/2 pound of ground beef

- 1 lightly beaten, large egg, it's optional

- 1/4 tsp. of pepper, divided

- 1/4 tsp. of salt

- 1 tube (having 4 ounces) crescent rolls refrigerated

- 2 tbsp. onion finely chopped

- 1/2 cup of half & half cream

Instructions:

1. Preheat the fryer to 300 degrees. Heat the butter over a moderate flame in a saucepan. Include mushrooms; stir, and cook for 5-6 minutes, until tender. Add flour & 1/8 of a tsp. of pepper when mixed. Add cream steadily. Boil it; stir and cook until thickened, for about 2 minutes. Take it out from heat & make it aside.

2. Combine 2 tbsp. of mushroom sauce, 1/8 tsp. of the remaining pepper, onion and egg yolk in a tub. Crumble over the mixture of beef and blend properly. Shape it into two loaves. Unroll and divide the crescent dough into two rectangles; push the perforations to close. Put meatloaf over every rectangle. Bring together the sides and press to seal. Brush it with one beaten egg if necessary.

3. Place the wellingtons on the greased tray inside the basket of the air fryer in a single sheet. Cook till see the thermometer placed into the meatloaf measures 160 degrees, 18 to 22 minutes and until you see golden brown color.

 Meanwhile, under low pressure, warm the leftover sauce; mix in the parsley. Serve your sauce, adding wellington.

3. Air-fried burgers

Cook time: 10 mins

Serving: 4 people

Difficulty: easy

Ingredients:

• 500 g of raw ground beef (1 lb.)

• 1 tsp. of Maggi seasoning sauce

• 1/2 tsp. of ground black pepper

• 1 tsp. parsley (dried)

- Liquid smoke (some drops)

- 1/2 tsp. of salt (salt sub)

- 1 tbsp. of Worcestershire sauce

- 1/2 tsp. of onion powder

- 1/2 tsp. of garlic powder

Instructions:

1. Spray the above tray, and set it aside. You don't have to spray your basket if you are having an air fryer of basket-type. The cooking temperature for basket types will be around 180 c or 350 f.

2. Mix all the spice things together in a little tub, such as the sauce of Worcestershire and dried parsley.

2. In a huge bowl, add it inside the beef.

3. Mix properly, and make sure to overburden the meat as this contributes to hard burgers.

4. Divide the mixture of beef into four, & the patties are to be shape off. Place your indent in the middle with the thumb to keep the patties from scrunching up on the center.

5. Place tray in the air fry; gently spray the surfaces of patties.

6. Cook for around 10 minutes over medium heat (or more than that to see that your food is complete). You don't have to turn your patties.

7. Serve it hot on a pan with your array of side dishes.

4. Air fryer meatloaf

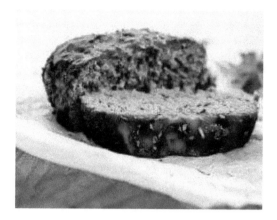

Cook time: 25 mins

Serving: 4 people

Difficulty: easy

Ingredients:

- 1/2 tsp. of Salt

- 1 tsp. of Worcestershire sauce

- 1/2 finely chopped, small onion

- 1 tbsp. of Yellow mustard

- 2 tbsp. of ketchup, divided

- 1 lb. Lean ground beef

- 1/2 tsp. Garlic powder

- 1/4 cup of dry breadcrumbs

- 1 egg, lightly beaten

- 1/4 tsp. Pepper

- 1 tsp. Italian seasoning

Instructions:

1. Put the onion, 1 tbsp. Ketchup, garlic powder, pepper, ground beef, egg, salt, breadcrumbs, Italian seasoning and Worcestershire sauce in a huge bowl.

2. Use hands to blend your spices with the meat equally, be careful you don't over-mix as it would make it difficult to over mix.

3. Shape meat having two inches height of 4 by 6, loaf. Switch your air fryer to a degree of 370 f & Put that loaf inside your air fryer.

4. Cook for fifteen min at a degree of 370 f.

5. In the meantime, mix the leftover 1 tbsp. of ketchup & the mustard in a tiny bowl.

6. Take the meatloaf out of the oven & spread the mixture of mustard over it.

7. Return the meatloaf to your air fryer & begin to bake at a degree of 370 degrees f till the thermometer placed inside the loaf measures 160 degrees f, around 8 to 10 further minutes.

8. Remove the basket from your air fryer when the meatloaf has touched 160 degrees f & then make the loaf stay inside the air fryer basket for around 5 to 10 minutes, after that slice your meatloaf.

5. Air fryer hamburgers

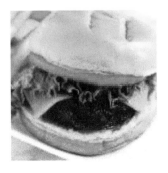

Cook time: 16 mins

Serving: 4 people

Difficulty: easy

Ingredients:

- 1 tsp. of onion powder

- 1 pound of ground beef (we are using 85/15)

- 4 pieces burger buns

- 1 tsp. salt

- 1/4 tsp. of black pepper

- 1 tsp. of garlic powder

- 1 tsp. of Worcestershire sauce

Instructions:

1. Method for standard ground beef:

2. Your air fryer must be preheated to 360 °.

3. In a bowl, put the unprocessed ground beef & add the seasonings.

4. To incorporate everything, make the of use your hands (or you can use a fork) & then shape the mixture in a ball shape (still inside the bowl).

5. Score the mixture of ground beef into 4 equal portions by having a + mark to split it.

Scoop out and turn each segment into a patty.

6. Place it in the air fryer, ensuring each patty has plenty of room to cook (make sure not to touch). If required, one can perform this in groups. We've got a bigger (5.8 quart) air fryer, and we did all of ours in a single batch.

7. Cook, turning half-way back, for 16 minutes. (Note: for bigger patties, you may have a need to cook longer.)

Process for Patties (pre-made):

1. In a tiny bowl, mix onion powder, pepper, garlic powder and salt, then stir till well mixed.

2. In a tiny bowl, pour in a few quantities of Worcestershire sauce. You may require A little more than one teaspoon (such as 1.5 tsp.), as some of it will adhere in your pastry brush.

3. Put patties on a tray & spoon or brush on a thin layer of your Worcestershire sauce.

4. Sprinkle with seasoning on every patty, saving 1/2 for another side.

5. With your hand, rub the seasoning to allow it to stick better.

6. Your air fryer should be preheated to 360 ° f.

7. Take out the basket when it's preheated & gently place your patties, seasoned one down, inside the basket.

8. Side 2 of the season, which is facing up the exact way as per above.

9. In an air fryer, put the basket back and cook for around 16 minutes, tossing midway through.

6. Air Fryer Meatloaf

Cook time: 25 mins

Serving: 4 people

Difficulty: Easy

Ingredients:

- Ground black pepper for taste

- 1 tbsp. of olive oil, or as required

- 1 egg, lightly beaten

- 1 tsp. of salt

- 1 pound of lean ground beef

- 1 tbsp. fresh thyme chopped

- 3 tbsp. of dry bread crumbs

- 1 finely chopped, small onion

- 2 thickly sliced mushrooms

Instructions:

1. Preheat your air fryer to a degree of 392 f (200°C).

2. Mix together egg, onion, salt, ground beef, pepper, bread crumbs and thyme in a tub. 3. Thoroughly knead & mix.

4. Transfer the mixture of beef in your baking pan & smooth out the surface. The mushrooms are to be pressed from the top & coated with the olive oil. Put the pan inside the basket of the air fryer & slide it inside your air fryer.

5. Set the timer of the air fryer for around 25 minutes & roast the meatloaf till it is nicely browned.

6. Make sure that the meatloaf stays for a minimum of 10 minutes, and after that, you can slice and serve.

7. Air Fryer Beef Kabobs

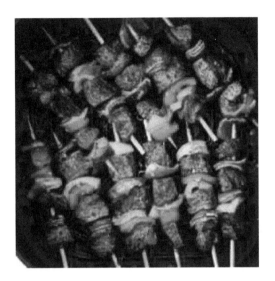

Cook time: 8 mins

Serving: 4 people

Difficulty: Easy

Ingredients:

- 1 big onion in red color or onion which you want

- 1.5 pounds of sirloin steak sliced into one-inch chunks

- 1 large bell pepper of your choice

For the marinade:

- 1 tbsp. of lemon juice

- Pinch of Salt & pepper

- 4 tbsp. of olive oil

- 1/2 tsp. of cumin

- 1/2 tsp. of chili powder

- 2 cloves garlic minced

Ingredients:

1. In a huge bowl, mix the beef & ingredients to marinade till fully mixed. Cover & marinate for around 30 minutes or up to 24 hours inside the fridge.

2. Preheat your air fryer to a degree of 400 f until prepared to cook. Thread the onion, pepper and beef onto skewers.

3. Put skewers inside the air fryer, which is already heated and the air fryer for about 8 to 10 minutes, rotating half-way until the outside is crispy and the inside is tender.

8. Air-Fried Beef and Vegetable Skewers

Cook time: 8 mins

Serving: 2

Difficulty: easy

Ingredients:

- 2 tbs. of olive oil

- 2 tsp. of fresh cilantro chopped

- Kosher salt & freshly black pepper ground

- 1 tiny yellow summer squash, sliced into one inch (of 2.5-cm) pieces

- 1/4 tsp. of ground coriander

- Lemon wedges to serve (optional)

- 1/8 tsp. of red pepper flakes

- 1 garlic clove, minced

- 1/2 tsp. of ground cumin

- 1/2 yellow bell pepper, sliced into one inch (that's 2.5-cm) pieces

- 1/2 red bell pepper, sliced into one inch (that's 2.5-cm) pieces

- 1/2 lb. (that's 250 g) boneless sirloin, sliced into one inch (of 2.5-cm) cubes

- 1 tiny zucchini, sliced into one inch (that's 2.5-cm) pieces

- 1/2 red onion, sliced into one inch (that's 2.5-cm) pieces

Ingredients:

1. Preheat your air fryer at 390 degrees f (199-degree c).

2. In a tiny bowl, mix together one tablespoon of cumin, red pepper flakes and coriander. Sprinkle the mixture of spices generously over the meat.

3. In a tub, mix together zucchini, oil, cilantro, bell peppers, summer squash, cilantro, onion and garlic. Season with black pepper and salt to taste.

4. Tightly thread the vegetables and meat onto the four skewers adding two layers rack of air fryer, rotating the bits and equally splitting them. Put the skewers over the rack & carefully set your rack inside the cooking basket. Put the basket inside the air fryer. Cook, without covering it for around 7 - 8 minutes, till the vegetables are crispy and tender & your meat is having a medium-rare.

5. Move your skewers to a tray, and if you want, you can serve them with delicious lemon wedges.

9. Air fryer taco calzones

Cook time: 10 mins

Serving: 2 people

Difficulty: easy

Ingredients:

- 1 cup of taco meat

- 1 tube of Pillsbury pizza dough thinly crust

- 1 cup of shredded cheddar

Instructions:

1. Spread out the layer of your pizza dough over a clean table. Slice the dough into four squares with the help of a pizza cutter.

2. By the use of a pizza cutter, cut every square into a big circle. Place the dough pieces aside to create chunks of sugary cinnamon.

3. Cover 1/2 of every dough circle with around 1/4 cup of taco meat & 1/4 cup of shredded cheese.

4. To seal it firmly, fold the remaining over the cheese and meat and push the sides of your dough along with the help of a fork so that it can be tightly sealed. Repeat for all 4 calzones.

5. Each calzone much is gently picked up & spray with olive oil or pan spray. Organize them inside the basket of Air Fryer.

Cook your calzones at a degree of 325 for almost 8 to 10 minutes. Monitor them carefully when it reaches to 8 min mark. This is done so that there is no chance of overcooking.

6. Using salsa & sour cream to serve.

7. For the making of cinnamon sugary chunks, split the dough pieces into pieces having equal sides of around 2 inches long. Put them inside the basket of the air

fryer & cook it at a degree of 325 for around 5 minutes. Instantly mix with the one ratio four sugary cinnamon mixtures.

10. Air Fryer Pot Roast

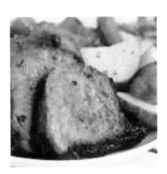

Cook time: 30 mins

Serving: 2 people

Difficulty: Medium

Ingredients:

- 1 tsp. of salt

- 3 tbsp. of brown sugar

- 1/2 cup of orange juice

- 1 tsp. of Worcestershire sauce

- 1/2 tsp. of pepper

- 3-4 pound thawed roast beef chuck roast

- 3 tbsp. of soy sauce

Instructions:

1. Combine brown sugar, Worcestershire sauce, soy sauce and orange juice.

2. Mix till the sugar is completely dissolved.

3. Spillover the roast & marinade for around 8 to 24 hours.

4. Put the roast in the basket of an air fryer.

5. Sprinkle the top with pepper and salt.

6. Air fry it at a degree of 400 f for around 30 minutes, turning it half-way through.

7. Allow it to pause for a period of 3 minutes.

8. Slice and serve into thick cuts.

Chapter 4: midnight snacks

1. Air fryer onion rings

Cook time: 7 mins

Serving: 2 people

Difficulty: easy

Ingredients:

- 2 beaten, large eggs

- Marinara sauce for serving

- 1 ½ tsp. of kosher salt

- ½ tsp. of garlic powder

- 1 medium yellow onion, cut into half in about (1 1/4 cm)

- 1 cup of flour for all-purpose (125 g)

- 1 ½ cups of panko breadcrumbs (172 g)

- 1 tsp. of paprika

- ⅛ tsp. of cayenne

- ½ tsp. of onion powder

- ½ tsp. black pepper freshly ground

Instructions:

1. Preheat your air fryer to 190°c (375°f).

2. Use a medium-size bowl to mix together onion powder, salt, paprika, cayenne, pepper, flour and garlic powder.

3. In 2 separate small cups, add your panko & eggs.

4. Cover onion rings with flour, then with the eggs, and afterward with the panko.

Working in lots, put your onion rings in one layer inside your air fryer & "fry" for 5 to 7 minutes or till you see golden brown color.

5. Using warm marinara sauce to serve.

2. Air fryer sweet potato chips

Cook time: 15 mins

Serving: 2

Difficulty: easy

Ingredients:

- 1 ½ tsp. of kosher salt

- 1 tsp. of dried thyme

- 1 large yam or sweet potato

- ½ tsp. of pepper

- 1 tbsp. of olive oil

Instructions:

1. Preheat your air fryer to a degree of 350 f (180 c).

2. Slice your sweet potato have a length of 3- to 6-mm (1/8-1/4-inch). In a medium tub, mix your olive oil with slices of sweet potato until well-seasoned. Add some pepper, thyme and salt to cover.

3. Working in groups, add your chips in one sheet & fry for around 14 minutes till you see a golden brown color and slightly crisp.

Fun.

3. Air fryer tortilla chips

Cook time: 5 mins

Serving: 2 people

Difficulty: easy

Ingredients:

• 1 tbsp. of olive oil

• Guacamole for serving

• 2 tsp. of kosher salt

• 12 corn of tortillas

• 1 tbsp. of McCormick delicious jazzy spice blend

Instructions:

1. Preheat your air fryer at a degree of 350 f (180 c).

2. Gently rub your tortillas with olive oil on every side.

3. Sprinkle your tortillas with delicious jazzy spice and salt mix on every side.

Slice every tortilla into six wedges.

4. Functioning in groups, add your tortilla wedges inside your air fryer in one layer & fry it for around 5 minutes or until you see golden brown color and crispy texture.

Serve adding guacamole

4. Air fryer zesty chicken wings

Cook time: 20 mins

Serving: 2 people

Difficulty: easy

Ingredients:

- 1 ½ tsp. of kosher salt

- 1 ½ lb. of patted dry chicken wings (of 680 g)

- 1 tbsp. of the delicious, zesty spice blend

Instructions:

1. Preheat your air fryer at 190°c (375°f).

2. In a tub, get your chicken wings mixed in salt & delicious zesty spice, which must be blend till well-seasoned.

3. Working in lots, add your chicken wings inside the air fryer in one layer & fry it for almost 20 minutes, turning it halfway through.

4. Serve it warm

5. Air fryer sweet potato fries

Cook time: 15 mins

Serving: 2 people

Difficulty: easy

Ingredients:

- 1/4 tsp. of sea salt

- 1 tbsp. of olive oil

- 2 (having 6-oz.) sweet potatoes, cut & peeled into sticks of 1/4-inch

- Cooking spray

- 1/4 tsp. of garlic powder

- 1 tsp. fresh thyme chopped

Instructions:

1. Mix together thyme, garlic powder, olive oil and salt in a bowl. Put sweet potato inside the mixture and mix well to cover.

2. Coat the basket of the air fryer gently with the help of cooking spray. Place your sweet potatoes in one layer inside the basket & cook in groups at a degree of 400 f until soft inside & finely browned from outside for around 14 minutes, rotating the fries halfway through the cooking process.

6. Air fryer churros with chocolate sauce

Cook time: 30 mins

Serving: 12

Difficulty: easy

Ingredients:

- 1/4 cup, adding 2 tbsp. Unsalted butter that's divided into half-cup (around 2 1/8 oz.)

- 3 tbsp. of heavy cream

- Half cup water

- 4 ounces of bitter and sweet finely chopped baking chocolate

- Flour for All-purpose

- 2 tsp. of ground cinnamon

- 2 large eggs

- 1/4 tsp. of kosher salt

- 2 tbsp. of vanilla kefir

- 1/3 cup of granulated sugar

Instruction:

1. Bring salt, water & 1/4 cup butter and boil it in a tiny saucepan with a medium-high flame. Decrease the heat to around medium-low flame; add flour & mix actively with a spoon made up of wood for around 30 seconds.

2. Stir and cook continuously till the dough is smooth. Do this till you see your dough continues to fall away from the sides of the pan & a film appears on the bottom of the pan after 2 to 3 minutes. Move the dough in a medium-sized bowl. Stir continuously for around 1 minute until slightly cooled. Add one egg from time to time while stirring continuously till you see it gets smoother after every addition. Move the mixture in the piping bag, which is fitted with having star tip of medium size. Chill it for around 30 minutes.

3. Pipe 6 (3" long) bits in one-layer inside a basket of the air fryer. Cook at a degree of 380 f for around 10 minutes. Repeat this step for the leftover dough.

4. Stir the sugar & cinnamon together inside a medium-size bowl. Use 2 tablespoons of melted butter to brush the cooked churros. Cover them with the sugar mixture.

5. Put the cream and chocolate in a tiny, microwaveable tub. Microwave with a high temperature for roughly 30 seconds until molten and flat, stirring every 15 seconds. Mix in kefir.

6. Serve the churros, including chocolate sauce.

7. Whole-wheat pizzas in an air fryer

Cook time: 10 mins

Serving: 2 people

Difficulty: easy

Ingredients:

- 1 small thinly sliced garlic clove

- 1/4 ounce of Parmigiano-Reggiano shaved cheese (1 tbsp.)

- 1 cup of small spinach leaves (around 1 oz.)

- 1/4 cup marinara sauce (lower-sodium)

- 1-ounce part-skim pre-shredded mozzarella cheese (1/4 cup)

- 1 tiny plum tomato, sliced into 8 pieces

- 2 pita rounds of whole-wheat

Instructions:

1. Disperse marinara sauce equally on one side of every pita bread. Cover it each with half of the tomato slices, cheese, spinach leaves and garlic.

2. Put 1 pita in the basket of air-fryer & cook it at a degree of 350 f until the cheese is melted and the pita is crispy. Repeat with the leftover pita.

8. Air-fried corn dog bites

Cook time: 15 mins

Serving: 4 people

Difficulty: easy

Ingredients:

- 2 lightly beaten large eggs

- 2 uncured hot dogs of all-beef

- Cooking spray

- 12 bamboo skewers or craft sticks

- 8 tsp. of yellow mustard

- 1 1/2 cups cornflakes cereal finely crushed

- 1/2 cup (2 1/8 oz.) Flour for All-purpose

Instructions:

1. Split lengthwise every hot dog. Cut every half in three same pieces. Add a bamboo skewer or the craft stick inside the end of every hot dog piece.

2. Put flour in a bowl. Put slightly beaten eggs in another shallow bowl. Put crushed cornflakes inside another shallow bowl. Mix the hot dogs with flour; make sure to shake the surplus. Soak in the egg, helping you in dripping off every excess. Dredge inside the cornflakes crumbs, pushing to stick.

3. Gently coat the basket of the air fryer with your cooking spray. Put around six bites of corn dog inside the basket; spray the surface lightly with the help of cooking spray. Now cook at a degree of 375 f till the coating shows a golden

brown color and is crunchy for about 10 minutes, flipping the bites of corn dog halfway in cooking. Do this step with other bites of the corn dog.

4. Put three bites of corn dog with 2 tsp. of mustard on each plate to, and then serve immediately.

9. Crispy veggie quesadillas in an air fryer

Cook time: 20 mins

Serving: 4 people

Difficulty: easy

Instructions:

- Cooking spray

- 1/2 cup refrigerated and drained pico de gallo

- 4 ounces far educing cheddar sharp cheese, shredded (1 cup)

- 1 tbsp. of fresh juice (with 1 lime)

- 4(6-in.) whole-grain Sprouted flour tortillas

- 1/4 tsp. ground cumin

- 2 tbsp. fresh cilantro chopped

- 1 cup red bell pepper sliced

- 1 cup of drained & rinsed black beans canned, no-salt-added

- 1 tsp. of lime zest plus

- 1 cup of sliced zucchini

- 2 ounces of plain 2 percent fat reduced Greek yogurt

Instructions:

1. Put tortillas on the surface of your work. Sprinkle two tbsp. Shredded cheese on the half of every tortilla. Each tortilla must be top with cheese, having a cup of 1/4 each black beans, slices of red pepper equally and zucchini slices. Sprinkle equally with the leftover 1/2 cup of cheese. Fold the tortillas making a shape of a half-moon. Coat quesadillas lightly with the help of cooking spray & protect them with toothpicks.

2. Gently spray the cooking spray on the basket of the air fryer. Cautiously put two quesadillas inside the basket & cook it at a degree of 400 f till the tortillas are of golden brown color & slightly crispy, vegetables get softened, and the cheese if finally melted for around 10 minutes, rotating the quesadillas halfway while cooking. Do this step again with the leftover quesadillas.

3. As the quesadillas are cooking, mix lime zest, cumin, yogurt and lime juice altogether in a small tub. For serving, cut the quesadilla in slices & sprinkle it with cilantro. Serve it with a tablespoon of cumin cream and around 2 tablespoons of pico de gallo.

10. Air-fried curry chickpeas

Cook time: 10 mins

Serving: 4 people

Difficulty: easy

Ingredients:

• 2 tbsp. of curry powder

• Fresh cilantro thinly sliced

• 1(15-oz.) Can chickpeas (like garbanzo beans), rinsed & drained (1 1/2 cups)

• 1/4 tsp. of kosher salt

- 1/2 tbsp. of ground turmeric

- 1/2 tsp. of Aleppo pepper

- 1/4 tsp. of ground coriander

- 2 tbsp. of olive oil

- 1/4 tsp. and 1/8 tsp. of Ground cinnamon

- 2 tbsp. of vinegar (red wine)

- 1/4 tsp. of ground cumin

Instructions:

1. Smash chickpeas softly inside a tub with your hands (don't crush); remove chickpea skins.

2. Apply oil and vinegar to chickpeas, & toss for coating. Add turmeric, cinnamon, cumin, curry powder and coriander; whisk gently so that they can be mixed together.

3. Put chickpeas in one layer inside the bask of air fryer & cook at a degree of 400 f till it's crispy for around 15 mins; shake the chickpeas timely while cooking.

4. Place the chickpeas in a tub. Sprinkle it with cilantro, Aleppo pepper and salt; blend to coat.

11. Air fry shrimp spring rolls with sweet chili sauce.

Cook time: 20 mins

Serving: 4

Difficulty: easy

Ingredients:

- 1 cup of matchstick carrots

- 8 (8" square) wrappers of spring roll

- 2 1/2 tbsp. of divided sesame oil

- 4 ounces of peeled, deveined and chopped raw shrimp

- 1/2 cup of chili sauce (sweet)

- 1 cup of (red) bell pepper julienne-cut

- 2 tsp. of fish sauce

- 3/4 cup snow peas julienne-cut

- 2 cups of cabbage, pre-shredded

- 1/4 tsp. of red pepper, crushed

- 1 tbsp. of lime juice (fresh)

- 1/4 cup of fresh cilantro (chopped)

Instructions:

1. In a large pan, heat around 1 1/2 tsp. of oil until softly smoked. Add carrots, bell pepper and cabbage; Cook, stirring constantly, for 1 to 1 1/2 minutes, until finely wilted. Place it on a baking tray; cool for 5 minutes.

2. In a wide tub, place the mixture of cabbage, snow peas, cilantro, fish sauce, red pepper, shrimp and lime juice; toss to blend.

3. Put the wrappers of spring roll on the surface with a corner that is facing you. Add a filling of 1/4 cup in the middle of every wrapper of spring roll, extending from left-hand side to right in a three-inch wide strip.

4. Fold each wrapper's bottom corner over the filling, stuffing the corner tip under the filling. Fold the corners left & right over the filling. Brush the remaining corner softly with water; roll closely against the remaining corner; press gently to cover. Use 2 teaspoons of the remaining oil to rub the spring rolls.

5. Inside the basket of air fryer, put four spring rolls & cook at a degree of 390 f till it's golden, for 6 - 7 minutes, rotating the spring rolls every 5 minutes. Repeat with the leftover spring rolls. Use chili sauce to serve.

Chapter 5: Dessert recipes

1. Air fryer mores

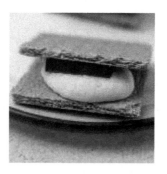

Cook time: 2 mins

Serving: 2 people

Difficulty: easy

Ingredients:

• 1 big marshmallow

• 2 graham crackers split in half

• 2 square, fine quality chocolate

Instructions:

1. Preheat the air fryer at a degree of 330 f.

2. When preheating, break 2 graham crackers into two to form four squares. Cut 1 big marshmallow into half evenly so that one side can be sticky.

3. Add every half of your marshmallow in a square of one graham cracker & push downwards to stick the marshmallow with graham cracker. You must now have two marshmallows coated with graham crackers & two regular graham crackers.

4. In one layer, put two graham crackers and marshmallows inside your air fryer & cook for about 2 minutes till you can see the marshmallow becoming toasted slightly.

5. Remove immediately and completely and add 1 chocolate square to the toasted marshmallow. Add the rest of the squares of the graham cracker and press down. Enjoy instantly.

2. Easy air fryer brownies

Cook time: 15 mins

Serving: 4 people

Difficulty: easy

Ingredients:

- 2 large eggs

- ½ cup flour for all-purpose

- ¼ cup melted unsalted butter

- 6 tbsp. of cocoa powder, unsweetened

- ¼ tsp. of baking powder

- ¾ cup of sugar

- ½ tsp. of vanilla extract

- 1 tbsp. of vegetable oil

- ¼ tsp. of salt

Instructions:

1. Get the 7-inch baking tray ready by gently greasing it with butter on all the sides and even the bottom. Put it aside

2. Preheat the air fryer by adjusting its temperature to a degree of 330 f & leaving it for around 5 minutes as you cook the brownie batter.

3. Add baking powder, cocoa powder, vanilla extract, flour for all-purpose, butter, vegetable oil, salt, eggs and sugar in a big tub & mix it unless well combined.

4. Add up all these for the preparation of the baking pan & clean the top.

5. Put it inside the air fryer & bake it for about 15 minutes or as long as a toothpick can be entered and comes out easily from the center.

6. Take it out and make it cool in the tray until you remove and cut.

3. Easy air fryer churros

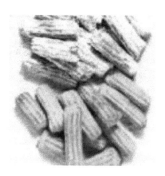

Cook time: 5 mins

Serving: 4 people

Difficulty: easy

Ingredients:

- 1 tbsp. of sugar

- Sifted powdered sugar & cinnamon or cinnamon sugar

- 1 cup (about 250ml) water

- 4 eggs

- ½ cup (113g) butter

- ¼ tsp. salt

- 1 cup (120g) all-purpose flour

Instructions:

1. Mix the ingredients bringing them to boil while stirring continuously.

2. Add flour & start mixing properly. Take it out from the heat & mix it till it gets smooth & the dough can be taken out from the pan easily.

3. Add one egg at one time and stir it until it gets smooth. Set it to cool.

4. Preheat your air fryer degree of 400 for 200 c.

5. Cover your bag of cake decorations with dough & add a star tip of 1/2 inch.

6. Make sticks which are having a length of 3 to 4 inches by moving your dough out from the bag in paper (parchment). You can now switch it inside your air fryer if you are ready to do so. If it is hard to handle the dough, put it inside the refrigerator for around 30 minutes.

7. Use cooking spray or coconut oil to spray the tray or the basket of your air fryer.

8. Add around 8 to 10 churros in a tray or inside the basket of the air fryer. Spray with oil.

9. Cook for 5 minutes at a degree of 400 for 200 c.

10. Until finished and when still hot, rill in regular sugar, cinnamon or sugar mixture.

11. Roll in the cinnamon-sugar blend, cinnamon or normal sugar until finished and when still high.

4. Air fryer sweet apples

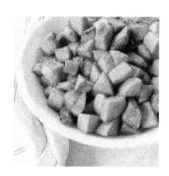

Cook time: 8 mins

Serving: 4 people

Difficulty: easy

Ingredients:

- ¼ cup of white sugar

- ⅓ Cup of water

- ¼ cup of brown sugar

- ½ tsp. of ground cinnamon

- 6 apples diced and cored

- ¼ tsp. of pumpkin pie spice

- ¼ tsp. of ground cloves

Instructions:

1. Put all the ingredients in a bowl that is oven safe & combine it with water and seasonings. Put the bowl inside the basket, oven tray or even in the toaster of an air fryer.

2. Air fry the mixture of apples at a degree of 350 f for around 6 minutes. Mix the apples & cook them for an extra 2 minutes. Serve it hot and enjoy.

5. Air fryer pear crisp for two

Cook time: 20 mins

Serving: 2

Difficulty: easy

Ingredients:

- ¾ tsp. of divided ground cinnamon

- 1 tbsp. of softened salted butter

- 1 tsp. of lemon juice

- 2 pears. Peeled, diced and cored

- 1 tbsp. of flour for all-purpose

- 2 tbsp. of quick-cooking oats

- 1 tbsp. of brown sugar

Instructions:

1. Your air fryer should be preheated at a degree of 360 f (180 c).

2. Mix lemon juice, 1/4 tsp. Cinnamon and pears in a bowl. Turn for coating and then split the mixture into 2 ramekins.

3. Combine brown sugar, oats, leftover cinnamon and flour in the tub. Using your fork to blend in the melted butter until the mixture is mushy. Sprinkle the pears.

4. Put your ramekins inside the basket of an air fryer & cook till the pears become bubbling and soft for around 18 - 20 minutes.

6. Keto chocolate cake – air fryer recipe

Cook time: 10 mins

Serving: 6 people

Difficulty: easy

Ingredients:

- 1 tsp. of vanilla extract

- 1/2 cup of powdered Swerve

- 1/3 cup of cocoa powder unsweetened

- 1/4 tsp. of salt

- 1 & 1/2 cups of almond flour

- 2 large eggs

- 1/3 cups of almond milk, unsweetened

- 1 tsp. of baking powder

Instructions:

1. In a big mixing tub, mix every ingredient until they all are well mixed.

2. Butter or spray your desired baking dish. We used bunt tins in mini size, but you can even get a 6-inch cake pan in the baskets of the air fryer.

3. Scoop batter equally inside your baking dish or dishes.

4. Set the temperature of the air fryer to a degree of 350 f & set a 10-minute timer. Your cake will be ready when the toothpick you entered comes out clear and clean.

Conclusion:

The air fryer seems to be a wonderful appliance that will assist you with maintaining your diet. You will also enjoy the flavor despite eating high amounts of oil if you prefer deep-fried food.

Using a limited quantity of oil, you will enjoy crunchy & crispy food without the additional adverse risk, which tastes exactly like fried food. Besides, the system is safe & easy to use. All you must do is choose the ingredients needed, and there will be nutritious food available for your family.

An air fryer could be something which must be considered if a person is attempting to eat a diet having a lower-fat diet, access to using the system to prepare a range of foods, & want trouble cooking experience.

Vegan Air Fryer Cookbook

Cook and Taste 50+ High-Protein Recipes. Kick start Muscles and Body Transformation, Kill Hunger and Feel More Energetic

By

Chef Carlo Leone

Contents

Introduction

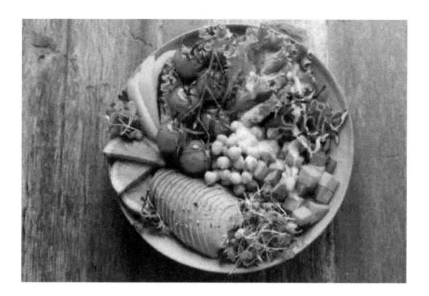

To have a good, satisfying life, a balanced diet is important. Tiredness and susceptibility to illnesses, many severe, arise from a lifestyle so full of junk food. Our community, sadly, does not neglect unsafe choices. People turn to immoral practices in order to satisfy desire, leading to animal torture. Two of the key explanations that people adhere to vegetarianism, a vegan-based diet that often excludes animal foods such as cheese, beef, jelly, and honey, are fitness and animal welfare.

It's essential for vegetarians to get the most nutrients out of any food, and that's where frying using an air fryer shines. The air fryer cooking will maintain as many nutrients as possible from beans and veggies, and the gadget makes it incredibly simple to cook nutritious food.

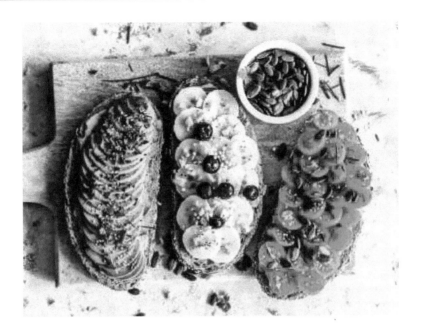

Although there are prepared vegan alternatives, the healthier choice, and far less pricey, is still to prepare your own recipes. This book provides the very first moves to being a vegan and offers 50 quick breakfast recipes, sides, snacks, and much more, so you have a solid base on which to develop.

This book will teach you all you need to thrive, whether you are either a vegan and only need more meal choices or have just begun contemplating transforming your diet.

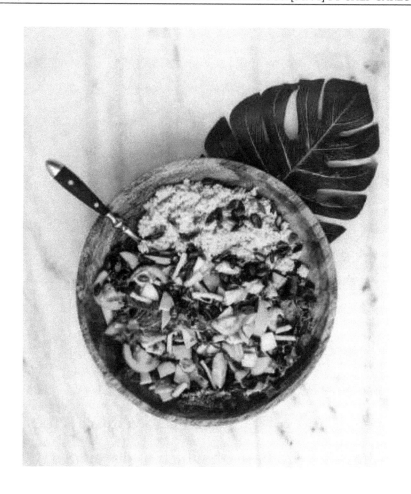

What is Cooking Vegan?

In recent decades, vegetarianism has become quite common, as individuals understand just how toxic the eating patterns of civilization have become. We are a society that enjoys meat, and, unfortunately, we go to dishonest measures to get the food we like. More citizens are choosing to give up beef and, unlike vegans, other livestock items due to various health issues, ethical issues, or both. Their diet moves to one focused on plants, whole grains, beans, fruit, seeds, nuts, and vegan varieties of the common dish.

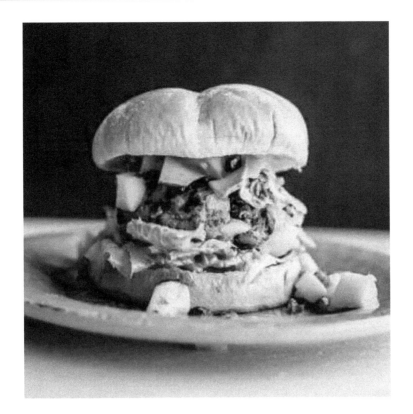

What advantages would veganism have?

There are a lot of advantages to a diet away from all animal items. Only a few includes:

- Healthier hair, skin, and nails

- High energy

- Fewer chances of flu and cold

- Fewer migraines

- Increased tolerance to cancer

- Strengthened fitness of the heart

Although research has proven that veganism will contribute to reducing BMI, it must not be followed for the mere sake of weight reduction. "Vegan" does not indicate "lower-calorie," and if you wish to reduce weight, other healthier activities, including exercising and consuming water, can complement the diet.

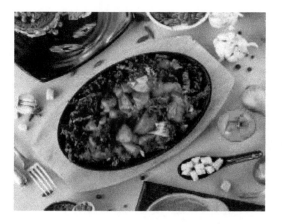

Air Fryer

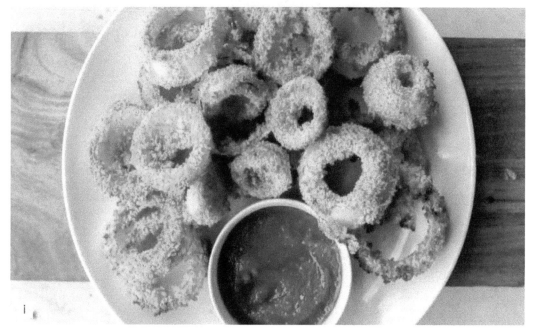

A common kitchen gadget used to create fried foods such as beef, baked goods and potato chips is an air fryer. It provides a crunchy, crisp coating by blowing hot air across the food. This also leads to a chemical reaction commonly known as the Maillard effect, which happens in the presence of heat in between reducing sugar and amino acid. This adds to shifts in food color and taste. Due to the reduced amount of calories and fat, air-fried items are marketed as a healthier substitute to deep-fried foods.

Rather than fully soaking the food in fat, air-frying utilizes just a teaspoon to create a flavor and feel equivalent to deep-fried foods.

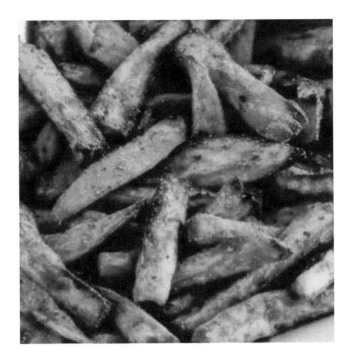

The flavor and appearance of the fried food in the air are similar to the deep fryer outcomes: On the surface, crispy; from the inside, soft. You do need to use a limited amount of oil, though, or any at all (based on what you're baking). But indeed, contrary to deep frying, if you agree to use only 1-2 teaspoons of plant-based oil with spices and you stuck to air-frying vegetables rather than anything else, air frying is certainly a better option.

The secret to weight loss, decreased likelihood of cardiovascular illness and better long-term wellbeing as we mature is any gadget that assists you and your friends in your vegetarian game.

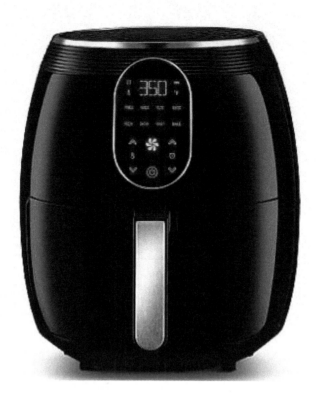

Air fryer's Working Process:

The air fryer is a worktop kitchen gadget that operates in the same manner as a traditional oven. To become acquainted with the operating theory of the traditional oven, you will need a little study. The air fryer uses rotating hot air to fry and crisp your meal, close to the convection oven. In a traditional convection oven, the airflow relies on revolving fans, which blast hot air around to produce an even or equalized temperature dispersal throughout the oven.

This is compared to the upward airflow of standard ovens, where the warm place is typically the oven's tip. And although the air fryer is not quite like the convection oven, it is a great approximation of it in the field of airflow for most components. The gadget has an air inlet at the top that lets air in and a hot air outlet at the side. All of these features are used to monitor the temperature within the air fryer. Temperatures will rise to 230 ° C, based on the sort of air fryer you're buying.

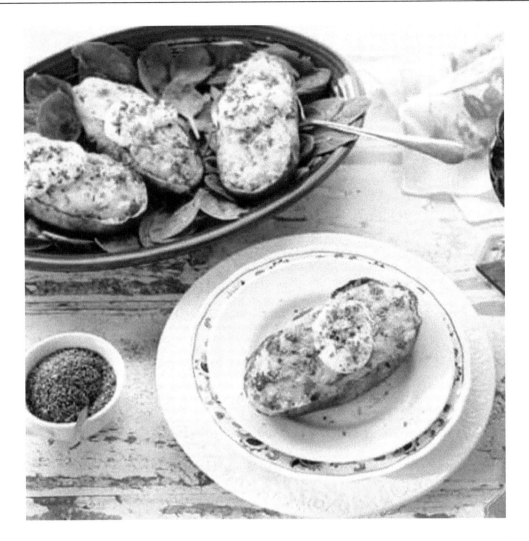

In conjunction with any grease, this hot air is used for cooking the food in the bowl within the device, if you like. Yes, if you want a taste of the oil, you should apply more oil. To jazz up the taste of the meal, simply add a little more to the blend. But the key concept behind the air fryer is to reduce the consumption of calories and fat without reducing the amount of taste.

Using air frying rather than deep frying saves between 70-80 calories, according to researchers. The growing success of recipes for air fryers is simply attributed to its impressive performance. It is simple to use and less time-consuming than conventional ovens.

This is more or less a lottery win for people searching for healthy alternative to deep-frying, as demonstrated by its widespread popularity in many homes today.

In contrast to conventional ovens or deep frying, the air fryer creates crispy, crunchy, wonderful, and far fewer fatty foods in less duration. For certain individuals like us; this is what distinguishes air fryer recipes.

Tips for using an Air Fryer

1. The food is cooked easily. Air fried, unlike conventional cooking techniques, cut the cooking time a great deal. Therefore, to stop burning the food or getting a not-so-great flavor, it is best to hold a close eye on the gadget. Notice, remember that the smaller the food on the basket, the shorter the cooking period, which implies that the food cooks quicker.

2. You may need to reduce the temperature at first. Bear in mind that air fryers depend on the flow of hot air, which heats up rapidly. This ensures that it's better, to begin with, a low temperature so that the food cooks equally. It is likely that when the inside is already cooking, the exterior of the food is all cooked and begins to become dark or too dry.

3. When air fryers are in operation, they create some noise. If you are new to recipes for air fryers, you may have to realize that air fryers create noise while working. When it's in service, a whirring tone emanates from the device. However, the slight annoyance pales in contrast to the various advantages of having an air fryer.

4. Hold the grate within the container at all hours. As previously mentioned, the air fryer has a container inside it, where the food is put and permitted to cook. This helps hot air to flow freely around the food, allowing for even cooking.

5. Don't stuff the air fryer with so much food at once. If you plan to make a meal for one guy, with only one batch, you would most definitely be able to get your cooking right. If you're cooking for two or more individuals, you can need to plan

the food in groups. With a 4 - 5 quart air fryer, you can always need to cook in groups, depending on the size and sort of air fryer you have. This not only means that your device works longer but also keeps your food from cooking unevenly. You shouldn't have to turn the air fryer off as you pull out the basket since it simply turns off on its own until the basket is out. Often, make sure the drawer is completely retracted; otherwise, the fryer would not turn back on.

6. Take the basket out of the mix and mix the ingredients. You might need to move the food around or switch it over once every few minutes, based on the dish you're preparing and the time it takes to prepare your dinner.

The explanation for this is that even cooking can be done. Certain recipes involve the foods in the basket to shake and shuffle throughout the cooking phase. And an easy-to-understand checklist is given for each recipe to direct you thru the cycle.

7. The air fryer does not need cooking mist. It isn't needed. In order to prevent the urge to use non-stick frying spray in the container, you must deliberately take care of this. The basket is now coated with a non-stick covering, so what you need to do is fill your meal inside the container and push it back in.

Outcome
You can create nutritious meals very simply and fast, right in the comfort of your house. There are many excellent recipes for producing healthier meals and nutritious foods, which you can notice in the air fryer recipes illustrated in this book. However, you'll need to pay careful attention to the ingredients and know-how to easily use the air fryer to do this. To get straightforward guidance on installation and usage, you can need to refer to the company's manual.

CHAPTER 1: Breakfast Recipes

1. Toasted French toast

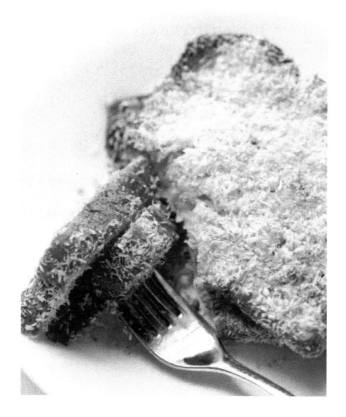

Preparation time: 2 minutes

Cooking time: 5 minutes

Servings: 1 people

Ingredients:

- ½ Cup of Unsweetened Shredded Coconut

- 1 Tsp. Baking Powder

- ½ Cup Lite Culinary Coconut Milk

- 2 Slices of Gluten-Free Bread (use your favorite)

Directions:

1. Stir together the baking powder and coconut milk in a large rimmed pot.

2. On a tray, layout your ground coconut.

3. Pick each loaf of your bread and dip it in your coconut milk for the very first time, and then pass it to the ground coconut, let it sit for a few minutes, then cover the slice entirely with the coconut.

4. Place the covered bread loaves in your air fryer, cover it, adjust the temperature to about 350 ° F and set the clock for around 4 minutes.

5. Take out from your air fryer until done, and finish with some maple syrup of your choice. French toast is done. Enjoy!

2. Vegan Casserole

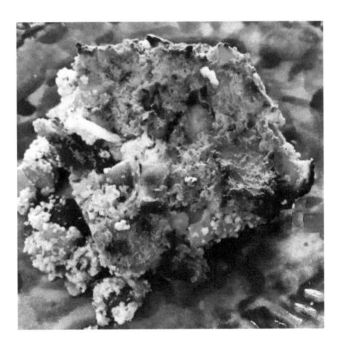

Preparation time: 10-12 minutes

Cooking time: 15-20 minutes

Servings: 2-3 people

Ingredients:

- 1/2 cup of cooked quinoa

- 1 tbsp. of lemon juice

- 2 tbsp. of water

- 2 tbsp. of plain soy yogurt

- 2 tbsp. of nutritional yeast

- 7 ounces of extra-firm tofu about half a block, drained but not pressed

- 1/2 tsp. of ground cumin

- 1/2 tsp. of red pepper flakes

- 1/2 tsp. of freeze-dried dill

- 1/2 tsp. of black pepper

- 1/2 tsp. of salt

- 1 tsp. of dried oregano

- 1/2 cup of diced shiitake mushrooms

- 1/2 cup of diced bell pepper I used a combination of red and green

- 2 small celery stalks chopped

- 1 large carrot chopped

- 1 tsp. of minced garlic

- 1 small onion diced

- 1 tsp. of olive oil

Directions:

1. Warm the olive oil over medium-low heat in a big skillet. Add your onion and garlic and simmer till the onion is transparent (for about 3 to 6 minutes). Add your bell pepper, carrot, and celery and simmer for another 3 minutes.

Mix the oregano, mushrooms, pepper, salt, cumin, dill, and red pepper powder. Mix completely and lower the heat to low. If the vegetables tend to cling, stir regularly and add in about a teaspoon of water.

2. Pulse the nutritional yeast, tofu, water, yogurt, and some lemon juice in a food mixer until fluffy. To your skillet, add your tofu mixture. Add in half a cup of cooked quinoa. Mix thoroughly.

3. Move to a microwave-proof plate or tray that works for your air fryer basket.

4. Cook for around 15 minutes at about 350°F (or 18 to 20 minutes at about 330°F, till it turns golden brown).

5. Please take out your plate or tray from your air fryer and let it rest for at least five minutes before eating.

3. Vegan Omelet

Preparation time: 15 minutes

Cooking time: 16 minutes

Servings: 3 people

Ingredients:

- ½ cup of grated vegan cheese

- 1 tbsp. of water

- 1 tbsp. of brags

- 3 tbsp. of nutritional yeast

- ¼ tsp. of basil

- ¼ tsp. of garlic powder

- ¼ tsp. of onion powder

- ¼ tsp. of pepper

- ½ tsp. of cumin

- ½ tsp. of turmeric

- ¼ tsp. of salt

- ¼ cup of chickpea flour (or you may use any bean flour)

- ½ cup of finely diced veggies (like chard, kale, dried mushrooms, spinach, watermelon radish etc.)

- half a piece of tofu (organic high in protein kind)

Directions:

4. Blend all your ingredients in a food blender or mixer, excluding the vegetables and cheese.

5. Move the batter from the blender to a container and combine the vegetables and cheese in it. Since it's faster, you could use both hands to combine it.

6. Brush the base of your air fryer bucket with some oil.

7. Put a couple of parchment papers on your counter. On the top of your parchment paper, place a cookie cutter of your desire.

8. In your cookie cutter, push 1/6 of the paste. Then raise and put the cookie cutter on a different section of your parchment paper.

9. Redo the process till you have about 6 pieces using the remainder of the paste.

10. Put 2 or 3 of your omelets at the base of your air fryer container. Using some oil, brush the topsides of the omelets.

11. Cook for around 5 minutes at about 370 °, turn and bake for another 4 minutes or more if needed. And redo with the omelets that remain.

12. Offer with sriracha mayo or whatever kind of dipping sauce you prefer. Or use them for a sandwich at breakfast.

4. Waffles with Vegan chicken

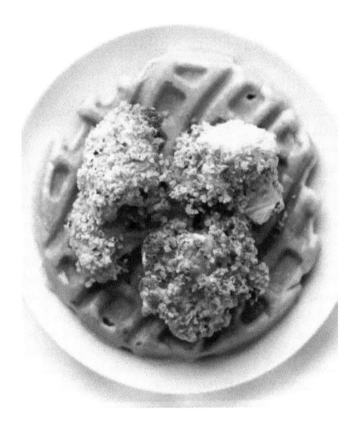

Preparation time: 10 minutes

Cooking time: 15 minutes

Servings: 2 people

Ingredients:

Fried Vegan Chicken:

- ¼ to ½ teaspoon of Black Pepper

- ½ teaspoon of Paprika

- ½ teaspoon of Onion Powder

- ½ teaspoon of Garlic Powder

- 2 teaspoon of Dried Parsley

- 2 Cups of Gluten-Free Panko

- ¼ Cup of Cornstarch

- 1 Cup of Unsweetened Non-Dairy Milk

- 1 Small Head of Cauliflower

Yummy Cornmeal Waffles:

- ½ teaspoon of Pure Vanilla Extract

- ¼ Cup of Unsweetened Applesauce

- ½ Cup of Unsweetened Non-Dairy Milk

- 1 to 2 TB Erythritol (or preferred sweetener)

- 1 teaspoon Baking Powder

- ¼ Cup of Stoneground Cornmeal

- ⅔ Cup of Gluten-Free All-Purpose Flour

Toppings:

- Vegan Butter

- Hot Sauce

- Pure Maple Syrup

Directions:

For making your Vegan Fried Chicken:

1. Dice the cauliflower (you wouldn't have to be careful in this) into big florets and put it aside.

2. Mix the cornstarch and milk in a tiny pot.

3. Throw the herbs, panko, and spices together in a big bowl or dish.

4. In the thick milk mixture, soak your cauliflower florets, then cover the soaked bits in the prepared panko mix before putting the wrapped floret into your air fryer bucket.

5. For the remaining of your cauliflower, redo the same process.

6. Set your air fryer clock for around 15 minutes to about 400 ° F and let the cauliflower air fry.

For making you're Waffles:

1. Oil a regular waffle iron and warm it up.

2. Mix all your dry ingredients in a pot, and then blend in your wet ingredients until you have a thick mixture.

3. To create a big waffle, utilize ½ of the mixture and redo the process to create another waffle for a maximum of two persons.

To Organize:

1. Put on dishes your waffles, place each with ½ of the cooked cauliflower, now drizzle with the hot sauce, syrup, and any extra toppings that you want. Serve warm!

5. Tempeh Bacon

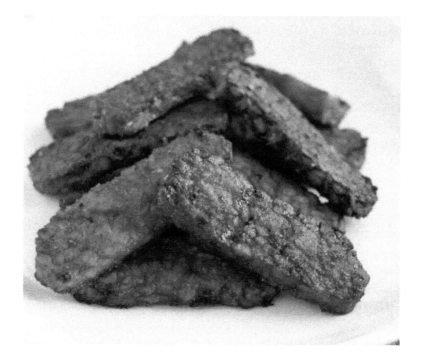

Preparation time: 15 minutes plus 2 hour marinating time

Cooking time: 10 minutes

Servings: 4 people

Ingredients:

- ½ teaspoon of freshly grated black pepper

- ½ teaspoon of onion powder

- ½ teaspoon of garlic powder

- 1 ½ teaspoon of smoked paprika

- 1 teaspoon of apple cider vinegar

- 1 tablespoon of olive oil (plus some more for oiling your air fryer)

- 3 tablespoon of pure maple syrup

- ¼ cup of gluten-free, reduced-sodium tamari

- 8 oz. of gluten-free tempeh

Directions:

1. Break your Tempeh cube into two parts and boil for about 10 minutes, some more if required. To the rice cooker bowl, add a cup of warm water. Then, put the pieces of tempeh into the steamer basket of the unit. Close the cover, push the button for heat or steam cooking (based on your rice cooker's type or brand), and adjust the steaming timer for around 10 minutes.

2. Let the tempeh cool completely before taking it out of the rice cooker or your steamer basket for around 5 minutes.

3. Now make the sauce while cooking the tempeh. In a 9" x 13" baking tray, incorporate all the rest of your ingredients and mix them using a fork. Then set it aside and ready the tempeh.

4. Put the tempeh steamed before and cooled on a chopping board, and slice into strips around 1/4' wide. Put each slice gently in the sauce. Then roll over each slice gently. Seal and put in the fridge for two to three hours or even overnight, rotating once or twice during the time.

5. Turn the bits gently one more time until you are about to create the tempeh bacon. And if you would like, you may spoon over any leftover sauce.

6. Put your crisper plate/tray into the air fryer if yours came with one instead of a built-in one. Oil the base of your crisper tray or your air fryer basket slightly with some olive oil or using an olive oil spray that is anti-aerosol.

7. Put the tempeh slices in a thin layer gently in your air fryer bucket. If you have a tiny air fryer, you will have to air fry it in two or multiple rounds. Air fry for around 10-15 minutes at about 325 ° F before the slices are lightly

golden but not burnt. You may detach your air fryer container to inspect it and make sure it's not burnt. It normally takes about 10 minutes.

6. Delicious Potato Pancakes

Preparation time: 5 minutes

Cooking time: 15 minutes

Servings: 4 people

Ingredients:

- black pepper according to taste
- 3 tablespoon of flour
- ¼ teaspoon of pepper
- ¼ teaspoon of salt
- ½ teaspoon of garlic powder
- 2 tablespoon of unsalted butter
- ¼ cup of milk
- 1 beaten egg
- 1 medium onion, chopped

Directions:

1. Preheat the fryer to about 390° F and combine the potatoes, garlic powder, eggs, milk, onion, pepper, butter, and salt in a small bowl; add in the flour and make a batter.

2. Shape around 1/4 cup of your batter into a cake.

3. In the fryer's cooking basket, put the cakes and cook for a couple of minutes.

4. Serve and enjoy your treat!

CHAPTER 2: Air Fryer Main Dishes

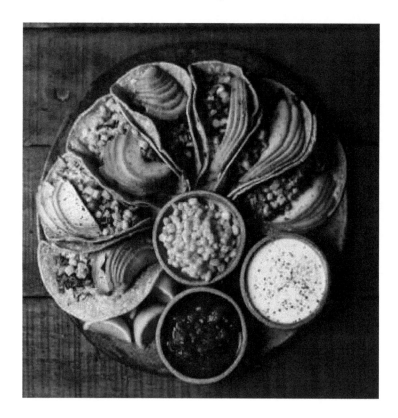

1. Mushroom 'n Bell Pepper Pizza

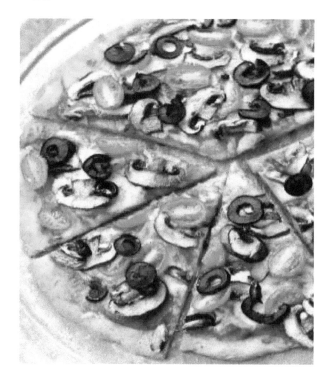

Preparation time: 5 minutes

Cooking time: 10 minutes

Servings: 10 people

Ingredients:

- salt and pepper according to taste

- 2 tbsp. of parsley

- 1 vegan pizza dough

- 1 shallot, chopped

- 1 cup of oyster mushrooms, chopped

- ¼ red bell pepper, chopped

Directions:

1. Preheat your air fryer to about 400°F.

2. Cut the pie dough into small squares. Just set them aside.

3. Put your bell pepper, shallot, oyster mushroom, and parsley all together into a mixing dish.

4. According to taste, sprinkle with some pepper and salt.

5. On top of your pizza cubes, put your topping.

6. Put your pizza cubes into your air fryer and cook for about 10 minutes.

2. Veggies Stuffed Eggplants

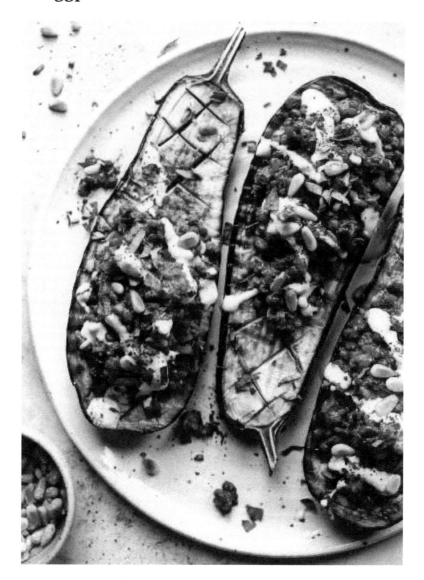

Preparation time: 5 minutes

Cooking time: 14 minutes

Servings: 5 people

Ingredients:

- 2 tbsp. of tomato paste

- Salt and ground black pepper, as required

- ½ tsp. of garlic, chopped

- 1 tbsp. of vegetable oil

- 1 tbsp. of fresh lime juice

- ½ green bell pepper, seeded and chopped

- ¼ cup of cottage cheese, chopped

- 1 tomato, chopped

- 1 onion, chopped

- 10 small eggplants, halved lengthwise

Directions:

1. Preheat your air fryer to about 320°F and oil the container of your air fryer.

2. Cut a strip longitudinally from all sides of your eggplant and scrape out the pulp in a medium-sized bowl.

3. Add lime juice on top of your eggplants and place them in the container of your Air Fryer.

4. Cook for around a couple of minutes and extract from your Air Fryer.

5. Heat the vegetable oil on medium-high heat in a pan and add the onion and garlic.

6. Sauté for around 2 minutes and mix in the tomato, salt, eggplant flesh, and black pepper.

7. Sauté and add bell pepper, tomato paste, cheese, and cilantro for roughly 3 minutes.

8. Cook for around a minute and put this paste into your eggplants.

9. Shut each eggplant with its lids and adjust the Air Fryer to 360°F.

10. Organize and bake for around 5 minutes in your Air Fryer Basket.

11. Dish out on a serving tray and eat hot.

3. Air-fried Falafel

Preparation time: 10 minutes

Cooking time: 25 minutes

Servings: 6 people

Ingredients:

- Salt and black pepper according to taste

- 1 teaspoon of chili powder

- 2 teaspoon of ground coriander

- 2 teaspoon of ground cumin

- 1 onion, chopped

- 4 garlic cloves, chopped

- Juice of 1 lemon

- 1 cup of fresh parsley, chopped

- ½ cup of chickpea flour

Directions:

1. Add flour, coriander, chickpeas, lemon juice, parsley, onion, garlic, chili, cumin, salt, turmeric, and pepper to a processor and mix until mixed, not too battery; several chunks should be present.

2. Morph the paste into spheres and hand-press them to ensure that they are still around.

3. Spray using some spray oil and place them in a paper-lined air fryer bucket; if necessary, perform in groups.

4. Cook for about 14 minutes at around 360°F, rotating once mid-way through the cooking process.

5. They must be light brown and crispy.

4. Almond Flour Battered Wings

Preparation time: 10 minutes

Cooking time: 25 minutes

Servings: 4 people

Ingredients:

- Salt and pepper according to taste

- 4 tbsp. of minced garlic

- 2 tbsp. of stevia powder

- 16 pieces of vegan chicken wings

- ¾ cup of almond flour

- ¼ cup of butter, melted

Directions:

1. Preheat your air fryer for about 5 minutes.

2. Mix the stevia powder, almond flour, vegan chicken wings, and garlic in a mixing dish. According to taste, sprinkle with some black pepper and salt.

3. Please put it in the bucket of your air fryer and cook at about 400°F for around 25 minutes.

4. Ensure you give your fryer container a shake midway through the cooking process.

5. Put in a serving dish after cooking and add some melted butter on top. Toss it to coat it completely.

5. Spicy Tofu

Preparation time: 5 minutes

Cooking time: 13 minutes

Servings: 3 people

Ingredients:

- Salt and black pepper, according to taste

- 1 tsp. of garlic powder

- 1 tsp. of onion powder

- 1½ tsp. of paprika

- 1½ tbsp. of avocado oil

- 3 tsp. of cornstarch

- 1 (14-ounces) block extra-firm tofu, pressed and cut into ¾-inch cubes

Directions:

1. Preheat your air fryer to about 390°F and oil the container of your air fryer with some spray oil.

2. In a medium-sized bowl, blend the cornstarch, oil, tofu, and spices and mix to cover properly.

3. In the Air Fryer basket, place the tofu bits and cook for around a minute, flipping twice between the cooking times.

4. On a serving dish, spread out the tofu and enjoy it warm.

6. Sautéed Bacon with Spinach

Preparation time: 5 minutes

Cooking time: 9 minutes

Servings: 2 people

Ingredients:

- 1 garlic clove, minced

- 2 tbsp. of olive oil

- 4-ounce of fresh spinach

- 1 onion, chopped

- 3 meatless bacon slices, chopped

Directions:

1. Preheat your air fryer at about 340° F and oil the air fryer's tray with some olive oil or cooking oil spray.

2. In the Air Fryer basket, put garlic and olive oil.

3. Cook and add in the onions and bacon for around 2 minutes.

4. Cook and mix in the spinach for approximately 3 minutes.

5. Cook for 4 more minutes and plate out in a bowl to eat.

7. Garden Fresh Veggie Medley

Preparation time: 5 minutes

Cooking time: 15 minutes

Servings: 4 people

Ingredients:

- 1 tbsp. of balsamic vinegar

- 1 tbsp. of olive oil

- 2 tbsp. of herbs de Provence

- 2 garlic cloves, minced

- 2 small onions, chopped

- 3 tomatoes, chopped

- 1 zucchini, chopped

- 1 eggplant, chopped

- 2 yellow bell peppers seeded and chopped

- Salt and black pepper, according to taste.

Directions:

1. Preheat your air fryer at about 355° F and oil up the air fryer basket.

2. In a medium-sized bowl, add all the ingredients and toss to cover completely.

3. Move to the basket of your Air Fryer and cook for around 15 minutes.

4. After completing the cooking time, let it sit in the air fryer for around 5 minutes and plate out to serve warm.

8. Colorful Vegetable Croquettes

Preparation time: 5 minutes

Cooking time: 10 minutes

Servings: 4 people

Ingredients:

- 1/2 cup of parmesan cheese, grated

- 2 eggs

- 1/4 cup of coconut flour

- 1/2 cup of almond flour

- 2 tbsp. of olive oil

- 3 tbsp. of scallions, minced

- 1 clove garlic, minced

- 1 bell pepper, chopped

- 1/2 cup of mushrooms, chopped

- 1/2 tsp. of cayenne pepper

- Salt and black pepper, according to taste.

- 2 tbsp. of butter

- 4 tbsp. of milk

- 1/2 pound of broccoli

Directions:

1. Boil your broccoli in a medium-sized saucepan for up to around 20 minutes. With butter, milk, black pepper, salt, and cayenne pepper, rinse the broccoli and mash it.

2. Add in the bell pepper, mushrooms, garlic, scallions, and olive oil and blend properly. Form into patties with the blend.

3. Put the flour in a deep bowl; beat your eggs in a second bowl; then put the parmesan cheese in another bowl.

4. Dip each patty into your flour, accompanied by the eggs and lastly the parmesan cheese, push to hold the shape.

5. Cook for around 16 minutes, turning midway through the cooking period, in the preheated Air Fryer at about 370° F. Bon appétit!

9. Cheesy Mushrooms

Preparation time: 3 minutes

Cooking time: 8 minutes

Servings: 4 people

Ingredients:

- 1 tsp. of dried dill

- 2 tbsp. of Italian dried mixed herbs

- 2 tbsp. of olive oil

- 2 tbsp. of cheddar cheese, grated

- 2 tbsp. of mozzarella cheese, grated

- Salt and freshly ground black pepper, according to taste

- 6-ounce of button mushrooms stemmed

Directions:

Preheat the air fryer at around 355° F and oil your air fryer basket.

In a mixing bowl, combine the Italian dried mixed herbs, mushrooms, salt, oil, and black pepper and mix well to cover.

In the Air Fryer bucket, place the mushrooms and cover them with some cheddar cheese and mozzarella cheese.

To eat, cook for around 8 minutes and scatter with dried dill.

10. Greek-style Roasted Vegetables

Preparation time: 10 minutes

Cooking time: 25 minutes

Servings: 3 people

Ingredients:

- 1/2 cup of Kalamata olives, pitted

- 1 (28-ounce) canned diced tomatoes with juice

- 1/2 tsp. of dried basil

- Sea salt and freshly cracked black pepper, according to taste

- 1 tsp. of dried rosemary

- 1 cup of dry white wine

- 2 tbsp. of extra-virgin olive oil

- 2 bell peppers, cut into 1-inch chunks

- 1 red onion, sliced

- 1/2 pound of zucchini, cut into 1-inch chunks

- 1/2 pound of cauliflower, cut into 1-inch florets

- 1/2 pound of butternut squash, peeled and cut into 1-inch chunks

Directions:

1. Add some rosemary, wine, olive oil, black pepper, salt, and basil along with your vegetables toss until well-seasoned.

2. Onto a lightly oiled baking dish, add 1/2 of the canned chopped tomatoes; scatter to fill the base of your baking dish.

3. Add in the vegetables and add the leftover chopped tomatoes to the top. On top of tomatoes, spread the Kalamata olives.

4. Bake for around 20 minutes at about 390° F in the preheated Air Fryer, turning the dish midway through your cooking cycle. Serve it hot and enjoy it!

11. Vegetable Kabobs with Simple Peanut Sauce

Preparation time: 10 minutes

Cooking time: 30 minutes

Servings: 4 people

Ingredients:

- 1/3 tsp. of granulated garlic

- 1 tsp. of dried rosemary, crushed

- 1 tsp. of red pepper flakes, crushed

- Sea salt and ground black pepper, according to your taste.

- 2 tbsp. of extra-virgin olive oil

- 8 small button mushrooms, cleaned

- 8 pearl onions, halved

- 2 bell peppers, diced into 1-inch pieces

- 8 whole baby potatoes, diced into 1-inch pieces

Peanut Sauce:

- 1/2 tsp. of garlic salt

- 1 tbsp. of soy sauce

- 1 tbsp. of balsamic vinegar

- 2 tbsp. of peanut butter

Directions:

1. For a few minutes, dunk the wooden chopsticks in water.

2. String the vegetables onto your chopsticks; drip some olive oil all over your chopsticks with the vegetables on it; dust with seasoning.

3. Cook for about 1 minute at 400°F in the preheated Air Fryer.

Peanut Sauce:

1. In the meantime, mix the balsamic vinegar with some peanut butter, garlic salt and some soy sauce in a tiny dish. Offer the kabobs with a side of peanut sauce. Eat warm!

12. Hungarian Mushroom Pilaf

Preparation time: 10 minutes

Cooking time: 50 minutes

Servings: 4 people

Ingredients:

- 1 tsp. of sweet Hungarian paprika

- 1/2 tsp. of dried tarragon

- 1 tsp. of dried thyme

- 1/4 cup of dry vermouth

- 1 onion, chopped

- 2 garlic cloves

- 2 tbsp. of olive oil

- 1 pound of fresh porcini mushrooms, sliced

- 2 tbsp. of olive oil

- 3 cups of vegetable broth

- 1 ½ cups of white rice

Directions:

1. In a wide saucepan, put the broth and rice, add some water, and bring it to a boil.

2. Cover with a lid and turn the flame down to a low temperature and proceed to cook for the next 18 minutes or so. After cooking, let it rest for 5 to 10 minutes, and then set aside.

3. Finally, in a lightly oiled baking dish, mix the heated, fully cooked rice with the rest of your ingredients.

4. Cook at about 200° degrees for around 20 minutes in the preheated Air Fryer, regularly monitoring to even cook.

5. In small bowls, serve. Bon appétit!

13. Chinese cabbage Bake

Preparation time: 15 minutes

Cooking time: 35 minutes

Servings: 4 people

Ingredients:

- 1 cup of Monterey Jack cheese, shredded

- 1/2 tsp. of cayenne pepper

- 1 cup of cream cheese

- 1/2 cup of milk

- 4 tbsp. of flaxseed meal

- 1/2 stick butter

- 2 garlic cloves, sliced

- 1 onion, thickly sliced

- 1 jalapeno pepper, seeded and sliced

- Sea salt and freshly ground black pepper, according to taste.

- 2 bell peppers, seeded and sliced

- 1/2 pound of Chinese cabbage, roughly chopped

Directions:

1. Heat the salted water in a pan and carry it to a boil. For around 2 to 3 minutes, steam the Chinese cabbage. To end the cooking process, switch the Chinese cabbage to cold water immediately.

2. Put your Chinese cabbage in a lightly oiled casserole dish. Add in the garlic, onion, and peppers.

3. Next, over low fire, melt some butter in a skillet. Add in your flaxseed meal steadily and cook for around 2 minutes to create a paste.

4. Add in the milk gently, constantly whisking until it creates a dense mixture. Add in your cream cheese. Sprinkle some cayenne pepper, salt, and black pepper. To the casserole tray, transfer your mixture.

5. Cover with some Monterey Jack cheese and cook for about 2 minutes at around 390° F in your preheated Air Fryer. Serve it warm.

14. Brussels sprouts With Balsamic Oil

Preparation time: 5 minutes

Cooking time: 15 minutes

Servings: 4 people

Ingredients:

- 2 tbsp. of olive oil

- 2 cups of Brussels sprouts, halved

- 1 tbsp. of balsamic vinegar

- ¼ tsp. of salt

Directions:

1. For 5 minutes, preheat your air fryer.

2. In a mixing bowl, blend all of your ingredients to ensure the zucchini fries are very well coated. Put the fries in the basket of an air fryer.

3. Close it and cook it at about 350°F for around 15 minutes.

15. Aromatic Baked Potatoes with Chives

Preparation time: 15 minutes

Cooking time: 45 minutes

Servings: 2 people

Ingredients:

- 2 tbsp. of chives, chopped

- 2 garlic cloves, minced

- 1 tbsp. of sea salt

- 1/4 tsp. of smoked paprika

- 1/4 tsp. of red pepper flakes

- 2 tbsp. of olive oil

- 4 medium baking potatoes, peeled

Directions:

1. Toss the potatoes with your seasoning, olive oil, and garlic.

2. Please put them in the basket of your Air Fryer. Cook at about 400° F for around 40 minutes just until the potatoes are fork soft in your preheated Air Fryer.

3. Add in some fresh minced chives to garnish. Bon appétit!

16. Easy Vegan "chicken"

Preparation time: 10 minutes

Cooking time: 20 minutes

Servings: 4 people

Ingredients:

- 1 tsp. of celery seeds

- 1/2 tsp. of mustard powder

- 1 tsp. of cayenne pepper

- 1/4 cup of all-purpose flour

- 1/2 cup of cornmeal

- 8 ounces of soy chunks

- Sea salt and ground black pepper, according to taste.

Directions:

1. In a skillet over medium-high flame, cook the soya chunks in plenty of water. Turn off the flame and allow soaking for several minutes. Drain the remaining water, wash, and strain it out.

2. In a mixing bowl, combine the rest of the components. Roll your soy chunks over the breading paste, pressing lightly to stick.

3. In the slightly oiled Air Fryer basket, place your soy chunks.

4. Cook at about 390° for around 10 minutes in your preheated Air Fryer, rotating them over midway through the cooking process; operate in batches if required. Bon appétit!

17. Paprika Vegetable Kebab's

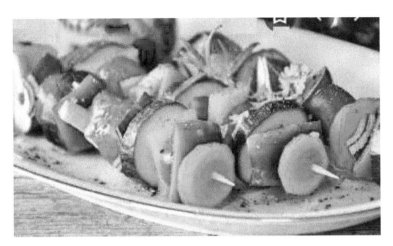

Preparation time: 10 minutes

Cooking time: 20 minutes

Servings: 4 people

Ingredients:

- 1/2 tsp. of ground black pepper

- 1 tsp. of sea salt flakes

- 1 tsp. of smoked paprika

- 1/4 cup of sesame oil

- 2 tbsp. of dry white wine

- 1 red onion, cut into wedges

- 2 cloves garlic, pressed

- 1 tsp. of whole grain mustard

- 1 fennel bulb, diced

- 1 parsnip, cut into thick slices

- 1 celery, cut into thick slices

Directions:

1. Toss all of the above ingredients together in a mixing bowl to uniformly coat. Thread the vegetables alternately onto the wooden skewers.

2. Cook for around 15 minutes at about 380° F on your Air Fryer grill plate.

3. Turn them over midway during the cooking process.

4. Taste, change the seasonings if needed and serve steaming hot.

18. Spiced Soy Curls

Preparation time: 5 minutes

Cooking time: 10 minutes

Servings: 2 people

Ingredients:

- 1 tsp. of poultry seasoning

- 2 tsp. of Cajun seasoning

- ¼ cup of fine ground cornmeal

- ¼ cup of nutritional yeast

- 4 ounces of soy curls

- 3 cups of boiling water

- Salt and ground white pepper, as needed

Directions:

1. Dip the soy curls for around a minute or so in hot water in a heat-resistant tub.

2. Drain your soy coils using a strainer and force the excess moisture out using a broad spoon.

3. Mix the cornmeal, nutritional yeast, salt, seasonings, and white pepper well in a mixing bowl.

4. Transfer your soy curls to the bowl and coat well with the blend. Let the air-fryer temperature to about 380° F. Oil the basket of your air fryers.

5. Adjust soy curls in a uniform layer in the lined air fryer basket. Cook for about 10 minutes in the air fryer, turning midway through the cycle.

6. Take out the soy curls from your air fryer and put them on a serving dish. Serve it steaming hot.

19. Cauliflower & Egg Rice Casserole

Preparation time: 5 minutes

Cooking time: 15 minutes

Servings: 4 people

Ingredients:

- 2 eggs, beaten

- 1 tablespoon of soy sauce

- Salt and black pepper according to taste.

- ½ cup of chopped onion

- 1 cup of okra, chopped

- 1 yellow bell pepper, chopped

- 2 teaspoon of olive oil

Directions:

1. Preheat your air fryer to about 380° F. Oil a baking tray with spray oil. Pulse the cauliflower till it becomes like thin rice-like capsules in your food blender.

2. Now add your cauliflower rice to a baking tray mix in the okra, bell pepper, salt, soy sauce, onion, and pepper and combine well.

3. Drizzle a little olive oil on top along with the beaten eggs. Put the tray in your air fryer and cook for about a minute. Serve it hot.

20.Hollandaise Topped Grilled Asparagus

Preparation time: 2 minutes

Cooking time: 15 minutes

Servings: 6 people

Ingredients:

- A punch of ground white pepper

- A pinch of mustard powder

- 3 pounds of asparagus spears, trimmed

- 3 egg yolks

- 2 tbsp. of olive oil

- 1 tsp. of chopped tarragon leaves

- ½ tsp. of salt

- ½ lemon juice

- ½ cup of butter, melted

- ¼ tsp. of black pepper

Directions:

1. Preheat your air fryer to about 330° F. In your air fryer, put the grill pan attachment.

2. Mix the olive oil, salt, asparagus, and pepper into a Ziploc bag. To mix all, give everything a quick shake. Load onto the grill plate and cook for about 15 minutes.

3. In the meantime, beat the lemon juice, egg yolks, and salt in a double boiler over a moderate flame until velvety.

4. Add in the melted butter, mustard powder, and some white pepper. Continue whisking till the mixture is creamy and thick. Serve with tarragon leaves as a garnish.

5. Pour the sauce over the asparagus spears and toss to blend.

21. Crispy Asparagus Dipped In Paprika-garlic Spice

Preparation time: 2 minutes

Cooking time: 15 minutes

Servings: 5 people

Ingredients:

- ¼ cup of almond flour

- ½ tsp. of garlic powder

- ½ tsp. of smoked paprika

- 10 medium asparagus, trimmed

- 2 large eggs, beaten

- 2 tbsp. of parsley, chopped

- Salt and pepper according to your taste

Directions:

1. For about 5 minutes, preheat your air fryer.

2. Mix the almond flour, garlic powder, parsley, and smoked paprika in a mixing dish. To taste, season with some salt and black pepper.

3. Soak your asparagus in the beaten eggs, and then dredge it in a combination of almond flour.

4. Put in the bowl of your air fryer. Close the lid. At about 350°F, cook for around a minute.

22. Eggplant Gratin with Mozzarella Crust

Preparation time: 10 minutes

Cooking time: 30 minutes

Servings: 2 people

Ingredients:

- 1 tablespoon of breadcrumbs

- ¼ cup of grated mozzarella cheese

- Cooking spray

- Salt and pepper according to your taste

- ¼ teaspoon of dried marjoram

- ¼ teaspoon of dried basil

- 1 teaspoon of capers

- 1 tablespoon of sliced pimiento-stuffed olives

- 1 clove garlic, minced

- ⅓ cup of chopped tomatoes

- ¼ cup of chopped onion

- ¼ cup of chopped green pepper

- ¼ cup of chopped red pepper

Directions:

1. Put the green pepper, eggplant, onion, red pepper, olives, tomatoes, basil marjoram, garlic, salt, capers, and pepper in a container and preheat your air fryer to about 300° F.

2. Lightly oil a baking tray with a spray of cooking olive oil.

3. Fill your baking with the eggplant combination and line it with the vessel.

4. Place some mozzarella cheese on top of it and top with some breadcrumbs. Put the dish in the frying pan and cook for a few minutes.

23. Asian-style Cauliflower

Preparation time: 10 minutes

Cooking time: 25 minutes

Servings: 4 people

Ingredients:

- 2 tbsp. of sesame seeds

- 1/4 cup of lime juice

- 1 tbsp. of fresh parsley, finely chopped

- 1 tbsp. of ginger, freshly grated

- 2 cloves of garlic, peeled and pressed

- 1 tbsp. of sake

- 1 tbsp. of tamari sauce

- 1 tbsp. of sesame oil

- 1 onion, peeled and finely chopped

- 2 cups of cauliflower, grated

Directions:

1. In a mixing bowl, mix your onion, cauliflower, tamari sauce, sesame oil, garlic, sake, and ginger; whisk until all is well integrated.

2. Air-fry it for around a minute at about 400° F.

3. Pause your Air Fryer. Add in some parsley and lemon juice.

4. Cook for an extra 10 minutes at about 300° degrees F in the air fryer.

5. In the meantime, in a non-stick pan, toast your sesame seeds; swirl them continuously over medium-low heat. Serve hot on top of the cauliflower with a pinch of salt and pepper.

24. Two-cheese Vegetable Frittata

Preparation time: 15 minutes

Cooking time: 35 minutes

Servings: 2 people

Ingredients:

- ⅓ cup of crumbled Feta cheese

- ⅓ cup of grated Cheddar cheese

- Salt and pepper according to taste

- ⅓ cup of milk

- 4 eggs, cracked into a bowl

- 2 teaspoon of olive oil

- ¼ lb. of asparagus, trimmed and sliced thinly

- ¼ cup of chopped chives

- 1 small red onion, sliced

- 1 large zucchini, sliced with a 1-inch thickness

- ⅓ cup of sliced mushrooms

Directions:

1. Preheat your air fryer to about 380° F. Set aside your baking dish lined with some parchment paper. Put salt, milk, and pepper into the egg bowl; whisk evenly.

2. Put a skillet on the stovetop over a moderate flame, and heat your olive oil. Add in the zucchini, asparagus, baby spinach, onion, and mushrooms; stir-fry for around 5 minutes. Transfer the vegetables into your baking tray, and finish with the beaten egg.

3. Put the tray into your air fryer and finish with cheddar and feta cheese.

4. For about 15 minutes, cook. Take out your baking tray and add in some fresh chives to garnish.

25. Rice & Beans Stuffed Bell Peppers

Preparation time: 10 minutes

Cooking time: 15 minutes

Servings: 5 people

Ingredients:

- 1 tbsp. of Parmesan cheese, grated

- ½ cup of mozzarella cheese, shredded

- 5 large bell peppers, tops removed and seeded

- 1½ tsp. of Italian seasoning

- 1 cup of cooked rice

- 1 (15-ounces) can of red kidney beans, rinsed and drained

- 1 (15-ounces) can of diced tomatoes with juice

- ½ small bell pepper, seeded and chopped

Directions:

1. Combine the tomatoes with juice, bell pepper, rice, beans, and Italian seasoning in a mixing dish. Using the rice mixture, fill each bell pepper uniformly.

2. Preheat the air fryer to 300° F. Oil the basket of your air fryer with some spray oil. Put the bell peppers in a uniform layer in your air fryer basket.

3. Cook for around 12 minutes in the air fryer. In the meantime, combine the Parmesan and mozzarella cheese in a mixing dish.

4. Remove the peppers from the air fryer basket and top each with some cheese mix. Cook for another 3 -4 minutes in the air fryer

5. Take the bell peppers from the air fryer and put them on a serving dish. Enable to cool slowly before serving. Serve it hot.

26. Parsley-loaded Mushrooms

Preparation time: 5 minutes

Cooking time: 15 minutes

Servings: 2 people

Ingredients:

- 2 tablespoon of parsley, finely chopped

- 2 teaspoon of olive oil

- 1 garlic clove, crushed

- 2 slices white bread

- salt and black pepper according to your taste

Directions:

1. Preheat the air fryer to about 360° F. Crush your bread into crumbs in a food blender. Add the parsley, garlic, and pepper; blend with the olive oil and mix.

2. Remove the stalks from the mushrooms and stuff the caps with breadcrumbs. In your air fryer basket, position the mushroom heads. Cook for a few minutes, just until golden brown and crispy.

27. Cheesy Vegetable Quesadilla

Preparation time: 2 minutes

Cooking time: 15 minutes

Servings: 1 people

Ingredients:

- 1 teaspoon of olive oil

- 1 tablespoon of cilantro, chopped

- ½ green onion, sliced

- ¼ zucchini, sliced

- ¼ yellow bell pepper, sliced

- ¼ cup of shredded gouda cheese

Directions:

1. Preheat your air fryer to about 390° F. Oil a basket of air fryers with some cooking oil.

2. Put a flour tortilla in your air fryer basket and cover it with some bell pepper, Gouda cheese, cilantro, zucchini, and green onion. Take the other tortilla to cover and spray with some olive oil.

3. Cook until slightly golden brown, for around 10 minutes. Cut into 4 slices for serving when ready. Enjoy!

28. Creamy 'n Cheese Broccoli Bake

Preparation time: 10 minutes

Cooking time: 30 minutes

Servings: 2 people

Ingredients:

- 1/4 cup of water

- 1-1/2 teaspoons of butter, or to taste

- 1/2 cup of cubed sharp Cheddar cheese

- 1/2 (14 ounces) can evaporate milk, divided

- 1/2 large onion, coarsely diced

- 1 tbsp. of dry bread crumbs, or to taste

- salt according to taste

- 2 tbsp. of all-purpose flour

- 1-pound of fresh broccoli, coarsely diced

Directions:

1. Lightly oil the air-fryer baking pan with cooking oil. Add half of the milk and flour into a pan and simmer at about 360° F for around 5 minutes.

2. Mix well midway through the cooking period. Remove the broccoli and the extra milk. Cook for the next 5 minutes after fully blending.

3. Mix in the cheese until it is fully melted. Mix the butter and bread crumbs well in a shallow tub. Sprinkle the broccoli on top.

4. At about 360° F, cook for around 20 minutes until the tops are finely golden brown. Enjoy and serve warm.

29. Sweet & Spicy Parsnips

Preparation time: 12 minutes

Cooking time: 44 minutes

Servings: 6 people

Ingredients:

- ¼ tsp. of red pepper flakes, crushed
- 1 tbsp. of dried parsley flakes, crushed
- 2 tbsp. of honey
- 1 tbsp. of n butter, melted
- 2 pounds of a parsnip, peeled and cut into 1-inch chunks
- Salt and ground black pepper, according to your taste.

Directions:

1. Let the air-fryer temperature to about 355° F. Oil the basket of your air fryers. Combine the butter and parsnips in a big dish.

2. Transfer the parsnip pieces into the lined air fryer basket arranges them in a uniform layer. Cook for a few minutes in the fryer.

3. In the meantime, combine the leftover ingredients in a large mixing bowl.

4. Move the parsnips into the honey mixture bowl after around 40 minutes and toss them to coat properly.

5. Again, in a uniform layer, organize the parsnip chunks into your air fryer basket.

6. Air-fry for another 3-4 minutes. Take the parsnip pieces from the air fryer and pass them onto the serving dish. Serve it warm.

30. Zucchini with Mediterranean Dill Sauce

Preparation time: 20 minutes

Cooking time: 60 minutes

Servings: 4 people

Ingredients:

- 1/2 tsp. of freshly cracked black peppercorns

- 2 sprigs thyme, leaves only, crushed

- 1 sprig rosemary, leaves only, crushed

- 1 tsp. of sea salt flakes

- 2 tbsp. of melted butter

- 1 pound of zucchini, peeled and cubed

For your Mediterranean Dipping:

- 1 tbsp. of olive oil

- 1 tbsp. of fresh dill, chopped

- 1/3 cup of yogurt

- 1/2 cup of mascarpone cheese

Directions:

1. To start, preheat your Air Fryer to 350° F. Now, add ice cold water to the container with your potato cubes and let them sit in the bath for about 35 minutes.

2. Dry your potato cubes with a hand towel after that. Whisk together the sea salt flakes, melted butter, thyme, rosemary, and freshly crushed peppercorns in a mixing container. This butter/spice mixture can be rubbed onto the potato cubes.

3. In the cooking basket of your air fryer, air-fry your potato cubes for around 18 to 20 minutes or until cooked completely; ensure you shake the potatoes at least once during cooking to cook them uniformly.

4. In the meantime, by mixing the rest of the ingredients, create the Mediterranean dipping sauce. To dip and eat, serve warm potatoes with Mediterranean sauce!

31. Zesty Broccoli

Preparation time: 10 minutes

Cooking time: 15 minutes

Servings: 4 people

Ingredients:

- 1 tbsp. of butter

- 1 large crown broccoli, chopped into bite-sized pieces

- 1 tbsp. of white sesame seeds

- 2 tbsp. of vegetable stock

- ½ tsp. of red pepper flakes, crushed

- 3 garlic cloves, minced

- ½ tsp. of fresh lemon zest, grated finely

- 1 tbsp. of pure lemon juice

Directions:

1. Preheat the Air fryer to about 355° F and oil an Air fryer pan with cooking spray. In the Air fryer plate, combine the vegetable stock, butter, and lemon juice.

2. Move the mixture and cook for about 2 minutes into your Air Fryer. Cook for a minute after incorporating the broccoli and garlic.

3. Cook for a minute with lemon zest, sesame seeds, and red pepper flakes. Remove the dish from the oven and eat immediately.

32. Chewy Glazed Parsnips

Preparation time: 15 minutes

Cooking time: 44 minutes

Servings: 6 people

Ingredients:

- ¼ tsp. of red pepper flakes, crushed

- 1 tbsp. of dried parsley flakes, crushed

- 2 tbsp. of maple syrup

- 1 tbsp. of butter, melted

- 2 pounds of parsnips, skinned and chopped into 1-inch chunks

Directions:

1. Preheat the Air fryer to about 355° F and oil your air fryer basket. In a wide mixing bowl, combine the butter and parsnips and toss well to cover. Cook for around 40 minutes with the parsnips in the Air fryer basket.

2. In the meantime, combine in a wide bowl the rest of your ingredients. Move this mix to your basket of the air fryer and cook for another 4 minutes or so. Remove the dish from the oven and eat promptly.

33. Hoisin-glazed Bok Choy

Preparation time: 5 minutes

Cooking time: 10 minutes

Servings: 4 people

Ingredients:

- 1 tbsp. of all-purpose flour

- 2 tbsp. of sesame oil

- 2 tbsp. of hoisin sauce

- 1/2 tsp. of sage

- 1 tsp. of onion powder

- 2 garlic cloves, minced

- 1 pound of baby Bok choy, roots removed, leaves separated

Directions:

1. In a lightly oiled Air Fryer basket, put the onion powder, garlic, Bok Choy, and sage. Cook for around 3 minutes at about 350° F in a preheated Air Fryer.

2. Whisk together the sesame oil, hoisin sauce, and flour in a deep mixing dish. Drizzle over the Bok choy with the gravy. Cook for an extra minute. Bon appétit!

34. Green Beans with Okra

Preparation time: 10 minutes

Cooking time: 20 minutes

Servings: 2 people

Ingredients:

- 3 tbsp. of balsamic vinegar

- ¼ cup of nutritional yeast

- ½ (10-ounces) of bag chilled cut green beans

- ½ (10-ounces) of bag chilled cut okra

- Salt and black pepper, according to your taste.

Directions:

1. Preheat your Air fryer to about 400° F and oil the air fryer basket.

2. In a wide mixing bowl, toss together the salt, green beans, okra, vinegar, nutritional yeast, and black pepper.

3. Cook for around 20 minutes with the okra mixture in your Air fryer basket. Dish out into a serving plate and eat warm.

35.Celeriac with some Greek Yogurt Dip

Preparation time: 12 minutes

Cooking time: 25 minutes

Servings: 2 people

Ingredients:

- 1/2 tsp. of sea salt

- 1/2 tsp. of ground black pepper, to taste

- 1 tbsp. of sesame oil

- 1 red onion, chopped into 1 1/2-inch piece

- 1/2 pound of celeriac, chopped into 1 1/2-inch piece

Spiced Yogurt:

- 1/2 tsp. of chili powder

- 1/2 tsp. of mustard seeds

- 2 tbsp. of mayonnaise

- 1/4 cup of Greek yogurt

Directions:

1. In the slightly oiled cooking basket, put the veggies in one uniform layer. Pour sesame oil over the veggies.

2. Season with a pinch of black pepper and a pinch of salt. Cook for around 20 minutes at about 300° F, tossing the basket midway through your cooking cycle.

3. In the meantime, whisk all the leftover ingredients into the sauce. Spoon the sauce over the veggies that have been cooked. Bon appétit!

36. Wine & Garlic Flavored Vegetables

Preparation time: 7-10 minutes

Cooking time: 15 minutes

Servings: 4 people

Ingredients:

- 4 cloves of garlic, minced

- 3 tbsp. of red wine vinegar

- 1/3 cup of olive oil

- 1 red onion, diced

- 1 package frozen diced vegetables

- 1 cup of baby Portobello mushrooms, diced

- 1 tsp. of Dijon mustard

- 1 ½ tbsp. of honey

- Salt and pepper according to your taste

- ¼ cup of chopped fresh basil

Directions:

1. Preheat the air fryer to about 330° F. In the air fryer, put the grill pan attachment.

2. Combine the veggies and season with pepper, salt, and garlic in a Ziploc container. To mix all, give everything a strong shake. Dump and cook for around 15 minutes on the grill pan.

3. Additionally, add the remainder of the ingredients into a mixing bowl and season with some more salt and pepper. Drizzle the sauce over your grilled vegetables.

37. Spicy Braised Vegetables

Preparation time: 10 minutes

Cooking time: 25 minutes

Servings: 4 people

Ingredients:

- 1/2 cup of tomato puree

- 1/4 tsp. of ground black pepper

- 1/2 tsp. of fine sea salt

- 1 tbsp. of garlic powder

- 1/2 tsp. of fennel seeds

- 1/4 tsp. of mustard powder

- 1/2 tsp. of porcini powder

- 1/4 cup of olive oil

- 1 celery stalk, chopped into matchsticks

- 2 bell peppers, deveined and thinly diced

- 1 Serrano pepper, deveined and thinly diced

- 1 large-sized zucchini, diced

Directions:

1. In your Air Fryer cooking basket, put your peppers, zucchini, sweet potatoes, and carrot.

2. Drizzle with some olive oil and toss to cover completely; cook for around 15 minutes in a preheated Air Fryer at about 350°F.

3. Make the sauce as the vegetables are frying by quickly whisking the remaining ingredients (except the tomato ketchup). Slightly oil up a baking dish that fits your fryer.

4. Add the cooked vegetables to the baking dish, along with the sauce, and toss well to cover.

5. Turn the Air Fryer to about 390° F and cook for 2-4 more minutes with the vegetables. Bon appétit!

CHAPTER 3: Air Fryer Snack Side Dishes and Appetizer Recipes

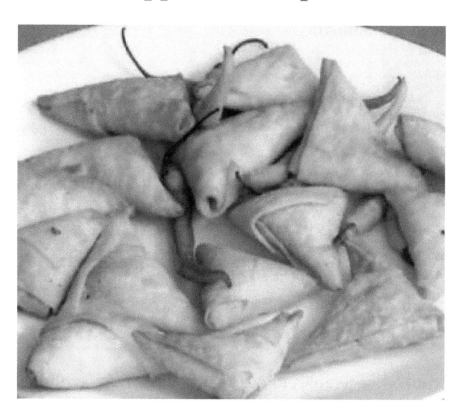

1. Crispy 'n Tasty Spring Rolls

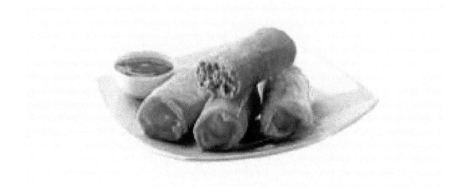

Preparation time: 5 minutes

Cooking time: 15 minutes

Servings: 4 people

Ingredients:

- 8 spring roll wrappers

- 1 tsp. of nutritional yeast

- 1 tsp. of corn starch + 2 tablespoon water

- 1 tsp. of coconut sugar

- 1 tbsp. of soy sauce

- 1 medium carrot, shredded

- 1 cup of shiitake mushroom, sliced thinly

- 1 celery stalk, chopped

- ½ tsp. of ginger, finely chopped

Directions:

1. Mix your carrots, celery stalk, soy sauce, coconut sugar, ginger, and nutritional yeast with each other in a mixing dish.

2. Have a tbsp. of your vegetable mix and put it in the middle of your spring roll wrappers.

3. Roll up and secure the sides of your wraps with some cornstarch.

4. Cook for about 15 minutes or till your spring roll wraps is crisp in a preheated air fryer at 200F.

2. Spinach & Feta Crescent Triangles

Preparation time: 10 minutes

Cooking time: 20 minutes

Servings: 4 people

Ingredients:

- ¼ teaspoon of salt

- 1 teaspoon of chopped oregano

- ¼ teaspoon of garlic powder

- 1 cup of crumbled feta cheese

- 1 cup of steamed spinach

Directions:

1. Preheat your air fryer to about 350 F, and then roll up the dough over a level surface that is gently floured.

2. In a medium-sized bowl, mix the spinach, feta, salt, oregano, and ground garlic cloves. Split your dough into four equal chunks.

3. Split the mix of feta/spinach among the four chunks of dough. Fold and seal your dough using a fork.

4. Please put it on a baking tray covered with parchment paper, and then put it in your air fryer.

5. Cook until nicely golden, for around 1 minute.

3. Healthy Avocado Fries

Preparation time: 5 minutes

Cooking time: 20 minutes

Servings: 2 people

Ingredients:

- ¼ cup of aquafaba

- 1 avocado, cubed

- Salt as required

Directions:

1. Mix the aquafaba, crumbs, and salt in a mixing bowl.

2. Preheat your air fryer to about 390°F and cover the avocado pieces uniformly in the crumbs blend.

3. Put the ready pieces in the cooking bucket of your air fryer and cook for several minutes.

4. Twice-fried Cauliflower Tater Tots

Preparation time: 5 minutes

Cooking time: 16 minutes

Servings: 12 people

Ingredients:

- 3 tbsp. Of oats flaxseed meal + 3 tbsp. of water)

- 1-pound of cauliflower, steamed and chopped

- 1 tsp. of parsley, chopped

- 1 tsp. of oregano, chopped

- 1 tsp. of garlic, minced

- 1 tsp. of chives, chopped

- 1 onion, chopped

- 1 flax egg (1 tablespoon 3 tablespoon desiccated coconuts)

- ½ cup of nutritional yeast

- salt and pepper according to taste

- ½ cup of bread crumbs

Directions:

1. Preheat your air fryer to about 390 degrees F.

2. To extract extra moisture, place the steamed cauliflower onto a ring and a paper towel.

3. Put and mix the remainder of your ingredients, excluding your bread crumbs, in a small mixing container.

4. Use your palms, blend it until well mixed and shapes into a small ball.

5. Roll your tater tots over your bread crumbs and put them in the bucket of your air fryer.

6. For a minute, bake. Raise the cooking level to about 400 F and cook for the next 10 minutes.

5. Cheesy Mushroom & Cauliflower Balls

Preparation time: 10 minutes

Cooking time: 50 minutes

Servings: 4 people

Ingredients:

- Salt and pepper according to taste

- 2 sprigs chopped fresh thyme

- ¼ cup of coconut oil

- 1 cup of Grana Padano cheese

- 1 cup of breadcrumbs

- 2 tablespoon of vegetable stock

- 3 cups of cauliflower, chopped

- 3 cloves garlic, minced

- 1 small red onion, chopped

- 3 tablespoon of olive oil

Directions:

1. Over moderate flame, put a pan. Add some balsamic vinegar. When the oil is heated, stir-fry your onion and garlic till they become transparent.

2. Add in the mushrooms and cauliflower and stir-fry for about 5 minutes. Add in your stock, add thyme and cook till your cauliflower has consumed the stock. Add pepper, Grana Padano cheese, and salt.

3. Let the mix cool down and form bite-size spheres of your paste. To harden, put it in the fridge for about 30 minutes.

4. Preheat your air fryer to about 350°F.

5. Add your coconut oil and breadcrumbs into a small bowl and blend properly.

6. Take out your mushroom balls from the fridge, swirl the breadcrumb paste once more, and drop the balls into your breadcrumb paste.

7. Avoid overcrowding, put your balls into your air fryer's container and cook for about 15 minutes, flipping after every 5 minutes to ensure even cooking.

8. Serve with some tomato sauce and brown sugar.

6. Italian Seasoned Easy Pasta Chips

Preparation time: 5 minutes

Cooking time: 10 minutes

Servings: 2 people

Ingredients:

- 2 cups of whole wheat bowtie pasta

- 1 tbsp. of olive oil

- 1 tbsp. of nutritional yeast

- 1 ½ tsp. of Italian seasoning blend

- ½ tsp. of salt

Directions:

1. Put the accessory for the baking tray into your air fryer.

2. Mix all the ingredients in a medium-sized bowl, offer it a gentle stir.

3. Add the mixture to your air fryer basket.

4. Close your air fryer and cook at around 400°degrees F for about 10 minutes.

7. Thai Sweet Potato Balls

Preparation time: 10 minutes

Cooking time: 50 minutes

Servings: 4 people

Ingredients:

- 1 cup of coconut flakes

- 1 tsp. of baking powder

- 1/2 cup of almond meal

- 1/4 tsp. of ground cloves

- 1/2 tsp. of ground cinnamon

- 2 tsp. of orange zest

- 1 tbsp. of orange juice

- 1 cup of brown sugar

- 1 pound of sweet potatoes

Directions:

1. Bake your sweet potatoes for around 25 to 30 minutes at about 380° F till they become soft; peel and mash them in a medium-sized bowl.

2. Add orange zest, orange juice, brown sugar, ground cinnamon, almond meal, cloves, and baking powder. Now blend completely.

3. Roll the balls around in some coconut flakes.

4. Bake for around 15 minutes or until fully fried and crunchy in the preheated Air Fryer at about 360° F.

5. For the rest of the ingredients, redo the same procedure. Bon appétit!

8. Barbecue Roasted Almonds

Preparation time: 5 minutes

Cooking time: 20 minutes

Servings: 6 people

Ingredients:

- 1 tbsp. of olive oil

- 1/4 tsp. of smoked paprika

- 1/2 tsp. of cumin powder

- 1/4 tsp. of mustard powder

- 1/4 tsp. of garlic powder

- Sea salt and ground black pepper, according to taste

- 1 ½ cups of raw almonds

Directions:

1. In a mixing pot, mix all your ingredients.

2. Line the container of your Air Fryer with some baking parchment paper. Arrange the covered almonds out in the basket of your air fryer in a uniform layer.

3. Roast for around 8 to 9 minutes at about 340°F, tossing the bucket once or twice. If required, work in groups.

4. Enjoy!

9. Croissant Rolls

Preparation time: 2 minutes

Cooking time: 6 minutes

Servings: 8 people

Ingredients:

- 4 tbsp. of butter, melted

- 1 (8-ounces) can croissant rolls

Directions:

1. Adjust the air-fryer temperature to about 320°F. Oil the basket of your air fryers.

2. Into your air fryer basket, place your prepared croissant rolls.

3. Airs fry them for around 4 minutes or so.

4. Flip to the opposite side and cook for another 2-3 minutes.

5. Take out from your air fryer and move to a tray.

6. Glaze with some melted butter and eat warm.

10. Curry' n Coriander Spiced Bread Rolls

Preparation time: 5 minutes

Cooking time: 15 minutes

Servings: 5 people

Ingredients:

- salt and pepper according to taste

- 5 large potatoes, boiled

- 2 sprigs, curry leaves

- 2 small onions, chopped

- 2 green chilies, seeded and chopped

- 1 tbsp. of olive oil

- 1 bunch of coriander, chopped

- ½ tsp. of turmeric

- 8 slices of vegan wheat bread, brown sides discarded

- ½ tsp. of mustard seeds

Directions:

1. Mash your potatoes in a bowl and sprinkle some black pepper and salt according to taste. Now set aside.

2. In a pan, warm up the olive oil over medium-low heat and add some mustard seeds. Mix until the seeds start to sputter.

3. Now add in the onions and cook till they become transparent. Mix in the curry leaves and turmeric powder.

4. Keep on cooking till it becomes fragrant for a couple of minutes. Take it off the flame and add the mixture to the potatoes.

5. Mix in the green chilies and some coriander. This is meant to be the filling.

6. Wet your bread and drain excess moisture. In the center of the loaf, put a tbsp. of the potato filling and gently roll the bread so that the potato filling is fully enclosed within the bread.

7. Brush with some oil and put them inside your air fryer basket.

8. Cook for around 15 minutes in a preheated air fryer at about 400°F.

9. Ensure that the air fryer basket is shaken softly midway through the cooking period for an even cooking cycle.

11. Scrumptiously Healthy Chips

Preparation time: 5 minutes

Cooking time: 10 minutes

Servings: 2 people

Ingredients:

- 2 tbsp. of olive oil

- 2 tbsp. of almond flour

- 1 tsp. of garlic powder

- 1 bunch kale

- Salt and pepper according to taste

Directions:

1. For around 5 minutes, preheat your air fryer.

2. In a mixing bowl, add all your ingredients, add the kale leaves at the end and toss to completely cover them.

3. Put in the basket of your fryer and cook until crispy for around 10 minutes.

12. Kid-friendly Vegetable Fritters

Preparation time: 5 minutes

Cooking time: 20 minutes

Servings: 4 people

Ingredients:

- 2 tbsp. of olive oil

- 1/2 cup of cornmeal

- 1/2 cup of all-purpose flour

- 1/2 tsp. of ground cumin

- 1 tsp. of turmeric powder

- 2 garlic cloves, pressed

- 1 carrot, grated

- 1 sweet pepper, seeded and chopped

- 1 yellow onion, finely chopped

- 1 tbsp. of ground flaxseeds

- Salt and ground black pepper, according to taste

- 1 pound of broccoli florets

Directions:

1. In salted boiling water, blanch your broccoli until al dente, for around 3 to 5 minutes. Drain the excess water and move to a mixing bowl; add in the rest of your ingredients to mash the broccoli florets.

2. Shape the paste into patties and position them in the slightly oiled Air Fryer basket.

3. Cook for around 6 minutes at about 400° F, flipping them over midway through the cooking process; if needed, operate in batches.

4. Serve hot with some Vegenaise of your choice. Enjoy it!

13. Avocado Fries

Preparation time: 10 minutes

Cooking time: 50 minutes

Servings: 4 people

Ingredients:

- 2 avocados, cut into wedges

- 1/2 cup of parmesan cheese, grated

- 2 eggs

- Sea salt and ground black pepper, according to taste.

- 1/2 cup of almond meal

- 1/2 head garlic (6-7 cloves)

Sauce:

- 1 tsp. of mustard

- 1 tsp. of lemon juice

- 1/2 cup of mayonnaise

Directions:

1. On a piece of aluminum foil, put your garlic cloves and spray some cooking spray on it. Wrap your garlic cloves in the foil.

2. Cook for around 1-2 minutes at about 400°F in your preheated Air Fryer. Inspect the garlic, open the foil's top end, and keep cooking for an additional 10-12 minutes.

3. Once done, let them cool for around 10 to 15 minutes; take out the cloves by pressing them out of their skin; mash your garlic and put them aside.

4. Mix the salt, almond meal, and black pepper in a small dish.

5. Beat the eggs until foamy in a separate bowl.

6. Put some parmesan cheese in the final shallow dish.

7. In your almond meal blend, dip the avocado wedges, dusting off any excess.

8. In the beaten egg, dunk your wedges; eventually, dip in some parmesan cheese.

9. Spray your avocado wedges on both sides with some cooking oil spray.

10. Cook for around 8 minutes in the preheated Air Fryer at about 395° F, flipping them over midway thru the cooking process.

11. In the meantime, mix the ingredients of your sauce with your cooked crushed garlic.

12. Split the avocado wedges between plates and cover with the sauce before serving. Enjoy!

14. Crispy Wings with Lemony Old Bay Spice

Preparation time: 10 minutes

Cooking time: 25 minutes

Servings: 4 people

Ingredients:

- Salt and pepper according to taste

- 3 pounds of vegan chicken wings

- 1 tsp. of lemon juice, freshly squeezed

- 1 tbsp. of old bay spices

- ¾ cup of almond flour

- ½ cup of butter

Directions:

1. For about 5 minutes, preheat your air fryer. Mix all your ingredients in a mixing dish, excluding the butter. Put in the bowl of an air fryer.

2. Preheat the oven to about 350°F and bake for around 25 minutes. Rock the fryer container midway thru the cooking process, also for cooking.

3. Drizzle with some melted butter when it's done frying. Enjoy!

15. Cold Salad with Veggies and Pasta

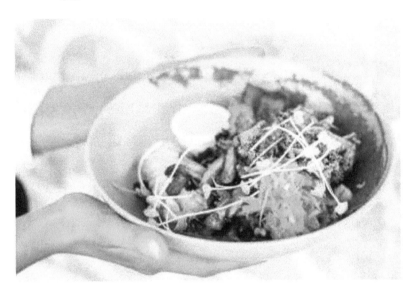

Preparation time: 30 minutes

Cooking time: 1 hour 35 minutes

Servings: 12 people

Ingredients:

- ½ cup of fat-free Italian dressing

- 2 tablespoons of olive oil, divided

- ½ cup of Parmesan cheese, grated

- 8 cups of cooked pasta

- 4 medium tomatoes, cut in eighths

- 3 small eggplants, sliced into ½-inch thick rounds

- 3 medium zucchinis, sliced into ½-inch thick rounds

- Salt, according to your taste.

Directions:

1. Preheat your Air fryer to about 355° F and oil the inside of your air fryer basket. In a dish, mix 1 tablespoon of olive oil and zucchini and swirl to cover properly.

2. Cook for around 25 minutes your zucchini pieces in your Air fryer basket. In another dish, mix your eggplants with a tablespoon of olive oil and toss to coat properly.

3. Cook for around 40 minutes your eggplant slices in your Air fryer basket. Re-set the Air Fryer temperature to about 320° F and put the tomatoes next in the ready basket.

4. Cook and mix all your air-fried vegetables for around 30 minutes. To serve, mix in the rest of the ingredients and chill for at least 2 hours, covered.

16. Zucchini and Minty Eggplant Bites

Preparation time: 15 minutes

Cooking time: 35 minutes

Servings: 8 people

Ingredients:

- 3 tbsp. of olive oil

- 1 pound of zucchini, peeled and cubed

- 1 pound of eggplant, peeled and cubed

- 2 tbsp. of melted butter

- 1 ½ tsp. of red pepper chili flakes

- 2 tsp. of fresh mint leaves, minced

Directions:

1. In a large mixing container, add all of the ingredients mentioned above.

2. Roast the zucchini bites and eggplant in your Air Fryer for around 30 minutes at about 300° F, flipping once or twice during the cooking cycle. Serve with some dipping sauce that's homemade.

17. Stuffed Potatoes

Preparation time: 15 minutes

Cooking time: 31 minutes

Servings: 4 people

Ingredients:

- 3 tbsp. of canola oil

- ½ cup of Parmesan cheese, grated

- 2 tbsp. of chives, chopped

- ½ of brown onion, chopped

- 1 tbsp. of butter

- 4 potatoes, peeled

Directions:

1. Preheat the Air fryer to about 390° F and oil the air fryer basket. Coat the canola oil on the potatoes and place them in your Air Fryer Basket.

2. Cook for around 20 minutes before serving on a platter. Halve each potato and scrape out the middle from each half of it.

3. In a frying pan, melt some butter over medium heat and add the onions. Sauté in a bowl for around 5 minutes and dish out.

4. Combine the onions with the middle of the potato, chives and half of the cheese. Stir well and uniformly cram the onion potato mixture into the potato halves.

5. Top and layer the potato halves in your Air Fryer basket with the leftover cheese. Cook for around 6 minutes before serving hot.

18. Paneer Cutlet

Preparation time: 5 minutes

Cooking time: 15 minutes

Servings: 1 people

Ingredients:

- ½ teaspoon of salt

- ½ teaspoon of oregano

- 1 small onion, finely chopped

- ½ teaspoon of garlic powder

- 1 teaspoon of butter

- ½ teaspoon of chai masala

- 1 cup of grated cheese

Directions:

1. Preheat the air fryer to about 350° F and lightly oil a baking dish. In a mixing bowl, add all ingredients and stir well. Split the mixture into cutlets and put them in an oiled baking dish.

2. Put the baking dish in your air fryer and cook your cutlets until crispy, around a minute or so.

19. Spicy Roasted Cashew Nuts

Preparation time: 10 Minutes

Cooking time: 20 Minutes

Servings: 4

Ingredients:

- 1/2 tsp. of ancho chili powder

- 1/2 tsp. of smoked paprika

- Salt and ground black pepper, according to taste

- 1 tsp. of olive oil

- 1 cup of whole cashews

Directions:

1. In a mixing big bowl, toss all your ingredients.

2. Line parchment paper to cover the Air Fryer container. Space out the spiced cashews in your basket in a uniform layer.

3. Roast for about 6 to 8 minutes at 300 degrees F, tossing the basket once or twice during the cooking process. Work in batches if needed. Enjoy!

CHAPTER 4: Deserts

1. Almond-apple Treat

Preparation time: 5 minutes

Cooking time: 15 minutes

Servings: 4 people

Ingredients:

- 2 tablespoon of sugar

- ¾ oz. of raisins

- 1 ½ oz. of almonds

Directions:

1. Preheat your air fryer to around 360° F.

2. Mix the almonds, sugar, and raisins in a dish. Blend using a hand mixer.

3. Load the apples with a combination of the almond mixture. Please put them in the air fryer basket and cook for a few minutes. Enjoy!

2. Pepper-pineapple With Butter-sugar Glaze

Preparation time: 5 minutes

Cooking time: 10 minutes

Servings: 2 people

Ingredients:

- Salt according to taste.

- 2 tsp. of melted butter

- 1 tsp. of brown sugar

- 1 red bell pepper, seeded and julienned

- 1 medium-sized pineapple, peeled and sliced

Directions:

1. To about 390°F, preheat your air fryer. In your air fryer, put the grill pan attachment.

2. In a Ziploc bag, combine all ingredients and shake well.

3. Dump and cook on the grill pan for around 10 minutes to ensure you turn the pineapples over every 5 minutes during cooking.

3. True Churros with Yummy Hot Chocolate

Preparation time: 10 minutes

Cooking time: 25 minutes

Servings: 3 people

Ingredients:

- 1 tsp. of ground cinnamon

- 1/3 cup of sugar

- 1 tbsp. of cornstarch

- 1 cup of milk

- 2 ounces of dark chocolate

- 1 cup of all-purpose flour

- 1 tbsp. of canola oil

- 1 tsp. of lemon zest

- 1/4 tsp. of sea salt

- 2 tbsp. of granulated sugar

- 1/2 cup of water

Directions:

1. To create the churro dough, boil the water in a pan over a medium-high flame; then, add the salt, sugar, and lemon zest and fry, stirring continuously, until fully dissolved.

2. Take the pan off the heat and add in some canola oil. Stir the flour in steadily, constantly stirring until the solution turns to a ball.

3. With a broad star tip, pipe the paste into a piping bag. In the oiled Air Fryer basket, squeeze 4-inch slices of dough. Cook for around 6 minutes at a temperature of 300° F.

4. Make the hot cocoa for dipping in the meantime. In a shallow saucepan, melt some chocolate and 1/2 cup of milk over low flame.

5. In the leftover 1/2 cup of milk, mix the cornstarch and blend it into the hot chocolate mixture. Cook for around 5 minutes on low flame.

6. Mix the sugar and cinnamon; roll your churros in this combination. Serve with a side of hot cocoa. Enjoy!

Conclusion

These times, air frying is one of the most common cooking techniques and air fryers have become one of the chef's most impressive devices. In no time, air fryers can help you prepare nutritious and tasty meals! To prepare unique dishes for you and your family members, you do not need to be a master in the kitchen.

Everything you have to do is buy an air fryer and this wonderful cookbook for air fryers! Soon, you can make the greatest dishes ever and inspire those around you.

Cooked meals at home with you! Believe us! Get your hands on an air fryer and this handy set of recipes for air fryers and begin your new cooking experience. Have fun!

The Complete Air Fryer Cookbook with Pictures

70+ Perfectly Portioned Air Fryer Recipes for Busy People on a Budget

By Chef Carlo Leone

Contents

INTRODUCTION:

The aim of this cookbook is to provide the easiness for those who are professional or doing job somewhere. But with earning, it is also quite necessary to cook food easily & timely instead of ordering hygienic or costly junk food. As we know, after doing office work, no one can cook food with the great effort. For the ease of such people, there are a lot of latest advancements in kitchen accessories. The most popular kitchen appliances usually helps to make foods or dishes like chicken, mutton, beef, potato chips and many other items in less time and budget. There are a lot of things that should be considered when baking with an air fryer. One of the most important tips is to make sure you have all of your equipment ready for the bake. It is best to be prepared ahead of time and this includes having pans, utensils, baking bags, the air fryer itself, and the recipe book instead of using stove or oven. With the help of an air fryer, you can make various dishes for a single person as well as the entire family timely and effortlessly. As there is a famous proverb that "Nothing can be done on its own", it indicates that every task takes time for completion. Some tasks take more time and effort and some requires less time and effort for their completion. Therefore, with the huge range of advancements that come to us are just for our ease. By using appliances like an air fryer comes for the comfort of professional people who are busy in earning their livelihood. In this book, you can follow the latest, delicious, and quick, about 70 recipes that will save your time and provide you healthy food without any great effort.

Chapter # 1:

An Overview & Benefits of an Air Fryer

Introduction:

The most popular kitchen appliance that usually helps to make foods or dishes like chicken, mutton, beef, potato chips and many other items in less time and budget.

Today, everything is materialistic, every person is busy to earn great livelihood. Due to a huge burden of responsibilities, they have no time to cook food on stove after doing hard work. Because, traditionally cooking food on the stove takes more time and effort. Therefore, there are a vast variety of Kitchen appliances. The kitchen appliances are so much helpful in making or cooking food in few minutes and in less budget. You come to home from job, and got too much tired. So, you can cook delicious food in an Air Fryer efficiently and timely as compared to stove. You can really enjoy the food without great effort and getting so much tired.

The Air Fryer Usability:

Be prepared to explore all about frying foods that you learned. To crisp, golden brown excellence (yes, French-fried potatoes and potato chips!), air fryers will fry your favourite foods using minimum or no oil. You can not only make commonly fried foods such as chips and French fries of potatoes, however it is also ideal for proteins, vegetables such as drummettes and chicken wings, coquettes & feta triangles as well as appetizers. And cookies are perfectly cooked in an air fryer, such as brownies and blondies.

The Air Fryer Works as:

- Around 350-375°F (176-190°C) is the ideal temperature of an Air Fryer

- To cook the surface of the food, pour over a food oil at the temperature mentioned above. The oil can't penetrate because it forms a type of seal.
- Simultaneously, the humidity within the food turns into steam that helps to actually cook the food from the inside. It is cleared that the steam helps to maintain the oil out of the food.
- The oil flows into the food at a low temperature, rendering it greasy.
- It oxidizes the oil and, at high temperatures, food will dry out.

On the other hand, an air fryer is similar to a convection oven, but in a diverse outfit, food preparation done at very high temperatures whereas, inside it, dry air circulates around the food at the same time, while making it crisp without putting additional fat, it makes it possible for cooking food faster.

What necessary to Search for in an Air Fryer?

As we know, several different sizes and models of air fryers are available now. If you're cooking for a gathering, try the extra-large air fryer, that can prepare or fry a whole chicken, other steaks or six servings of French fries.

Suppose, you've a fixed counter space, try the Large Air Fryer that uses patented machinery to circulate hot air for sufficient, crispy results. The latest air fryer offers an extra compact size with identical capacity! and tar equipment, which ensures that food is cooking evenly (no further worries of build-ups). You will be able to try all the fried foods you enjoy, with no embarrassment.

To increase the functionality of an air fryer, much more, you can also purchase a wide range of different accessories, including a stand, roasting pan, muffin cups, and mesh baskets. Check out the ingredients of our air fryer we created, starting from buttermilk with black pepper seasoning to fry chicken or Sichuan garlic seasoning suitable for Chinese cuisine.

We will read about the deep fryer, with tips and our favourite recipes like burgers, chicken wings, and many more.

Most Common - Five Guidelines for an Air Fryer usage:

1. Shake the food.

Open the air fryer and shake the foods efficiently because the food is to "fry" in the machine's basket—Light dishes like Sweet French fries and Garlic chips will compress. Give Rotation to the food every 5-10 mins for better performance

2. Do not overload.

Leave enough space for the food so that the air circulates efficiently; so that's gives you crunchy effects. Our kitchen testing cooks trust that the snacks and small batches can fry in air fryer.

3. Slightly spray to food.

Gently spray on food by a cooking spray bottle and apply a touch of oil on food to make sure the food doesn't stick to the basket.

4. Retain an Air fry dry.

Beat food to dry before start cooking (even when marinated, e.g.) to prevent splashing & excessive smoke. Likewise, preparing high-fat foods such as chicken steaks or wings, be assured to remove the grease from the lower part of machine regularly.

5. Other Most Dominant cooking techniques.

The air fryer is not just for deep frying; It is also perfect for further safe methods of cooking like baking, grilling, roasting and many more. Our kitchen testing really loves using the unit for cooking salmon in air fryer!

An Air Fryer Helps to reduce fat content

Generally, food cooked in deep fryer contains higher fat level than preparing food in other cooking appliances. For Example; a fried chicken breast contains about 30% more fat just like a fat level in roasted chicken

Many Manufacturers claimed, an Air fryer can reduce fat from fried food items up-to 75%. So, an air fryer requires less amount of fat than a deep fryer. As, many dishes cooked in deep fryer consume 75% oil (equal to 3 cups) and an air fryer prepare food by applying the oil in just about 1 tablespoon (equal to 15ml).

One research tested the potato chips prepared in air fryer characteristics then observed: the air frying method produces a final product with slightly lower fat but same moisture content and color. So, there is a major impact on anyone's health, an excessive risk of illnesses such as inflammation, infection and heart disease has been linked to a greater fat intake from vegetable oils.

Air Fryer provides an Aid in Weight Loss

The dishes prepared deep fryer are not just having much fat but also more in calories that causes severe increase in weight. Another research of 33,542 Spanish grown-ups indicates that a greater usage of fried food linked with a higher occurrence of obesity. Dietetic fat has about twice like many calories per gram while other macro-nutrients such as carbohydrates, vitamins and proteins, averaging in at 9 calories throughout each and every gram of oil or fat.

By substituting to air fryer is an easy way to endorse in losing weight and to reduce calories and it will be done only by taking food prepared in air fryer.

Air Fried food may reduce the potentially harmful chemicals

Frying foods can produce potentially hazardous compounds such as acrylamide, in contrast to being higher in fat and calories. An acrylamide is a compound that is formed in carbohydrate- rich dishes or foods during highly-heated cooking methods such as frying. Acrylamide is known as a "probable carcinogen" which indicates as some research suggests that it could be associated with the development of cancer. Although the findings are conflicting, the link between dietary acrylamide and a greater risk of kidney, endometrial and ovarian cancers has been identified in some reports. Instead of cooking food in a deep fryer, air frying your food may aid the acrylamide content. Some researches indicates that air-frying method may cut the acrylamide by 90% by comparing deep frying method. All other extremely harmful chemicals produced by high-heat cooking are polycyclic aromatic hydrocarbons, heterocyclic amines and aldehydes and may be associated with a greater risk of cancer. That's why, the air fried food may help to reduce the chance of extremely dangerous chemicals or compounds and maintain your health.

Chapter # 2:

70 Perfectly Portioned Air Fryer Recipes for Busy People in Minimum Budget

1. Air fried corn, zucchini and haloumi fritters

Ingredients

- Coarsely grated block haloumi - 225g
- Coarsely grated Zucchini - 2 medium sized
- Frozen corn kernels - 150g (1 cup)
- Lightly whisked eggs - 2
- Self-raising flour - 100g
- Extra virgin olive oil - to drizzle
- Freshly chopped oregano leaves - 3 tablespoons
- Fresh oregano extra sprigs - to serve
- Yoghurt - to serve

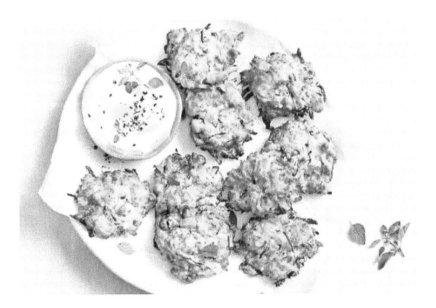

Method

1. Use your palms to squeeze out the extra liquid from the zucchini and place them in a bowl. Add the corn and haloumi and stir for combining them. Then add the eggs, oregano and flour. Add seasoning and stir until fully mixed.

2. Set the temperature of an air fryer to 200 C. Put spoonsful of the mixture of zucchini on an air fryer. Cook until golden and crisp, for 8 minutes. Transfer to a dish that is clean. Again repeat this step by adding the remaining mixture in 2 more batches.

3. Take a serving plate and arrange soft fritters on it. Take yoghurt in a small serving bowl. Add seasoning of black pepper on the top of yoghurt. Drizzle with olive oil. At the end, serve this dish with extra oregano.

2. Air fryer fried rice

Ingredients

- Microwave long grain rice - 450g packet
- Chicken tenderloins - 300g
- Rindless bacons - 4 ranchers
- Light Soy sauce - 2 tablespoons
- Oyster sauce - 2 tablespoons
- Sesame oil - 1 tablespoon
- Fresh finely grated ginger - 3 tablespoons
- Frozen peas - 120g (3/4 cup)
- Lightly whisked eggs - 2
- Sliced green shallots - 2
- Thin sliced red chilli - 1
- Oyster sauce - to drizzle

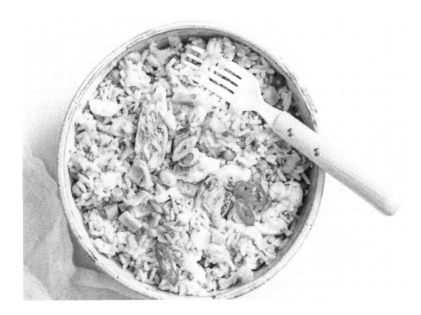

Method

1. Set the 180°C temperature of an air fryer. Bacon and chicken is placed on the rack of an air fryer. Cook them until fully cooked for 8-10 minutes. Shift it to a clean plate and set this plate aside to cool. Then, slice and chop the bacon and chicken.

2. In the meantime, separate the rice grains in the packet by using your fingers. Heat the rice for 60 seconds in a microwave. Shift to a 20cm ovenproof, round high-sided pan or dish. Apply the sesame oil, soy sauce, ginger, oyster sauce and 10ml water and mix well.

3. Put a pan/dish in an air fryer. Cook the rice for 5 minutes till them soft. Then whisk the chicken, half of bacon and peas in the eggs. Completely cook the eggs in 3 minutes. Mix and season the top of half shallot with white pepper and salt.

4. Serve with the seasoning of chilli, remaining bacon and shallot and oyster sauce.

3. Air fried banana muffins

Ingredients

- Ripe bananas - 2
- Brown sugar - 60g (1/3 cup)
- Olive oil - 60ml (1/4 cup)
- Buttermilk - 60ml (1/4 cup)

- Self-raising flour - 150g (1 cup)
- Egg - 1
- Maple syrup - to brush or to serve

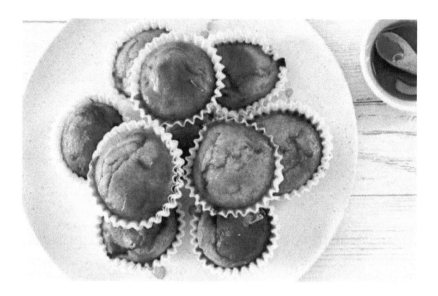

Method

1. Mash the bananas in a small bowl using a fork. Until needed, set aside.

2. In a medium cup, whisk the flour and sugar using a balloon whisk. In the middle, make a well. Add the buttermilk, oil and egg. Break up the egg with the help of a whisk. Stir by using wooden spoon until the mixture is mixed. Stir the banana through it.

3. Set the temperature of an air fryer at 180C. Splits half of the mixture into 9 cases of patties. Remove the rack from the air fryer and pass the cases to the rack carefully. Switch the rack back to the fryer. Bake the muffins completely by cooking them for 10 minutes. Move to the wire rack. Repeat this step on remaining mixture to produce 18 muffins.

4. Brush the muffin tops with maple syrup while they're still warm. Serve, if you like, with extra maple syrup.

4. Air fried Nutella brownies

Ingredients

- Plain flour - 150g (1 cup)

- Castor white sugar - 225g (1 cup)
- Lightly whisked eggs - 3
- Nutella - 300g (1 cup)
- Cocoa powder - to dust

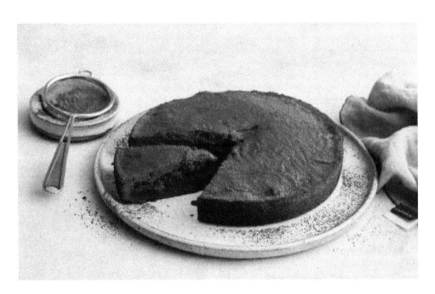

Method

1. Apply butter in a 20cm circular cake pan. Cover the base by using baking paper.

2. Whisk the flour and sugar together in a bowl by using balloon whisk. In the middle, make a well. Add the Nutella and egg in the middle of bowl by making a well. Stir with a large metal spoon until mixed. Move this mixture to the previously prepared pan and smooth the surface of the mixture by using metal spoon.

3. Pre - heat an air fryer to 160C. Bake the brownie about 40 minutes or until a few crumbs stick out of a skewer inserted in the middle. Fully set aside to cool.

4. Garnish the top of the cake by dusting them with cocoa powder, and cut them into pieces. Brownies are ready to be served.

5. Air fried celebration bites

Ingredients

- Frozen shortcrust partially thawed pastry - 4 sheets

- Lightly whisked eggs - 1
- Unrapped Mars Celebration chocolates - 24
- Icing sugar - to dust
- Cinnamon sugar - to dust
- Whipped cream - to serve

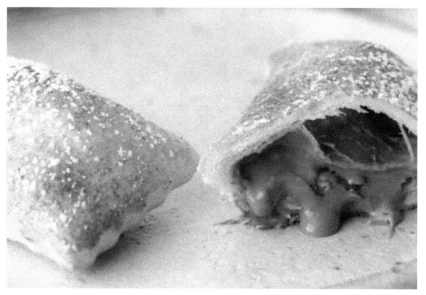

Method

1. Slice each pastry sheet into 6 rectangles. Brush the egg gently. One chocolate is placed in the middle of each rectangular piece of pastry. Fold the pastry over to cover the chocolate completely. Trim the pastry, press and seal the sides. Place it on a tray containing baking paper. Brush the egg on each pastry and sprinkle cinnamon sugar liberally.

2. In the air-fryer basket, put a sheet of baking paper, making sure that the paper is 1 cm smaller than the basket to allow airflow. Put six pockets in the basket by taking care not to overlap. Cook for 8-9 minutes at 190°C until pastries are completely cooked with golden color. Shift to a dish. Free pockets are then used again.

3. Sprinkle Icing sugar on the top of tasty bites. Serve them with a whipped cream to intensify its flavor.

6. Air fried nuts and bolts

Ingredients

- Dried farfalle pasta - 2 cups
- Extra virgin olive oil - 60ml (1/4th cup)
- Brown sugar - 2 tablespoons
- Onion powder - 1 tablespoon
- Smoked paprika - 2 tablespoons
- Chili powder - 1/2 tablespoon
- Garlic powder - 1/2 tablespoon
- Pretzels - 1 cup
- Raw macadamias - 80g (1/2 cup)
- Raw cashews - 80g (1/2 cup)
- Kellog's Nutri-grain cereal - 1 cup
- Sea salt - 1 tablespoon

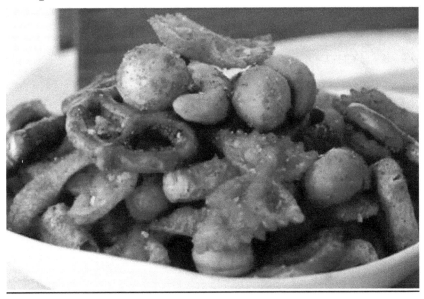

Method

1. Take a big saucepan of boiling salted water, cook the pasta until just ready and soft. Drain thoroughly. Shift pasta to a tray and pat with a paper towel to dry. Move the dried pasta to a wide pot.

2. Mix the sugar, oil, onion, paprika, chili and garlic powders together in a clean bowl. Add half of this mixture in the bowl containing pasta. Toss this bowl slightly for the proper coating of mixture over pasta.

3. Set the temperature at 200C of an Air Fryer. Put the pasta in air fryer's pot. After cooking for 5 minutes, shake the pot and cook for more 5-7 minutes, until they look golden and crispy. Shift to a wide bowl.

4. Take the pretzels in a bowl with the nuts and apply the remaining mixture of spices. Toss this bowl for the proper coating. Put in air fryer's pot and cook at 180C for 3-4 minutes. Shake this pot and cook for more 2-3 minutes until it's golden in color. First add pasta and then add the cereal. Sprinkle salt on it and toss to mix properly. Serve this dish after proper cooling.

7. Air fried coconut shrimps

Ingredients

- Plain flour - 1/2 cup
- Eggs - 2
- Bread crumbs - 1/2 cup
- Black pepper powder - 1.5 teaspoons
- Sweetless flaked coconut - 3/4 cup
- Uncooked, deveined and peeled shrimp - 12 ounces
- Salt - 1/2 teaspoon
- Honey - 1/4 cup
- Lime juice - 1/4 cup
- Finely sliced serrano chili - 1
- Chopped cilantro - 2 teaspoons
- Cooking spray

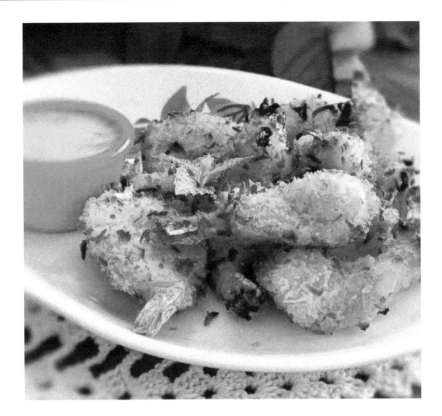

Method

1. Stir the pepper and flour in a clean bowl together. Whisk the eggs in another bowl and h panko and coconut in separate bowl. Coat the shrimps with flour mixture by holding each shrimp by tail and shake off the extra flour. Then coat the floured shrimp with egg and allow it to drip off excess. Give them the final coat of coconut mixture and press them to stick. Shift on a clean plate. Spray shrimp with cooking oil.

2. Set the temperature of the air-fryer to 200C. In an air fryer, cook half of the shrimp for 3 minutes. Turn the shrimp and cook further for more 3 minutes until color changes in golden. Use 1/4 teaspoon of salt for seasoning. Repeat this step for the rest of shrimps.

3. In the meantime, prepare a dip by stirring lime juice, serrano chili and honey in a clean bowl.

4. Serve fried shrimps with sprinkled cilantro and dip.

8. Air fried Roasted Sweet and Spicy Carrots

Ingredients

- Cooking oil
- Melted butter - 1 tablespoon
- Grated orange zest - 1 teaspoon
- Carrots - 1/2 pound
- Hot honey - 1 tablespoon
- Cardamom powder - 1/2 teaspoon
- Fresh orange juice - 1 tablespoon
- Black pepper powder - to taste
- Salt - 1 pinch

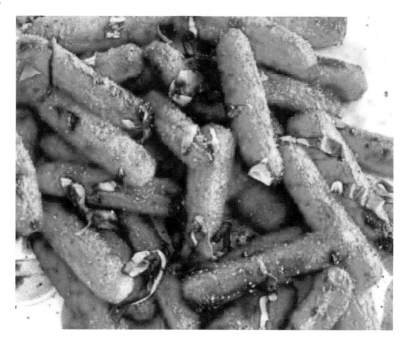

Method

1. Set the temperature of an air to 200C. Lightly coat its pot with cooking oil.

2. Mix honey, cardamom and orange zest in a clean bowl. Take 1 tablespoon of this sauce in another bowl and place aside. Coat carrots completely by tossing them in remaining sauce. Shift carrots to an air fryer pot.

3. Air fry the carrots and toss them after every 6 minutes. Cook carrots for 15-20 minutes until they are fully cooked and roasted. Combine honey butter sauce with orange juice to make sauce. Coat carrots with this sauce. Season with black pepper and salt and serve this delicious dish.

9. Air fried Chicken Thighs

Ingredients

- Boneless chicken thighs - 4
- Extra virgin olive oil - 2 teaspoons
- Smoked paprika - 1 teaspoon
- Salt - 1/2 teaspoon
- Garlic powder - 3/4 teaspoon
- Black pepper powder - 1/2 teaspoon

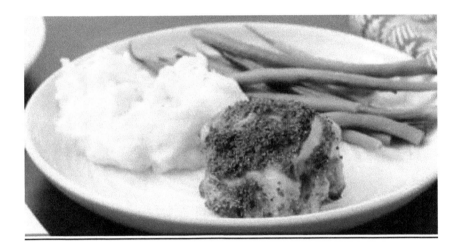

Method

1. Set the temperature of an air fryer to 200C.

2. Dry chicken thighs by using tissue paper. Brush olive oil on the skin side of each chicken thigh. Shift the single layer of chicken thighs on a clean tray.

3. Make a mixture of salt, black pepper, paprika and garlic powder in a clean bowl. Use a half of this mixture for the seasoning of 4 chicken thighs on both sides evenly. Then shift single layer of chicken thighs in an air fryer pot by placing skin side up.

4. Preheat the air fryer and maintain its temperature to 75C. Fry chicken for 15-18 minutes until its water become dry and its color changes to brown. Serve immediately.

10. Air fried French Fries

Ingredients

- Peeled Potatoes - 1 pound
- Vegetable oil - 2 tablespoon
- Cayenne pepper - 1 pinch
- Salt - 1/2 teaspoon

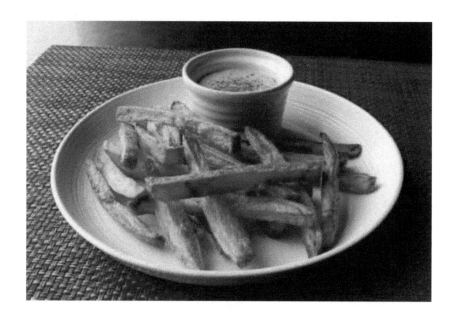

Method

1. Lengthwise cut thick slices of potato of 3/8 inches.

2. Soak sliced potatoes for 5 minutes in water. Drain excess starch water from soaked potatoes after 5 minutes. Place these potatoes in boiling water pan for 8-10 minutes.

3. Remove water from the potatoes and dry them completely. Cool them for 10 minutes and shift in a clean bowl. Add some oil and fully coat the potatoes with cayenne by tossing.

4. Set the temperature of an air fryer to 190C. Place two layers of potatoes in air fryer pot and cook them for 10-15 minutes. Toss fries continuously and cook for more 10 minutes until their color changes to golden brown. Season fries with salt and serve this appetizing dish immediately.

11. Air fried Mini Breakfast Burritos

Ingredients

- Mexican style chorizo - 1/4 cup
- Sliced potatoes - 1/2 cup
- Chopped serrano pepper - 1
- 8-inch flour tortillas - 4
- Bacon grease - 1 tablespoon
- Chopped onion - 2 tablespoon
- Eggs - 2
- Cooking avacado oil - to spray
- Salt - to taste
- Black pepper powder - to taste

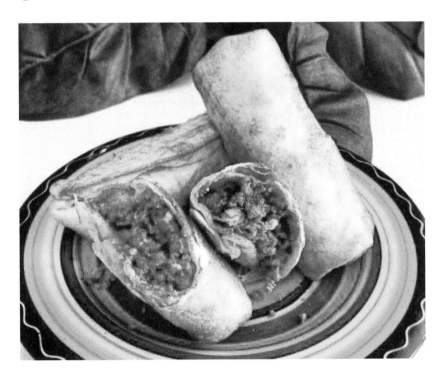

Method

1. Take chorizo in a large size pan and cook on medium flame for 8 minutes with continuous stirring until its color change into reddish brown. Shift chorizo in a clean plate and place separate.

2. Take bacon grease in same pan and melt it on medium flame. Place sliced potatoes and cook them for 10 minutes with constant stirring. Add serrano pepper and onion meanwhile. Cook for more 2-5 minutes until potatoes are fully cooked, onion and serrano pepper become soften. Then add chorizo and eggs and cook for more 5 minutes until potato mixture is fully incorporated. Use pepper and salt for seasoning.

3. In the meantime, heat tortillas in a large pan until they become soft and flexible. Put 1/3 cup of chorizo mixture at the center of each tortilla. Filling is covered by rolling the upper and lower side of tortilla and give shape of burrito. Spray cooking oil and place them in air fryer pot.

4. Fry these burritos at 200C for 5 minutes. Change the side's continuously and spray with cooking oil. Cook in air fryer for 3-4 minutes until color turns into light brown. Shift burritos in a clean dish and serve this delicious dish.

12. Air fried Vegan Tator Tots

Ingredients

- Frozen potato nuggets (Tator Tots) - 2 cups
- Buffalo wing sauce - 1/4 cup
- Vegan ranch salad - 1/4 cup

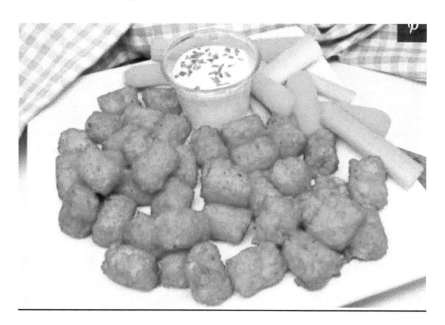

Method

1. Set the temperature of an air fryer to 175C.

2. Put frozen potato nuggets in air fryer pot and cook for 6-8 minutes with constant shake.

3. Shift potatoes to a large-sized bowl and add wing sauce. Combine evenly by tossing them and place them again in air fryer pot.

4. Cook more for 8-10 minutes without disturbance. Shift to a serving plate. Serve with ranch dressing and enjoy this dish.

13. Air fried Roasted Cauliflower

Ingredients

- Cauliflower florets - 4 cups
- Garlic - 3 cloves
- Smoked paprika - 1/2 teaspoon
- Peanut oil - 1 tablespoon
- Salt - 1/2 teaspoon

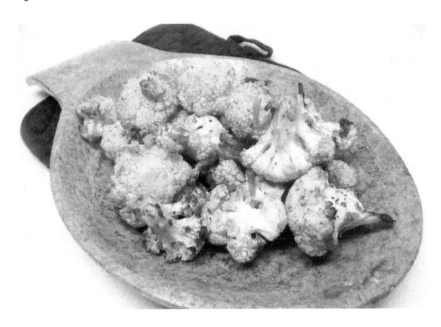

Method

1. Set the temperature of an air fryer to 200C.

2. Smash garlic cloves with a knife and mix with salt, oil and paprika. Coat cauliflower in this mixture.

3. Put coated cauliflower in air fryer pot and cook around 10-15 minutes with stirring after every 5 minutes. Cook according to desired color and crispiness and serve immediately.

14. Air fried Cinnamon-Sugar Doughnuts

Ingredients

- White sugar - 1/2 cup
- Brown sugar - 1/4 cup
- Melted butter - 1/4 cup
- Cinnamon powder - 1 teaspoon
- Ground nutmeg - 1/4 TEASPOON
- Packed chilled flaky biscuit dough - 1 (16.3 ounce)

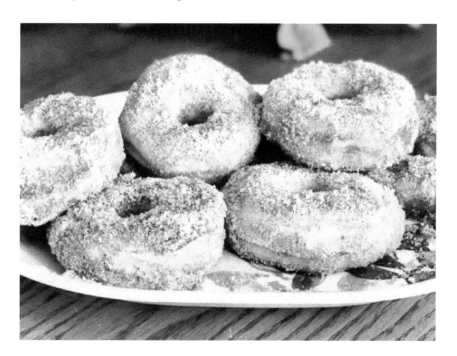

Method

1. Put melted butter in a clean bowl. Add brown sugar, white sugar, nutmeg and cinnamon and mix.

2. Divide and cut biscuit dough into many single biscuits and give them the shape of doughnuts using a biscuit cutter. Shift doughnuts in an air fryer pot.

3. Air fry the doughnuts for 5-6 minutes at 175C until color turns into golden brown. Turn the side of doughnuts and cook for more 1-3 minutes.

4. Shift doughnuts from air fryer to a clean dish and dip them in melted butter. Then completely coat these doughnuts in sugar and cinnamon mixture and serve frequently.

15. Air Fried Broiled Grapefruit

Ingredients

- Chilled red grapefruit - 1
- Melted butter - 1 tablespoon
- Brown sugar - 2 tablespoon
- Ground cinnamon - 1/2 teaspoon
- Aluminium foil

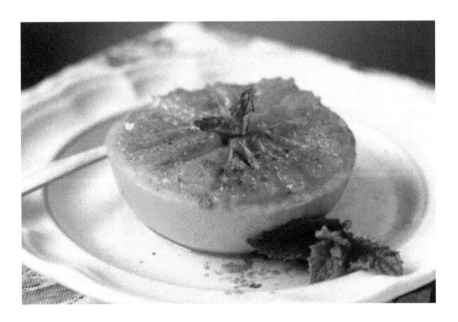

Method

1. Set the temperature of an air fryer to 200C.

2. Cut grapefruit crosswise to half and also cut a thin slice from one end of grapefruit for sitting your fruit flat on a plate.

3. Mix brown sugar in melted butter in a small sized bowl. Coat the cut side of the grapefruit with this mixture. Dust the little brown sugar over it.

4. Take 2 five inch pieces of aluminium foil and put the half grapefruit on each piece. Fold the sides evenly to prevent juice leakage. Place them in air fryer pot.

5. Broil for 5-7 minutes until bubbling of sugar start in an air fryer. Before serving, sprinkle cinnamon on grapefruit.

16. Air Fried Brown Sugar and Pecan Roasted Apples

Ingredients

- Apples - 2 medium
- Chopped pecans - 2 tablespoons
- Plain flour - 1 teaspoon
- Melted butter - 1 tablespoon
- Brown sugar - 1 tablespoon
- Apple pie spice - 1/4 teaspoon

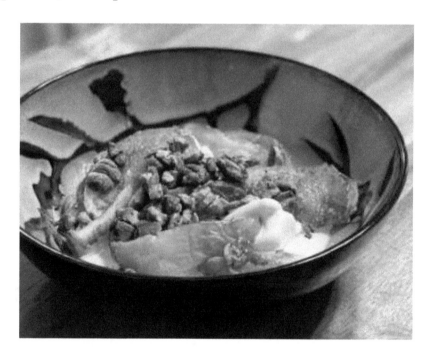

Method

1. Set the temperature of an air fryer to 180C.

2. Mix brown sugar, pecan, apple pie spice and flour in a clean bowl. Cut apples in wedges and put them in another bowl and coat them with melted butter by tossing. Place a single layer in an air fryer pot and add mixture of pecan on the top.

3. Cook apples for 12-15 minutes until they get soft.

17. Air Fried Breaded Sea Scallops

Ingredients

- Crushed butter crackers - 1/2 cup
- Seafood seasoning - 1/2 teaspoon
- Sea scallops - 1 pound
- Garlic powder - 1/2 teaspoon
- Melted butter - 2 tablespoons
- Cooking oil - for spray

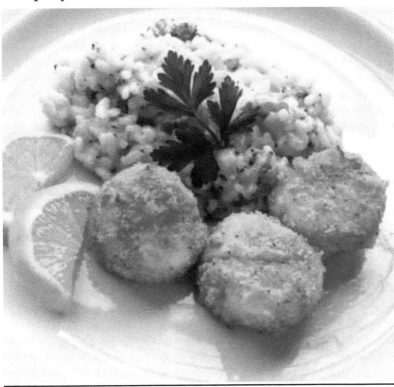

Method

1. Set the temperature of an air fryer to 198C.

2. Combine garlic powder, seafood seasoning and cracker crumbs in a clean bowl. Take melted butter in another bowl.

3. Coat each scallop with melted butter. Then roll them in breading until completely enclose. Place them on a clean plate and repeat this step with rest of the scallops.

4. Slightly spray scallops with cooking oil and place them on the air fryer pot at equal distance. You may work in 2-3 batches.

5. Cook them for 2-3 minutes in preheated air fryer. Use a spatula to change the side of each scallop. Cook for more 2 minutes until they become opaque. Dish out in a clean plate and serve immediately.

18. Air Fried Crumbed Fish

Ingredients

- Flounder fillets - 4
- Dry bread crumbs - 1 cup
- Egg - 1
- Sliced lemon - 1
- Vegetable oil - 1/4 cup

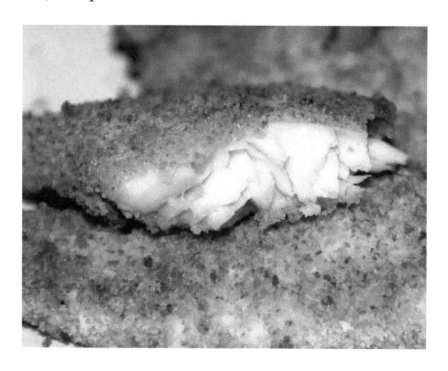

Method

1. Set the temperature of an air fryer to 180C.

2. Combine oil and bread crumbs in a clean bowl and mix them well.

3. Coat each fish fillets with beaten egg, then evenly dip them in the crumbs mixture.

4. Place coated fillets in preheated air fryer and cook for 10-12 minutes until fish easily flakes by touching them with fork. Shift prepared fish in a clean plate and serve with lemon slices.

19. Air Fried Cauliflower and Chickpea Tacos

Ingredients

- Cauliflower - 1 small
- Chickpeas - 15 ounce
- Chili powder - 1 teaspoon
- Cumin powder - 1 teaspoon
- Lemon juice - 1 tablespoon
- Sea salt - 1 teaspoon
- Garlic powder - 1/4 teaspoon
- Olive oil - 1 tablespoon

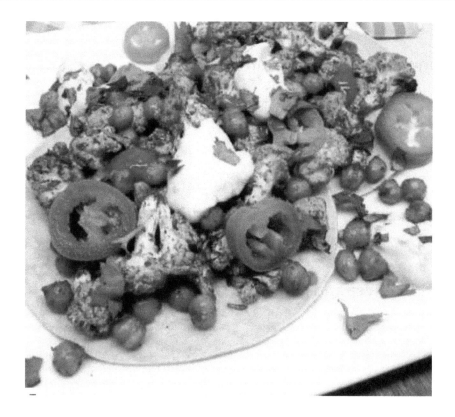

Method

1. Set the temperature of an air fryer to 190C.

2. Mix lime juice, cumin, garlic powder, salt, olive oil and chili powder in a clean bowl. Now coat well the cauliflower and chickpeas in this mixture by constant stirring.

3. Put cauliflower mixture in an air fryer pot. Cook for 8-10 minutes with constant stirring. Cook for more 10 minutes and stir for final time. Cook for more 5 minutes until desired crispy texture is attained.

5. Place cauliflower mixture by using spoon and serve.

20. Air Fried Roasted Salsa

Ingredients

- Roma tomatoes - 4
- Seeded Jalapeno pepper - 1

- Red onion - 1/2
- Garlic - 4 cloves
- Cilantro - 1/2 cup
- Lemon juice - 1
- Cooking oil - to spray
- Salt - to taste

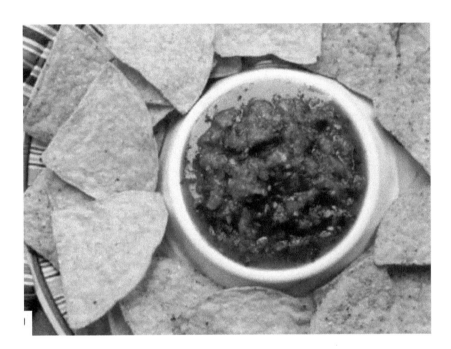

Method

1. Set the temperature of an air fryer to 200C.

2. Put tomatoes, red onion and skin side down of jalapeno in an air fryer pot. Brush lightly these vegetables with cooking oil for roasting them easily.

3. Cook vegetables in an air fryer for 5 minutes. Then add garlic cloves and again spray with cooking oil and fry for more 5 minutes.

4. Shift vegetables to cutting board and allow them to cool for 8-10 minutes.

5. Separate skins of jalapeno and tomatoes and chop them with onion into large pieces. Add them to food processor bowl and add lemon juice, cilantro, garlic and

salt. Pulsing for many times until all the vegetables are evenly chopped. Cool them for 10-15 minutes and serve this delicious dish immediately.

21. Air Fried Flour Tortilla Bowls

Ingredients

- Flour tortilla - 1 (8 inch)
- Souffle dish - 1 (4 1/2 inch)

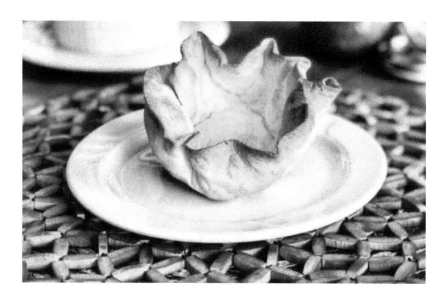

Method

1. Set the temperature of an air fryer to 190C.

2. Take tortilla in a large pan and heat it until it become soft. Put tortilla in the souffle dish by patting down side and fluting up from its sides of dish.

3. Air fry tortilla for 3-5 minutes until its color change into golden brown.

4. Take out tortilla bowl from the dish and put the upper side in the pot. Air fry again for more 2 minutes until its color turns into golden brown. Dish out and serve.

22. Air Fried Cheese and Mini Bean Tacos

Ingredients

- Can Refried beans - 16 ounce
- American cheese - 12 slices
- Flour tortillas - 12 (6 inch)
- Taco seasoning mix - 1 ounce
- Cooking oil - to spray

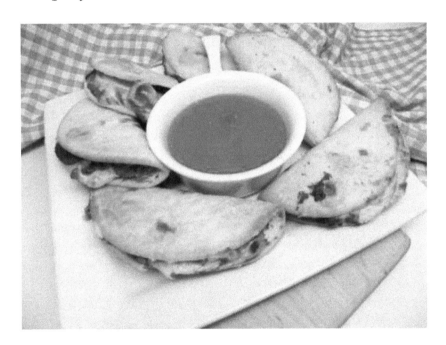

Method

1. Set the temperature of an air fryer to 200C.

2. Combine refried beans and taco seasoning evenly in a clean bowl and stir.

3. Put 1 slice of cheese in the center of tortilla and place 1 tablespoon of bean mixture over cheese. Again place second piece of cheese over this mixture. Fold tortilla properly from upper side and press to enclose completely. Repeat this step for the rest of beans, cheese and tortillas.

4. Spray cooking oil on the both sides of tacos. Put them in an air fryer at equal distance. Cook the tacos for 3 minutes and turn it side and again cook for more 3 minutes. Repeat this step for the rest of tacos. Transfer to a clean plate and serve immediately.

23. Air Fried Lemon Pepper Shrimp

Ingredients

- Lemon - 1
- Lemon pepper - 1 teaspoon
- Olive oil - 1 tablespoon
- Garlic powder - 1/4 teaspoon
- Paprika - 1/4 teaspoon
- Deveined and peeled shrimps - 12 ounces
- Sliced lemon – 1

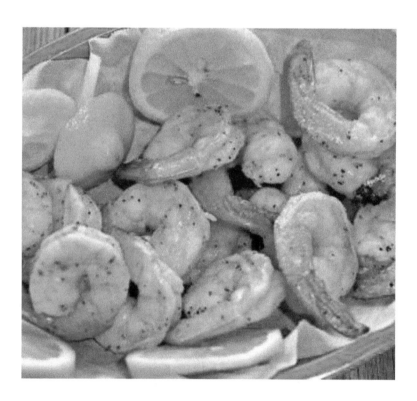

Method

1. Set the temperature of an air fryer to 200C.

2. Mix lemon pepper, garlic powder, and olive oil, paprika and lemon juice in a clean bowl. Coat shrimps by this mixture by tossing.

3. Put shrimps in an air fryer and cook for 5-8 minutes until its color turn to pink. Dish out cooked shrimps and serve with lemon slices.

24. Air Fried Shrimp a la Bang Bang

Ingredients

- Deveined raw shrimps - 1 pound
- Sweet chili sauce - 1/4 cup
- Plain flour - 1/4 cup
- Green onions - 2
- Mayonnaise - 1/2 cup
- Sriracha sauce - 1 tablespoon
- Bread crumbs - 1 cup
- Leaf lettuce - 1 head

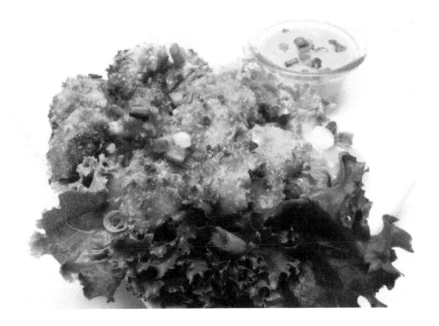

Method

1. Set the temperature of an air fryer to 200C

2. Make a bang bang sauce by mixing chili sauce, mayonnaise and sriracha sauce in a clean bowl. Separate some sauce for dipping in a separate small bowl.

3. Place bread crumbs and flour in two different plates. Coat shrimps with mayonnaise mixture, then with flour and then bread crumbs. Set coated shrimps on a baking paper.

4. Place them in an air fryer pot and cook for 10-12 minutes. Repeat this step for the rest of shrimps. Transfer shrimps to a clean dish and serve with green onions and lettuce.

25. Air Fried Spicy Bay Scallops

Ingredients

- Bay scallops - 1 pound
- Chili powder - 2 teaspoons
- Smoked paprika- 2 teaspoons
- Garlic powder - 1 teaspoon
- Olive oil - 2 teaspoons
- Black pepper powder - 1/4 teaspoon
- Cayenne red pepper - 1/8 teaspoon

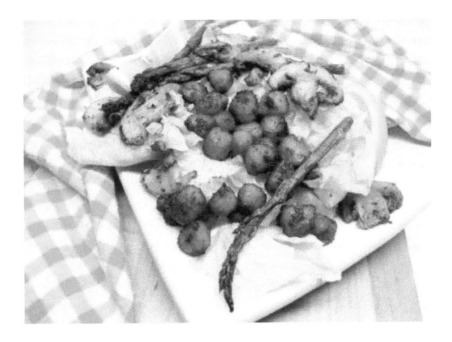

Method

1. Set the temperature of an air fryer to 200C

2. Mix smoked paprika, olive oil, bay scallops, garlic powder, pepper, chili powder and cayenne pepper in a clean bowl and stir properly. Shift this mixture to an air fryer.

3. Air fry for 6-8 minutes with constant shaking until scallops are fully cooked. Transfer this dish in a clean plate and serve immediately.

26. Air Fried Breakfast Fritatta

Ingredients

- Fully cooked breakfast sausages - 1/4 pound
- Cheddar Monterey Jack cheese - 1/2 cup
- Green onion - 1
- Cayenne pepper - 1 pinch
- Red bell pepper - 2 tablespoons
- Eggs - 4
- Cooking oil - to spray

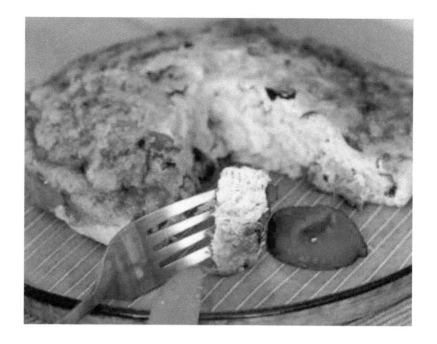

Method

1. Set the temperature of an air fryer to 180C.

2. Mix eggs, sausages, Cheddar Monterey Jack cheese, onion, bell pepper and cayenne in a clean bowl and stir to mix properly.

3. Spray cooking oil on a clean non-stick cake pan. Put egg mixture in the cake pan. Air fry for 15-20 minutes until fritatta is fully cooked and set. Transfer it in a clean plate and serve immediately.

27. Air Fried Roasted Okra

Ingredients

- Trimmed and sliced Okra - 1/2 pound
- Black pepper powder - 1/8 teaspoon
- Olive oil - 1 teaspoon
- Salt - 1/4 teaspoon

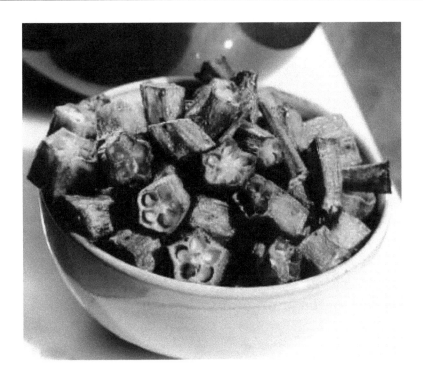

Method

1. Set the temperature of an air fryer to 175C.

2. Mix olive oil, black pepper, salt and okra in a clean bowl and stir to mix properly.

3. Make a single layer of this mixture in an air fryer pot. Air fry for 5-8 minutes with constant stirring. Cook for more 5 minutes and again toss. Cook for more 3 minutes and dish out in a clean plate and serve immediately.

28. Air Fried Rib-Eye Steak

Ingredients

- Rib-eye steak - 2 (1 1/2 inch thick)
- Olive oil - 1/4 cup
- Grill seasoning - 4 teaspoons
- Reduced sodium soy sauce - 1/2 cup

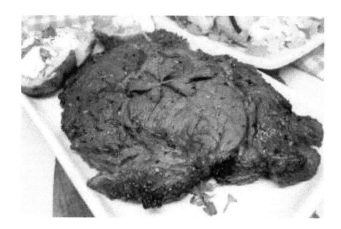

Method

1. Mix olive oil, soy sauce, seasoning and steaks in a clean bowl and set aside meat for marination.

2. Take out steaks and waste the remaining mixture. Remove excess oil from steak by patting.

3. Add 1 tablespoon water in an air fryer pot for the prevention from smoking during cooking of steaks.

3. Set the temperature of an air fryer to 200C. Place steaks in an air fryer pot. Air fry for 7-8 minutes and turn its side after every 8 minutes. Cook for more 7 minutes until it is rarely medium. Cook for final 3 minutes for a medium steak and dish out in a clean plate and serve immediately.

29. Air Fried Potato Chips

Ingredients

- Large potatoes - 2
- Olive oil - to spray
- Fresh parsley - optional
- Sea salt - 1/2 teaspoon

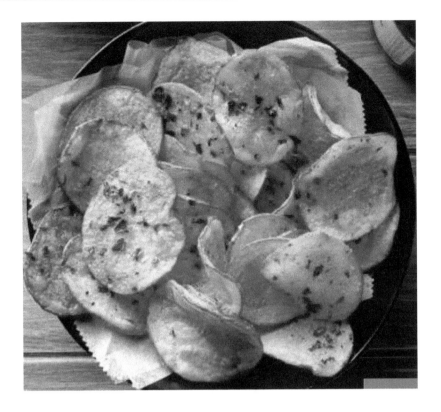

Method

1. Set the temperature of an air fryer to 180C.

2. Peel off the potatoes and cut them into thin slices. Shift the slices in a bowl containing ice chilled water and soak for 10 minutes. Drain potatoes, again add chilled water and soak for more 15 minutes.

3. Remove water from potatoes and allow to dry by using paper towel. Spray potatoes with cooking oil and add salt according to taste.

4. Place a single layer of potatoes slices in an oiled air fryer pot and cook for 15-18 minutes until color turns to golden brown and crispy. Stir constantly and turn its sides after every 5 minutes.

5. Dish out these crispy chips and serve with parsley.

30. Air Fried Tofu

Ingredients

- Packed tofu - 14 ounces
- Olive oil - 1/4 cup
- Reduced sodium soy sauce - 3 tablespoons
- Crushed red pepper flakes - 1/4 teaspoon
- Green onions - 2
- Cumin powder - 1/4 teaspoon
- Garlic - 2 cloves

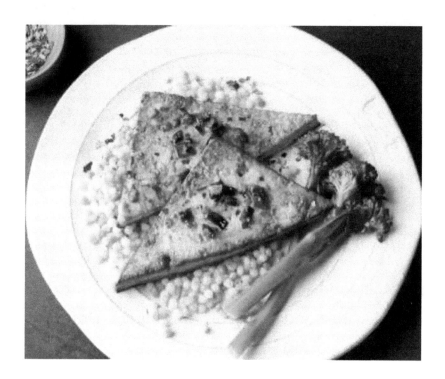

Method

1. Set the temperature of an air fryer to 200C.

2. Mix olive oil, soy sauce, onions, garlic, cumin powder and red pepper flakes in a deep bowl to make marinade mixture.

3. Cut 3/8 inches' thick slices of tofu lengthwise and then diagonally. Coat tofu with marinade mixture. Place them in refrigerate for 4-5 minutes and turn them after every 2 minutes.

4. Place tofu in buttered air fryer pot. Put remaining marinade over each tofu. Cook for 5-8 minutes until color turns to golden brown. Dish out cooked tofu and serve immediately.

31. Air Fried Acorn Squash Slices

Ingredients

- Medium sized acorn squash - 2
- Soft butter - 1/2 cup
- Brown sugar - 2/3 cup

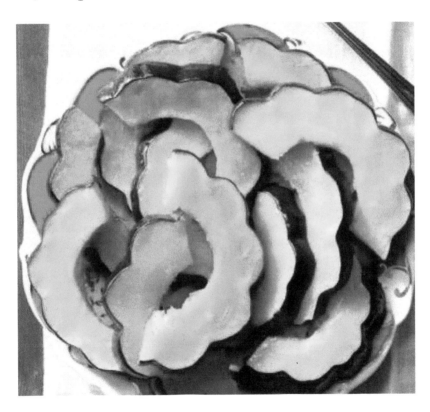

Method

1. Set the temperature of an air fryer to 160C.

2. Cut squash into two halves from length side and remove seeds. Again cut these halves into half inch slices.

3. Place a single layer of squash on buttered air fryer pot. Cook each side of squash for 5 minutes.

4. Mix butter into brown sugar and spread this mixture on the top of every squash. Cook for more 3 minutes. Dish out and serve immediately.

32. Air Fried Red Potatoes

Ingredients

- Baby potatoes - 2 pounds
- Olive oil - 2 tablespoons
- Fresh rosemary - 1 tablespoon
- Garlic - 2 cloves
- Salt - 1/2 teaspoon
- Black pepper - 1/4 teaspoon

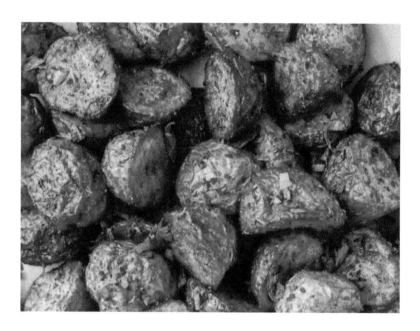

Method

1. Set the temperature of an air fryer to 198C.

2. Cut potatoes into wedges. Coat them properly with minced garlic, rosemary, black pepper and salt.

3. Place coated potatoes on buttered air fryer pot. Cook potatoes for 5 minutes until golden brown and soft. Stir them at once. Dish out in a clean plate and serve immediately.

33. Air Fried Butter Cake

Ingredients

- Melted butter - 7 tablespoons
- White sugar - 1/4 cup & 2 tablespoons
- Plain flour - 1 & 2/3 cup
- Egg - 1
- Salt - 1 pinch
- Milk - 6 tablespoons
- Cooking oil - to spray

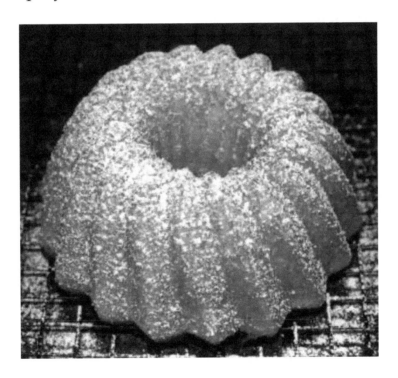

Method

1. Set the temperature of an air fryer to 180C and spray with cooking oil.

2. Beat white sugar, and butter together in a clean bowl until creamy and light. Then add egg and beautiful fluffy and smooth. Add salt and flour and stir. Then add milk and mix until batter is smooth. Shift batter to an preheated air fryer pot and level its surface by using spatula.

3. Place in an air fryer and set time of 15 minutes. Bake and check cake after 15 minutes by inserting toothpick in the cake. If toothpick comes out clean it means cake has fully baked.

4. Take out cake from air fryer and allow it to cool for 5-10 minutes. Serve immediately and enjoy.

34. Air Fried Jelly and Peanut Butter S'mores

Ingredients

- Chocolate topping peanut butter cup - 1
- Raspberry jam (seedless) - 1 teaspoon
- Marshmallow - 1 large
- Chocolate cracker squares – 2

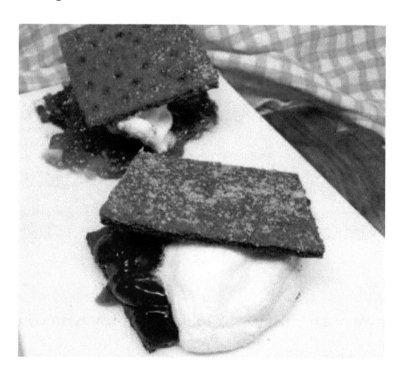

Method

1. Set the temperature of an air fryer to 200C.

2. Put peanut butter cup on one cracker square and topped with marshmallow and jelly. Carefully transfer it in the preheated air fryer.

3. Cook for 1 minute until marshmallow becomes soft and light brown. Remaining cracker squares is used for topping.

4. Shift this delicious in a clean plate and serve immediately.

35. Air Fried Sun-Dried Tomatoes

Ingredients

- Red grape tomatoes - 5 ounces
- Olive oil - 1/4 teaspoon
- Salt - to taste

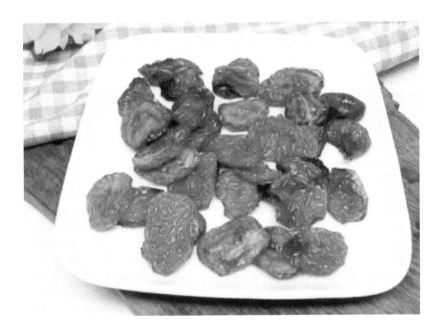

Method

1. Set the temperature of an air fryer to 115C.

2. Combine tomatoes halves, salt and olive oil evenly in a clean bowl. Shift tomatoes in an air fryer pot by placing skin side down.

3. Cook in air fryer for 45 minutes. Smash tomatoes by using spatula and cook for more 30 minutes. Repeat this step with the rest of tomatoes.

4. Shift this delicious dish in a clean plate and allow it to stand for 45 minutes to set. Serve this dish and enjoy.

36. Air Fried Sweet Potatoes Tots

Ingredients:

- Peeled Sweet Potatoes - 2 small (14oz.total)
- Garlic Powder - 1/8 tsp
- Potato Starch - 1 tbsp
- Kosher Salt, Divided - 11/4 tsp
- Unsalted Ketchup - 3/4 Cup
- Cooking Oil for spray

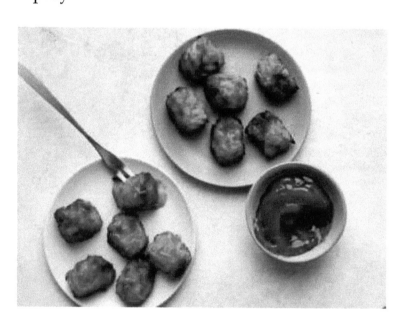

Method:

1. Take water in a medium pan and give a single boil over high flame. Then, add the sweet potatoes in the boiled water & cook for 15 minutes till potatoes becomes soft. Move the potatoes to a cooling plate for 15 minutes.

2. Rub potatoes using the wide hole's grater over a dish. Apply the potato starch, salt and garlic powder and toss gently. Make almost 24 shaped cylinders (1-inch) from the mixture.

3. Coat the air fryer pot gently with cooking oil. Put single layer of 1/2 of the tots in the pot and spray with cooking oil. Cook at 400 °F for about 12 to 14 minutes till lightly browned and flip tots midway. Remove from the pot and sprinkle with salt. Repeat with rest of the tots and salt left over. Serve with ketchup immediately.

37. Air Fried Banana Bread

Ingredients:

- White Whole Wheat Flour - 3/4 cup (3 oz.)
- Mashed Ripe Bananas - 2 medium or (about 3/4th cup)
- Cinnamon powder– 4 pinches
- Kosher Salt - 1/2 tsp
- Baking Soda - 1/4 tsp
- Large Eggs, Lightly Beaten - 2
- Regular Sugar - 1/2 cup
- Vanilla Essence - 1 tsp
- Vegetable Oil - 2 tbsp
- Roughly Chopped and toasted Walnuts - 2 table-spoons (3/4 oz.)
- Plain Non-Fat Yogurt - 1/3 cup
- Cooking Oil for Spray - as required

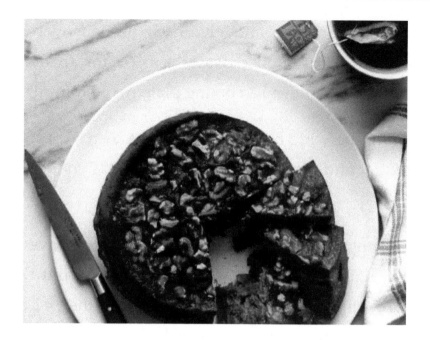

Method:

1. Cover the base of a 6-inches round cake baking pan with baking paper and lightly brush with melted butter. Beat the flour, baking soda, salt, and cinnamon together in a clean bowl and let it reserve.

2. Whisk the mashed bananas, eggs, sugar, cream, oil and vanilla together in a separate bowl. Stir the wet ingredients gently into the flour mixture until everything is blended. Pour the mixture in the prepared pan and sprinkle with the walnuts.

3. Set the temperature of an air fryer to 310 °F and put the pan in the air fryer. Cook until browned, about 30 to 35 minutes. Rotate the pan periodically until a wooden stick put in it and appears clean. Before flipping out & slicing, move the bread to a cooling rack for 15 minutes.

38. Air Fried Avocado Fries

Ingredients:

- Avocados --. 2 - Cut each into the 8 pieces
- All-purpose flour - 1/2 cup (about 21/8 oz.)

- Panko (Japanese Style Breadcrumbs) - 1/2 cup
- Large Eggs - 2
- Kosher Salt - 1/4 tsp
- Apple Cider - 1 tbsp
- Sriracha Chilli Sause - 1 tbsp
- Black pepper - 11/2 tsp
- Water - 1 tbsp
- Unsalted Ketchup - 1/2 cup
- Cooking spray

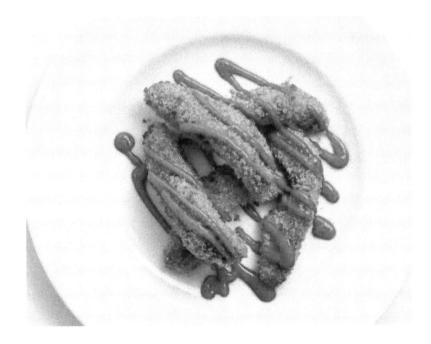

Method:

1. Mix flour and pepper collectively in a clean bowl. Whip eggs & water gently in another bowl. Take panko in a third bowl. Coat avocado slices in flour and remove extra flour by shaking. Then, dip the slices in the egg and remove any excess. Coat in panko by pushing to stick together. Spray well the avocado slices with cooking oil.

2. In the air fryer's basket, put avocado slices & fry at 400 ° F until it turns into golden for 7-8 minutes. Turn avocado wedges periodically while frying. Take out from an air fryer and use salt for sprinkling.

3. Mix the Sriracha, ketchup, vinegar, and mayonnaise together in a small bowl. Put two tablespoons of sauce on each plate with 4 avocado fries before serving.

39. "Strawberry Pop Tarts" in an Air Fryer

Ingredients:

- Quartered Strawberries - (about 13/4 cups equal to 8 ounces)
- White/Regular Sugar - 1/4 cup
- Refrigerated Piecrusts - 1/2(14.1-oz)
- Powdered Sugar - 1/2 cup (about 2-oz)
- Fresh Lemon Juice - 11/2 tsp
- Rainbow Candy Sprinkles - 1 tbsp(about 1/2 ounce)
- Cooking Spray

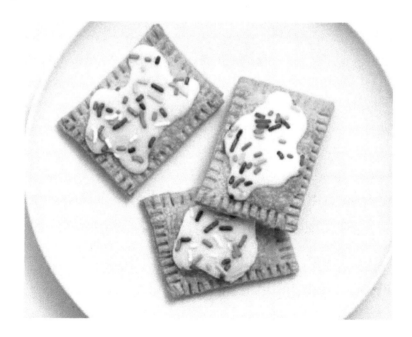

Method:

1. Mix strawberries & white sugar and stay for 15 minutes with periodically stirring. Air fryer them for 10 minutes until glossy and reduced with constant stirring. Let it cool for 30 minutes.

2. Use the smooth floured surface to roll the pie crust and make 12-inches round shape. Cut the dough into 12 rectangles of (2 1/2- x 3-inch), re-rolling strips if necessary. Leaving a 1/2-inch boundary, add the spoon around 2 tea-spoons of strawberry mixture into the middle of 6 of dough rectangles. Brush the edges of the rectangles of the filled dough with water. Then, press the edges of rest dough rectangles with a fork to seal. Spray the tarts very well with cooking oil.

3. In an air fryer pot, put 3 tarts in a single layer and cook them at 350 ° F for 10 minutes till golden brown. With the rest of the tarts, repeat the process. Set aside for cooling for 30 minutes.

4. In a small cup, whip the powdered sugar & lemon juice together until it gets smooth. Glaze the spoon over the cooled tarts and sprinkle equally with candy.

40. Lighten up Empanadas in an Air Fryer

Ingredients:

- Lean Green Beef - 3 ounces
- Cremini Mushrooms - Chopped finely - 3 ounces
- White onion - Chopped finely - 1/4th cup
- Garlic – Chopped finely - 2 tsp.
- Pitted Green Olives - 6
- Olive Oil - 1 table-spoon
- Cumin - 1/4th tsp
- Cinnamon - 1/8th tsp
- Chopped tomatoes - 1/2 cup
- Paprika - 1/4 tea-spoon
- Large egg lightly Beaten - 1

- Square gyoza wrappers - 8

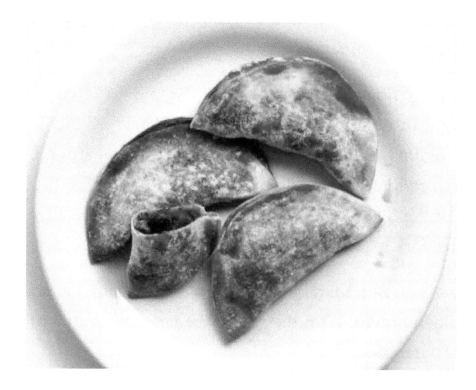

Method:

1. In a medium cooking pot, let heat oil on the medium/high temperature. Then, add beef & onion; for 3 minutes, cook them, mixing the crumble, until getting brown. Put the mushrooms; let them cook for 6 mins, till the mushrooms start to brown, stirring frequently. Add the paprika, olives, garlic, cinnamon, and cumin; cook for three minutes until the mushrooms are very tender and most of the liquid has been released. Mix in the tomatoes and cook, turning periodically, for 1 minute. Put the filling in a bowl and let it cool for 5 minutes.

2. Arrange 4 wrappers of gyoza on a worktop. In each wrapper, put around 1 1/2 tablespoons of filling in the middle. Clean the edges of the egg wrappers; fold over the wrappers and pinch the edges to seal. Repeat with the remaining wrappers and filling process.

3. Place the 4 empanadas in one single layer in an air-fryer basket and cook for 7 minutes at 400 °F until browned well. Repeat with the empanadas that remain.

41. Air Fried Calzones

Ingredients:

- Spinach Leaves --> 3 ounces (about 3 cups)
- Shredded Chicken breast --> 2 ounces (about 1/3 cup)
- Fresh Whole Wheat Pizza Dough --> 6 ounces
- Shredded Mozzarella Cheese --> 11/2 ounces (about 6 tbsp)
- Low Sodium Marinara Sauce --> 1/3 cup

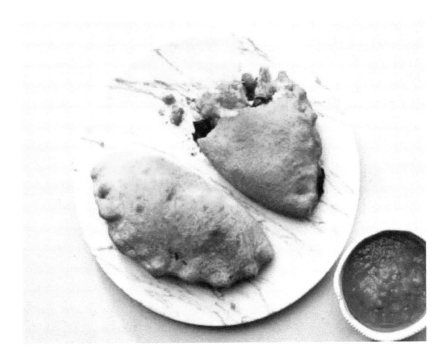

Method:

1. First of all, in a medium pan, let heat oil on medium/high temperature. Include onion & cook, continue mixing then well efficiently, for two min, till get soft. After that, add the spinach; then cover & cook it until softened. After that, take out the pan from the heat; mix the chicken & marinara sauce.

2. Divide the dough in to the four identical sections. Then, roll each section into a 6-inches circle on a gently floured surface. Place over half of each dough circular shape with one-fourth of the spinach mixture. Top with one-fourth of the cheese

each. Fold the dough to make half-moons and over filling, tightening the edges to lock. Coat the calzones well with spray for cooking

3. In the basket of an air fryer, put the calzones and cook them at 325 ° F until the dough becomes nicely golden brown, in 12 mins, changing the sides of the calzones after 8 mins.

42. Air Fried Mexican Style Corns

Ingredients:

- Unsalted Butter - 11/2 tbsp.
- Chopped Garlic -2 tsp
- Shucked Fresh Corns - 11/2 lb
- Fresh Chopped Cilantro - 2 tbsp.
- Lime zest - 1 tbsp.
- Lime Juice - 1 tsp
- Kosher Salt - 1/2 tsp
- Black Pepper - 1/2 tsp

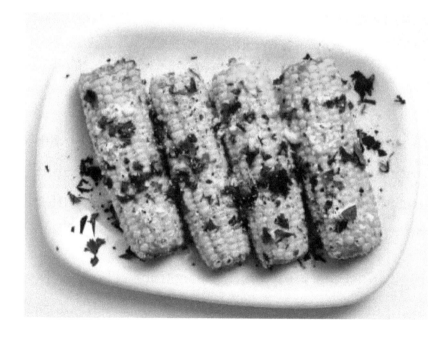

Method:

1. Coat the corn delicately with the cooking spray, and put the corn in the air fryer's basket in one single layer. Let it Cooking for 14 mins at 400 °F till tender then charred gently, changing the corn half the way via cooking.

2. In the meantime, whisk together all the garlic, lime juice, butter, & lime zest in the microwaveable pot. Let an air fryer on Fast, about 30 seconds, until the butter melts and the garlic is aromatic. Put the corn on the plate and drop the butter mixture on it. Using the salt, cilantro, and pepper to sprinkle. Instantly serve this delicious recipe.

43. Air Fryer Crunchy & Crispy Chocolate Bites

Ingredients:

- Frozen Shortcrust Pastry - Partially thawed -- 4
- Cinnamon for dusting -- as required
- Icing Sugar for dusting -- as required
- Mars Celebration Chocolates -- 24
- Whipped Cream - as required

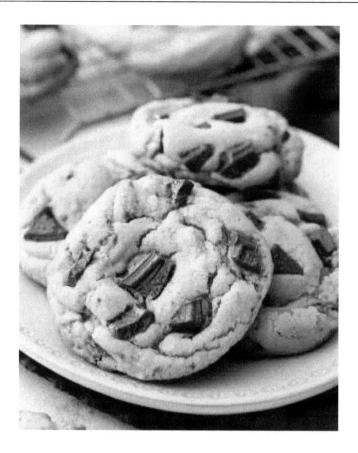

Method:

1. First of all, cut each pastry sheet into 6 equal rectangles. Brush the egg finely. In the centre of each piece of the pastry, place one chocolate. Fold the pastry over to seal the chocolate. Trim the extra pastry, then press and lock the corners. Put it on a tray lined with baking sheet. Brush the tops with an egg. Use the mixture of cinnamon and sugar to sprinkle liberally.

2. In the air-fryer basket, put a layer of the baking paper, ensuring that the paper is 1 cm smaller than that of the basket to permit air to circulate well. Place the 6 pockets in basket, taking care that these pockets must not to overlap. Then, cook them for 8-9 mins at 190 ° C till they become golden and the pastry are prepared thoroughly. As the pockets cooked, transfer them into a dish. Repeat the process with the pockets that remain.

3. After taking out from the air fryer, dust the Icing sugar and at last with whipped cream. Serve them warm.

44. Doritos-Crumbled Chicken tenders in an Air fryer

Ingredients:

- Buttermilk -- 1 cup (about 250ml)
- Doritos Nacho Cheese Corn Chips -- 170g Packet
- Halved Crossways Chicken Tenderloins -- 500g
- Egg -- 1
- Plain Flour -- 50g
- Mild Salsa -- for serving

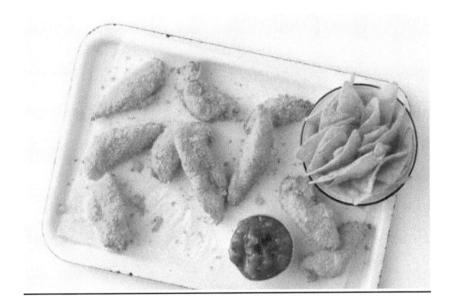

Method:

1.Take a ceramic bowl or glass and put the chicken in it. Then, c over the buttermilk with it. Wrap it and put it for 4 hours or may be overnight in the refrigerator to marinate.

2. Let Preheat an air fryer at 180C. Then, cover a Baking tray with grease-proof paper.

3. In a Chopper, add the corn chips then pulse them until the corn chips become coarsely chopped. Then, transfer the chopped chips to a dish. In a deep cup, put the egg and beat it. On another plate, put the flour.

4. Remove the unnecessary water from the chicken, and also discard the buttermilk. Then, dip the chicken in the flour mixture and wipe off the extra flour. After that, dip in the beaten egg and then into the chips of corn, press it firmly to coat well. Transfer it to the tray that made ready to next step.

5. In the air fryer, put half of the chicken and then, fry for 8 to 10 mins until they are golden as well as cooked completely. Repeat the process with the chicken that remain.

Transfer the chicken in the serving dish. Enjoy this delicious recipe with salsa.

45. Air Fryer Ham & Cheese Croquettes

Ingredients:

- Chopped White Potatoes -- 1 kg
- Chopped Ham -- 100g
- Chopped Green Shallots -- 2
- Grated Cheddar Cheese -- 80g (about 1 cup)
- All-purpose flour -- 50g
- eggs -- 2
- Breadcrumbs -- 100g
- Lemon Slices -- for serving
- Tonkatsu Sause -- for serving

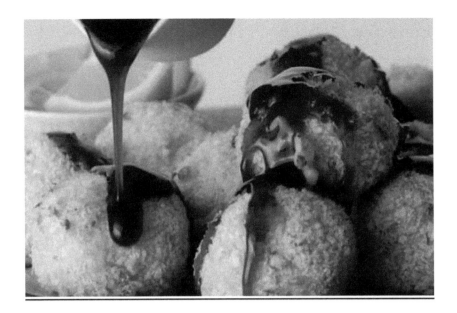

Method:

1. In a large-sized saucepan, put the potatoes. Cover with chill water. Carry it over high temperature to a boil. Boil till tender for 10 to 12 minutes. Drain thoroughly. Return over low heat to pan. Mix until it is smooth and has allowed to evaporate the certain water. Withdraw from the sun. Switch to a tub. Fully set aside to chill.

2. Then, add the shallot, Ham and cheese in the mashed potatoes also season with kosher salt. Mix it well. Take the 2 tablespoons of the mixture and make its balls. And repeat process for the rest of mixture.

3. Take the plain flour in a plate. Take another small bowl and beat the eggs. Take the third bowl and add the breadcrumbs in it. Toss the balls in the flour. Shake off the extra flour then in eggs and coat the breadcrumbs well. Make the balls ready for frying. Take all the coated balls in the fridge for about 15 minutes.

4. Preheat an air fryer at 200 ° C. Then, cook the croquettes for 8 to10 mints until they become nicely golden, in two rounds. Sprinkle the tonkatsu sauce and serve the croquettes with lemon slices.

46. Air Fryer Lemonade Scones

Ingredients:

- Self-raising flour -- 525g (about 3 1/2 cups)
- Thickened Cream -- 300ml
- Lemonade -- 185ml (about 3/4 cup)
- Caster Sugar -- 70g (1/3 cup)
- Vanilla Essence -- 1 tsp
- Milk -- for brushing
- Raspberry Jam -- for serving
- Whipped Cream -- for serving

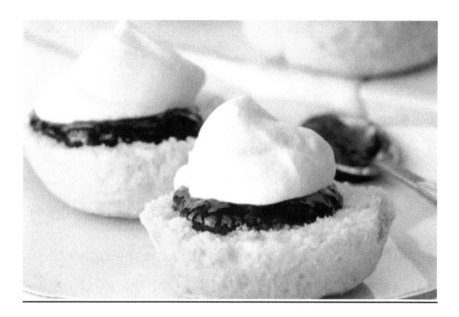

Method:

1. In a large-sized bowl, add the flour and sugar together. Mix it well. Add lemonade, vanilla and cream. In a big bowl, add the flour and sugar. Just make a well. Remove milk, vanilla and lemonade. Mix finely, by using a plain knife, till the dough comes at once.

2. Take out the dough on the flat surface and sprinkle the dry flour on the dough. Knead it gently for about 30 secs until the dough get smooth. On a floured surface, roll out the dough. Politely knead for thirty seconds, until it is just smooth. Form the dough into a round shape about 2.5 cm thick. Toss around 5.5 cm blade into

the flour. Cut the scones out. Push the bits of remaining dough at once gently and repeat the process to make Sixteen scones.

3. In the air fryer bucket, put a layer of baking paper, ensuring that the paper is 1 cm shorter than the bucket to allow air to flow uniformly. Put 5 to 6 scones on paper in the bucket, even hitting them. Finely brush the surfaces with milk. Let cook them for about 15 mins at 160 ° C or when they tapped on the top, until become golden and empty-sounding. Move it safely to a wire or cooling rack. Repeat the same process with the rest of scones and milk two more times.

4. Serve the lemonade scones warm with raspberry jam & whipped cream.

47. Air Fryer Baked Potatoes

Ingredients:

- Baby Potatoes -- Halved shape -- 650g
- Fresh rosemary sprigs-- 2 large
- Sour Cream -- for serving
- Sweet Chilli Sauce -- for serving
- Salt -- for seasoning

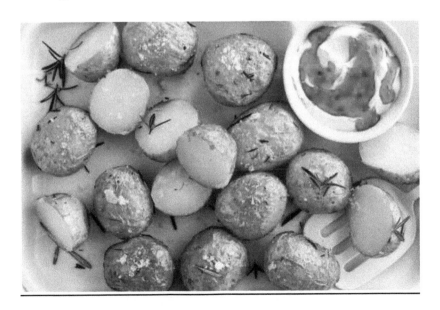

Method:

1. Firstly, at 180C, pre-heat the air fryer. In an air fryer, put the rosemary sprigs & baby potatoes. Use oil for spray and salt for seasoning. Then, cook them for fifteen min until become crispy and cooked completely, also turning partially.

2. Serve the baked potatoes sweet chilli Sause & sour cream to enhance its flavour.

48. Air Fryer Mozzarella Chips

Ingredients:

- All-purpose flour -- 1 tbsp
- Breadcrumbs -- 2/3 cup
- Garlic Powder -- 3 tbsp
- Lemon Juice -- 1/3 cup
- Avocado -- 1
- Basil Pesto -- 2 tbsp
- Plain Yogurt -- 1/4 cup
- Chopped Green Onion --1
- Cornflakes crumbs -- 1/4 cup
- Mozzarella block -- 550g
- Eggs – 2
- Olive Oil for spray

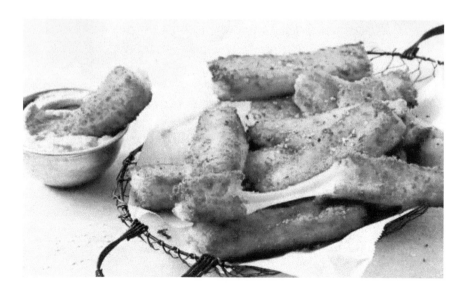

Method:

1. Start making Creamy and fluffy Avocado Dipped Sauce: In a small-sized food processor, put the yogurt, avocado, lemon juice, onion, and pesto. Also add the pepper & salt, blend properly. Process it well until it get mixed and smooth. Switch the batter to a bowl. Cover it. Place in the fridge, until It required.

2. Take a large-sized tray and place a baking sheet. In a large bowl, add the garlic powder & plain flour together. Also add the salt and season well. Take another medium bowl, whisk the eggs. Mix the breadcrumbs well in bowl.

3. Make the 2 cm thick wedges of mozzarella, then put them into the sticks. For coating, roll the cheese in the flour. Shake off the extra flour. Then, coat the sticks in the egg fusion, then in the breadcrumbs, operating in rounds. Place the prepared plate on it. Freeze till solid, or even for around 1 hour.

4. Spray the oil on the mozzarella lightly. Wrap the air fryer bucket with baking sheet, leaving an edge of 1 cm to enable air to flow. Then, cook at 180C, for 4 to 4 1/2 mins until the sticks become crispy & golden. Serve warm with sauce to dip.

49. Air Fryer Fetta Nuggets

Ingredients:

- All-purpose flour -- 1 tbsp.
- Chilli flakes -- 1 tsp
- Onion powder -- 1 tsp
- Sesame Seeds -- 1/4 cup
- Fetta Cheese Cubes -- Cut in 2 cm 180g
- Fresh Chives -- for serving
- Breadcrumbs -- 1/4 cup

BARBECUE SAUSE:

- apple cider -- 11/2 tsp
- Chilli Flakes -- 1/2 tsp
- Barbecue Sause -- 1//4 cup

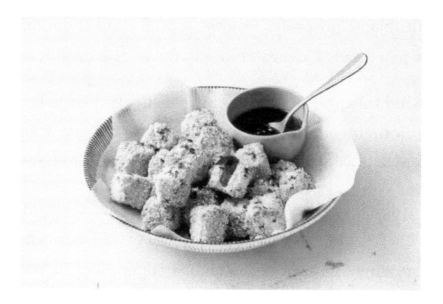

Method:

1. Mix the onion powder, flour and chilli flakes in a medium-sized bowl. Use pepper for seasoning. Take another bowl, and beat an egg. Take one more bowl and mix sesame seeds and breadcrumbs. Then, toss the fetta in the chilli flakes, onion powder & flour mixture. Dip the fetta in egg, and toss again in breadcrumbs fusion. Put them on a plate.

2. Pre- heat the air fryer at 180 °C. Put the cubes of fetta in a baking tray, in the basket of the air fryer. cook till fetta cubes become golden, or may be for 6 mins.

3. In the meantime, mix all the wet ingredients and create the Barbecue sauce.

4. Sprinkle the chives on the fetta and serve with Barbecue Sause.

50. Air Fryer Japanese Chicken Tender

Ingredients:

- McCormick Katsu Crumb for seasoning -- 25g

- Pickled Ginger -- 1 tbsp.
- Japanese-Style Mayonnaise -- 1/3 cup
- Chicken Tenderloins -- 500g
- Oil for spray

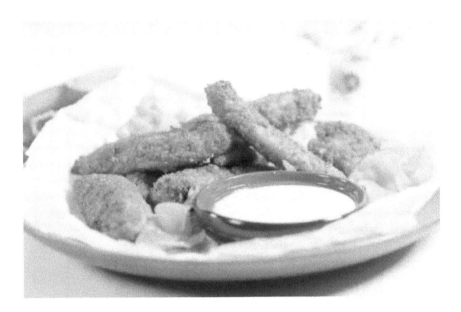

Method:

1. Put the chicken on tray in the form of single layer. Sprinkle the half seasoning on chicken. Then, turn chicken and sprinkle the seasoning again evenly. Use oil for spray on it.

2. Pre-heat at 180°C, an air fryer. Let the chicken cooking for about 12 - 14 mins until it becomes golden & cooked completely.

3. In the meantime, take a small-sized bowl, mix the mayonnaise and the remaining pickling sauce.

4. Serve the chicken with white sauce and put the ginger on the side, in a platter.

51. Whole-Wheat Pizzas in an Air Fryer

Ingredients:

- Low-sodium Marinara Sauce -- 1/4 cup

- Spinach leaves -- 1 cup
- Pita Breads -- 2
- Shredded Mozzarella Cheese -- 1/4 cup
- Parmigiano- Reggiano Cheese -- 1/4 ounces (about 1 tbsp.)
- Tomato slices -- 8
- Sliced Garlic Clove -- 1

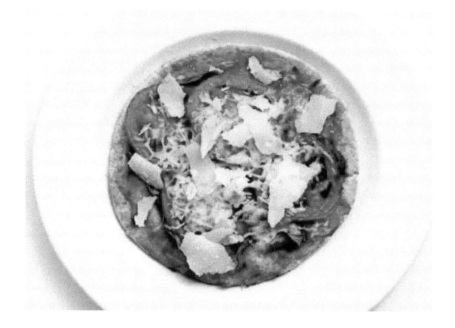

Method:

1. Spread the marinara sauce on 1 side of each pita bread uniformly. Cover the cheese spinach leaves, tomato slices and garlic, with half of each of these.

2. Put one pita bread in an air fryer pot, then cook it at 350°F till the cheese becomes melted and pita becomes crispy, 4 - 5 mins. Repeat the process with the pita leftover.

52. Air Fryer Crispy Veggie Quesadillas

Ingredients:

- 6 inches Whole Grain Flour Tortillas -- 4
- Full fat Cheddar Cheese -- 4 ounces (about 1 cup)

- Sliced Zucchini -- 1 cup
- Lime Zest -- 1 tbsp.
- Lime Juice -- 1 tsp.
- Fresh Cilantro -- 2 tbsp.
- Chopped Red Bell Pepper -- (about 1 cup)
- Cumin -- 1/4 tsp.
- Low-fat Yoghurt -- 2 ounces
- Refrigerated Pico de Gallo -- 1/2 cup
- Oil for spray

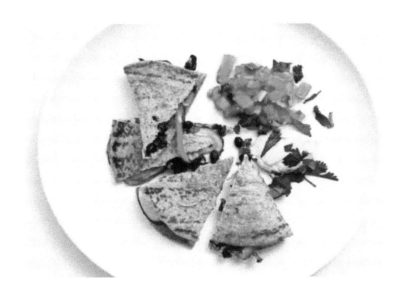

Method:

1. Put tortillas on the surface of the work. Sprinkle onto half of each tortilla with 2 tbsp. of grated cheese. Cover each tortilla with 1/4 cup of chopped red bell pepper, zucchini chunks & the black beans on the top of the cheese. Sprinkle finely with 1/2 cup of cheese left. Fold over the tortillas to create quesadillas form like half-moons. Coat the quesadillas slightly with a cooking spray, & lock them with match picks or toothpicks.

2. Lightly brush a bucket of air fryer with cooking oil spray. Place 2 quesadillas carefully in the basket. Cook at 400°F till the tortillas become golden brown & gently crispy. Melt the cheese & gradually tender the vegetables for ten mins,

tossing the quesadillas partially throughout the cooking period. Repeat the process with leftover quesadillas.

3. Mix together lime zest, yogurt, cumin, & lime juice, in a small-sized bowl since the quesadillas getting prepare. Break each quesadilla in-to the pieces to serve and then sprinkle the coriander. With one tbsp. of cumin cream and two tablespoons of pico de gallo, and serve each.

53. Air Fried Curry Chickpeas

Ingredients:

- Drained & Rinsed Un-Salted Chickpeas -- 11/2 cups (15-oz.)
- Olive Oil -- 2 tbsp.
- Curry Powder -- 2 tsp.
- Coriander -- 1/4 tsp.
- Cumin -- 1/4 tsp.
- Cinnamon -- 1/4 tsp.
- Turmeric -- 1/2 tsp.
- Aleppo Pepper -- 1/2 tsp.
- Red Wine Vinegar -- 2 tbsp.
- Kosher Salt -- 1/4 tsp.
- Sliced Fresh Cilantro -- as required

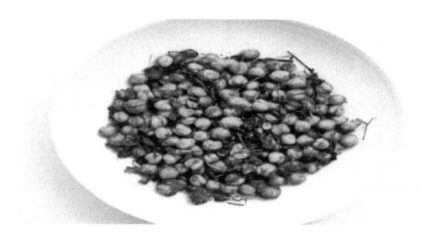

Method:

1. Break the chickpeas lightly in a medium-sized bowl with your hands (don't crush them); and then remove the skins of chickpea.

2. Add oil & vinegar to the chickpeas, and stir to coat. Then, add curry powder, turmeric, coriander, cumin, & cinnamon; mix gently to combine them.

3. In the air fryer bucket, put the chickpeas in one single layer & cook at 400°F temperature until becoming crispy, for about 15 min, stirring the chickpeas periodically throughout the cooking process.

4. Place the chickpeas in a dish. Sprinkle the salt, cilantro and Aleppo pepper on chickpeas; and cover it.

54. Air Fried Beet Chips

Ingredients:

- Canola Oil -- 1 tsp.
- Medium-sized Red Beets -- 3
- Black Pepper -- 1/4 tsp.
- Kosher Salt -- 3/4 tsp.

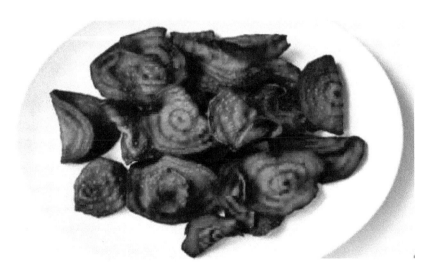

Method:

1. Cut and Peel the red beets. Make sure each beet cutted into 1/8-inch-thick slices. Take a large-sized bowl and toss the beets slices, pepper, salt and oil well.

2. Put half beets in air fryer bucket and then cook at the 320°F temperature about 25 - 30 mins or until they become crispy and dry. Flip the bucket about every 5 mins. Repeat the process for the beets that remain.

55. Double-Glazed Air Fried Cinnamon Biscuits

Ingredients:

- Cinnamon -- 1/4 tsp.
- Plain Flour -- 2/3 cup (about 27/8 oz.)
- Whole-Wheat Flour -- 2/3 cup (about22/3 oz.)
- Baking Powder -- 1 tsp.
- White Sugar -- 2 tbsp.
- Kosher Salt -- 1/4 tsp.
- Chill Salted Butter -- 4 tbsp.
- Powdered Sugar -- 2 cups (about 8-oz.)
- Water -- 3 tbsp.
- Whole Milk -- 1/3 cup
- Oil for spray -- as required

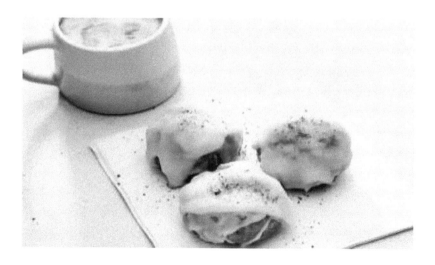

Method:

1. In a medium-sized bowl, stir together salt, plain flour, baking powder, white sugar cinnamon and butter. Use two knives or pastry cutter to cut mixture till butter becomes well mixed with the flour and the mixture seems to as coarse cornmeal. Add the milk, then mix well until the dough becomes a ball. Place the dough on a floury surface and knead for around 30 seconds until the dough becomes smooth. Break the dough into 16 identical parts. Roll each part carefully into a plain ball.

2. Coat the air fryer pot well with oil spray. Put 8 balls in the pot, by leaving the space between each one; spray with cooking oil. Cook them until get browned & puffed, for 10 - 12 mins at 350°F temperature. Take out the doughnut balls from the pot carefully and put them on a cooling rack having foil for five mins. Repeat the process with the doughnut balls that remain.

3. In a medium pot, mix water and powdered sugar together until smooth. Then, spoon half of the glaze carefully over the doughnut balls. Cool for five mins and let it glaze once and enabling to drip off extra glaze.

56. Lemon Drizzle Cake in an Air Fryer

Ingredients:

- Grated Lemon rind -- 2 tsp.
- Cardamom -- 1 tsp.
- Softened Butter -- 150g
- Eggs -- 3
- Honey-flavoured Yoghurt -- 3/4 cup
- Self-raising flour -- 11/2 cups
- Caster Sugar -- 2/3 cup (150g)
- Lemon Zest -- for serving

LEMON ICING:

- Icing Sugar -- 1 cup
- Lemon Juice -- 11/2 tbsps.
- Softened Butter -- 10g

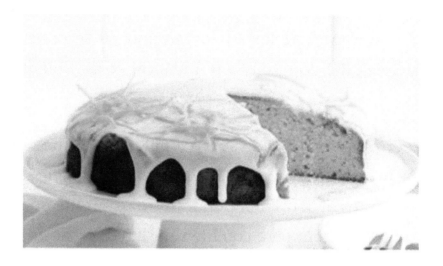

Method:

1. First, grease a 20 cm cake baking pan of round shape having butter paper. Take an electric beater and beat cardamom, sugar, lemon rind, and butter until the mixture becomes smooth & pale. Then, add the eggs one by one and beat well. Put the eggs in the flour and yoghurt. Fold by spatula and make the surface very smooth.

2. Pre-heat the air fryer at 180 C temperature. Put the pan in air fryer's pot. Bake it for about 35 mins. Check it by putting skewer in it that comes out clean without any sticky batter. Reserve it in the pan for 5 minutes to become cool before shifting it to a cooling rack.

3. Make the lemon glaze, add butter and icing sugar in a bowl. By adding lemon juice as required and form a smooth paste.

4. Put the cake on a plate to serve. Sprinkle the lemon zest and lemon icing to serve.

57. Air Fryer dukkah-Crumbed chicken

Ingredients:

- Chicken Thigh Fillets -- 8
- Herb or dukkah -- 45g packet
- Plain Flour -- 1/3 cup (about 50g)
- Kaleslaw kit -- 350g Packet
- Breadcrumbs -- 1 cup (about 80g)
- Eggs -- 2

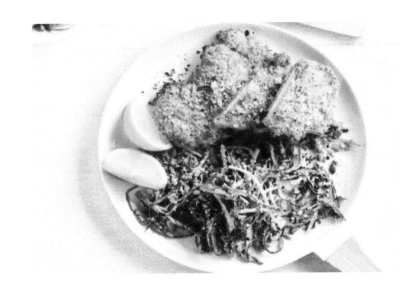

Method:

1. Put half of the chicken within 2 sheets of cling paper. Gently beat until it remains 2 cm thick by using a meat hammer or rolling pin. Repeat the process with the chicken that remains.

2. In a deep bowl, mix breadcrumbs and dukkah together. Beat an egg in medium bowl., Put the flour and all the seasoning on a tray. Coat chicken pieces one by one in the flour and shake off the extra. Dip chicken pieces into the egg, then in breadcrumbs for coating. Move them to a dish. Cover them with the plastic wrapper & leave it to marinate for 30 mins in the fridge.

3. Pre-heat air fryer at 200°C temperature. Use olive oil to spray the chicken pieces. Put half of the chicken in one single layer in the air fryer pot. Cook them for about 16 mins and turning partially until they become golden & get cooked completely. Move to a plate & wrap them with foil to stay warm. Repeat the process with the chicken pieces that remains.

4. After that, place the kaleslaw kit in a serving bowl by following instructions mentioned in the packets.

5. Divide the prepared chicken & the kaleslaw between serving platters, and season it.

58. Air Fryer Vietnamese-style spring roll salad

Ingredients:

- Rice Noodles -- 340g
- Crushed Garlic -- 1 clove
- Grated Ginger -- 2 tsp.
- Pork Mince -- 250g
- Lemongrass paste -- 1 tsp
- Cutted into matchsticks the Peeled Carrots -- 2
- Sliced Spring onion -- 3
- Fish sauce -- 2 tsp.
- Spring roll pastries -- 10 sheets
- Coriander -- 1/2 cup
- Sliced Red Chilli - 1 long
- Vietnamese-style Salad -- for dressing
- Mint Leaves -- 1/2
- Bean Sprouts -- 1 cup

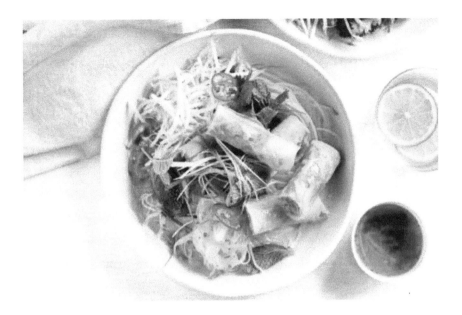

Method:

1. Take a large-sized saucepan and cook the noodles for about 4 mins until get soft. Take the cold water and discharge thoroughly. Cutting 1 cup of the boiled noodles into the short lengths, with the leftover noodles reserved.

2. Take a large-sized bowl, add the mince, lemongrass, ginger, garlic, half carrot, spring onion, and fish sauce together and mix them well.

3. On a clean surface, put one pastry paper. Add two tablespoons across 1 side of the mince fusion diagonally. With just a little spray, brush its opposite side. Fold and roll on the sides to completely cover the mince filling. Repeat the process with the sheets of pastry and fill the thin layer of mince mixture, that remain.

4. Pre-heat at 200°C, an air fryer. Use olive oil, spray on the spring rolls. Put in the bucket of air fryer and cook the spring rolls for fifteen mins until cooked completely. Change the sides half-way during cooking.

5. After that, equally split reserved noodles in the serving bowls. Place coriander, bean sprouts, mint and the remaining spring onion and carrots at the top of the serving bowl.

6. Then, break the spring rolls in the half and place them over the mixture of noodles. Sprinkle the chili and serve with Vietnamese-style salad dressing according to your taste.

59. Air Fryer Pizza Pockets

Ingredients:

- Olive oil - 2 tsp.
- Sliced Mushrooms - 6 (about 100g)
- Chopped Leg Ham - 50g
- Crumbled Fetta - 80g
- White Wraps - 4
- Basil Leaves - 1/4 cup
- Baby Spinach - 120g
- Tomato Paste - 1/3 cup
- Chopped Red Capsicum - 1/2
- Dried Oregano - 1/2 tsp
- Olive oil - for spray
- Green Salad - for serving

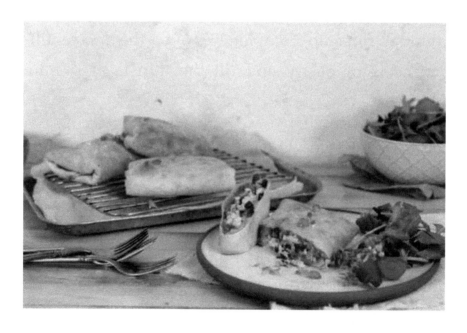

Method:

1. Heat oil on medium temperature in an air fryer. Cook capsicum for about five minutes until it starts to soften. Add mushrooms and cook them for another five mins until mushrooms become golden and evaporating any water left in the pan. Move mushrooms to another bowl. Leave them to cool for 10 mins.

2. Take a heatproof bowl and put spinach in it. Cover it with boiling water. Wait for 1 min until slightly wilted. Drain water and leave it to cool for about 10 mins.

3. Excessive spinach moisture is squeezed and applied to the capsicum mixture. Add the oregano, basil, ham and fetta. Season it with both salt & pepper. Mix it well to combine properly.

4. Put one wrapper on the smooth surface. Add 1 tbsp of tomato paste to the middle of the wrap. Cover it with a combination of 1-quarter of the capsicum. Roll up the wrap to completely enclose the filling, give it as the shape of parcel and folding the sides. To build four parcels, repeat the procedure with the remaining wraps, mixture of capsicum & tomato paste. Use oil spray on the tops.

5. Pre-heat the air fryer at 180 C temperature. Cook the parcels for 6 - 8 mins until they become golden & crispy, take out them and move to 2 more batches. Serve along with the salad.

60. Air Fryer Popcorn Fetta with Maple Hot Sauce

Ingredients:

- Marinated Fetta cubes - 265g
- Cajun for seasoning - 2 tsp.
- Breadcrumbs - 2/3 cups
- Corn flour - 2 tbsp.
- Egg - 1
- Chopped Fresh Coriander - 1 tbsp.

- Coriander leaves - for serving

Maple hot sauce:

- Maple syrup - 2 tbsp.
- Sriracha - 1 tbsps.

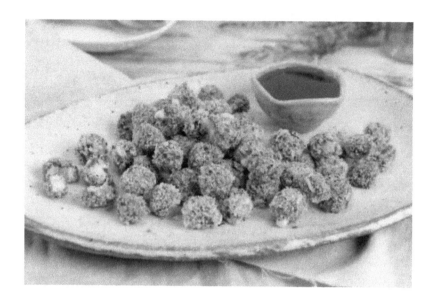

Method:

1. Drain the fetta, then reserve 1 tbsp of oil making sauce.

2. Take a bowl, mix the cornflour and the Cajun seasoning together. Beat the egg in another bowl. Take one more bowl and combine the breadcrumbs & cilantro in it. Season it with salt & pepper. Work in batches, coat the fetta in cornflour mixture, then dip in the egg. After that, toss them in breadcrumb mixture for coating. Place them on the plate and freeze them for one hour.

3. Take a saucepan, add Sriracha, reserved oil and maple syrup together and put on medium low heat. Stir it for 3 - 4 minutes continuously until sauce get start to thicken. Then, remove the maple sauce from heat.

4. Pre-heat the air fryer at 180C. Place the cubes of fetta in a single layer in the air fryer's pot. Cook them for 3 - 4 mins until just staring softened, and fettas

become golden. Sprinkled with extra coriander leaves and serve them with the maple hot sauce.

61. Air fryer Steak Fajitas

Ingredients:

- Chopped tomatoes - 2 large
- Minced Jalapeno pepper - 1
- Cumin - 2 tsp.
- Lime juice - 1/4 cup
- Fresh minced Cilantro - 3 tbsp.
- Diced Red Onion - 1/2 cup
- 8-inches long Whole-wheat tortillas - 6
- Large onion - 1 sliced
- Salt - 3/4 tsp divided
- Beef steak - 1

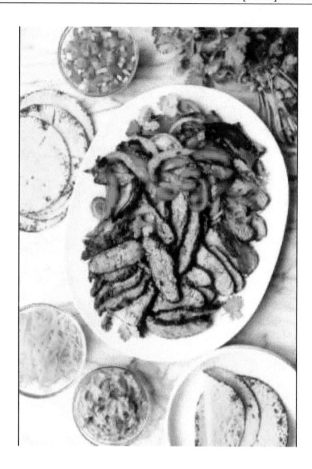

Method:

1. Mix first 5 ingredients in a clean bowl then stir in cumin and salt. Let it stand till before you serve.

2. Pre-heat the air fryer at 400 degrees. Sprinkle the cumin and salt with the steak that remain. Place them on buttered air-fryer pot and cook the steak until the meat reaches the appropriate thickness (a thermometer should read 135 ° for medium-rare; 140 °; moderate, 145 °), for 6 to 8 mins per side. Remove from the air fryer and leave for five min to stand.

3. Then, put the onion in the air-fryer pot. Cook it until get crispy-tender, stirring once for 2 - 3 mins. Thinly slice the steak and serve with onion & salsa in the tortillas. Serve it with avocado & lime slices if needed.

62. Air-Fryer Fajita-Stuffed Chicken

Ingredients:

- Boneless Chicken breast - 4
- Finely Sliced Onion - 1 small
- Finely Sliced Green pepper - 1/2 medium-sized
- Olive oil - 1 tbsp.
- Salt - 1/2 tsp.
- Chilli Powder - 1 tbsp.
- Cheddar Cheese - 4 ounces
- Cumin - 1 tsp.
- Salsa or jalapeno slices - optional

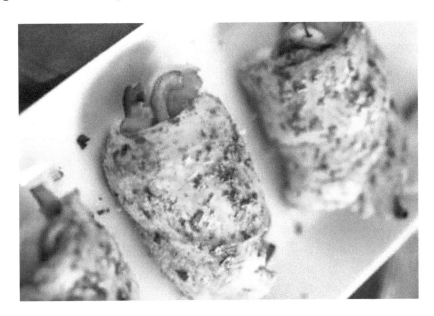

Method:

1. Pre-heat the air fryer at the 375 degrees. In the widest part of every chicken breast, cut a gap horizontally. Fill it with green pepper and onion. Combine olive oil and the seasonings in a clean bowl and apply over the chicken.

2. Place the chicken on a greased dish in the form of batches in an air-fryer pot. Cook it for 6 minutes. Stuff the chicken with cheese slices and secure the chicken pieces with toothpicks. Cook at 165° until for 6 to 8 minutes. Take off the toothpicks. Serve the delicious chicken with toppings of your choosing, if wanted.

63. Nashvilla Hot Chicken in an Air Fryer

Ingredients:

- Chicken Tenderloins - 2 pounds
- Plain flour - 1 cup
- Hot pepper Sauce - 2 tbsp.
- Egg - 1 large
- Salt - 1 tsp.
- Pepper - 1/2 tsp.
- Buttermilk - 1/2 cup
- Cayenne Pepper - 2 tbsp.
- Chilli powder - 1 tsp.
- Pickle Juice - 2 tbsp.
- Garlic Powder - 1/2 tsp.
- Paprika - 1 tsp.
- Brown Sugar - 2 tbsp.
- Olive oil - 1/2 cup
- Cooling oil for spray

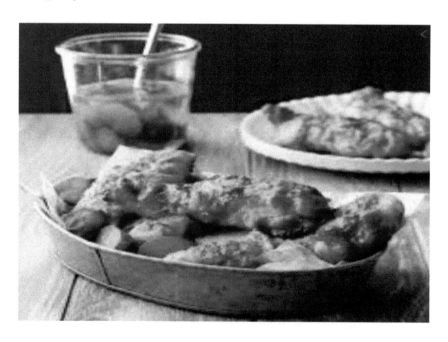

Method:

1. Combine pickle juice, hot sauce and salt in a clean bowl and coat the chicken on its both sides. Put it in the fridge, cover it, for a minimum 1 hour. Throwing away some marinade.

2. Pre-heat the air fryer at 375 degrees. Mix the flour, the remaining salt and the pepper in another bowl. Whisk together the buttermilk, eggs, pickle juice and hot sauce well. For coating the both sides, dip the chicken in plain flour; drip off the excess. Dip chicken in egg mixture and then again dip in flour mixture.

3. Arrange the single layer of chicken on a greased air-fryer pot and spray with cooking oil. Cook for 5 to 6 minutes until it becomes golden brown. Turn and spray well. Again, cook it until golden brown, for more 5-6 minutes.

4. Mix oil, brown sugar, cayenne pepper and seasonings together. Then, pour on the hot chicken and toss to cover. Serve the hot chicken with pickles.

64. Southern-style Chicken

Ingredients:

- Crushed Crackers - 2 cups (about 50)
- Fresh minced parsley - 1 tbsp.
- Paprika - 1 tsp.
- Pepper - 1/2 tsp.
- Garlic salt - 1 tsp.
- Fryer Chicken - 1
- Cumin - 1/4 tsp.
- Egg - 1
- Cooking Oil for spray

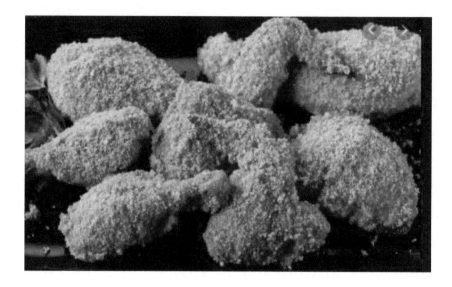

Method:

1. Set the temperature of an air fryer at 375 degrees. Mix the first 7 ingredients in a deep bowl. Beat an egg in deep bowl. Soak the chicken in egg, then pat in the cracker mixture for proper coat. Place the chicken in a single layer on the greased air-fryer pot and spray with cooking oil.

2. Cook it for 10 minutes. Change the sides of chicken and squirt with cooking oil spray. Cook until the chicken becomes golden brown & juices seem to be clear, for 10 - 20 minutes longer.

65. Chicken Parmesan in an Air Fryer

Ingredients:

- Breadcrumbs - 1/2 cup
- Pepper - 1/4 tsp.
- Pasta Sauce - 1 cup
- Boneless Chicken breast - 4
- Mozzarella Cheese - 1 cup
- Parmesan Cheese - 1/3 cup
- Large Eggs - 2
- Fresh basil - Optional

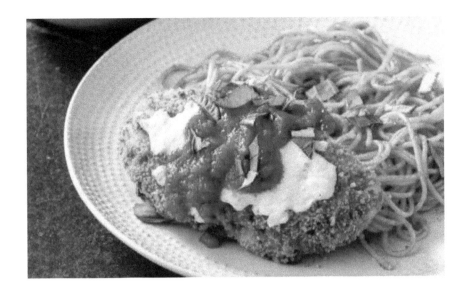

Method:

1. Set the temperature of an air-fryer at 375 degrees. In a deep bowl, beat the eggs gently. Combine the breadcrumbs, pepper and parmesan cheese in another bowl. Dip the chicken in beaten egg and coat the chicken parmesan with breadcrumbs mixture.

2. In an air-fryer pot, put the chicken in single layer. Cook the chicken for 10 to 12 mins with changing the sides partially. Cover the chicken with cheese and sauce. Cook it for 3 to 4 minutes until cheese has melted. Then, sprinkle with basil leaves and serve.

66. Lemon Chicken Thigh in an Air Fryer

Ingredients:

- Bone-in Chicken thighs- 4
- Pepper - 1/8 tsp.
- Salt - 1/8 tsp.
- Pasta Sauce - 1 cup
- Lemon Juice - 1 tbsp.
- Lemon Zest - 1 tsp.
- Minced Garlic - 3 cloves

- Butter - 1/4 cup
- Dried or Fresh Rosemary - 1 tsp.
- Dried or Fresh Thyme - 1/4 tsp.

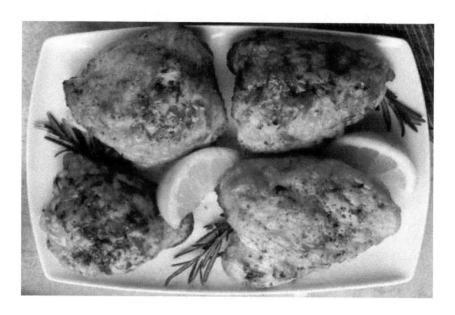

Method:

1. Pre-heat the air fryer at 400 degrees. Combine the butter, thyme, rosemary, garlic, lemon juice & zest in a clean bowl. Spread a mixture on each of the thigh's skin. Use salt and pepper to sprinkle.

2. Place the chicken, then side up the skin, in a greased air-fryer pot. Cook for 20 mins and flip once. Switch the chicken again (side up the skin) and cook it for about 5 mins until the thermometer will read 170 degrees to 175 degrees. Then, place in the serving plate and serve it.

67. Salmon with Maple-Dijon Glaze in air fryer

Ingredients:

- Salmon Fillets - 4 (about ounces)
- Salt - 1/4 tsp.
- Pepper - 1/4 tsp.
- Butter - 3 tbsp.

- Mustard - 1 tbsp.
- Lemon Juice - 1 medium-sized
- Garlic clove - 1 minced
- Olive oil

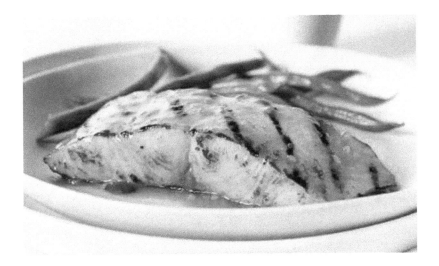

Method:

1. Pre-heat the air fryer at 400 degrees. Melt butter in a medium-sized pan on medium temperature. Put the mustard, minced garlic, maple syrup & lemon juice. Lower the heat and cook for 2 - 3 minutes before the mixture thickens significantly. Take off from the heat and set aside for few mins.

2. Brush the salmon with olive oil and also sprinkle the salt and pepper on it.

3. In an air fryer bucket, put the fish in a single baking sheet. Cook for 5 to 7 mins until fish is browned and easy to flake rapidly with help of fork. Sprinkle before to serve the salmon with sauce.

68. Air Fryer Roasted Beans

Ingredients:

- Fresh Sliced Mushrooms - 1/2 pounds
- Green Beans cut into 2-inch wedges - 1 pound
- Italian Seasoning - 1 tsp.

- Pepper - 1/8 tsp.
- Salt - 1/4 tsp.
- Red onion - 1 small
- Olive oil - 2 tbsp.

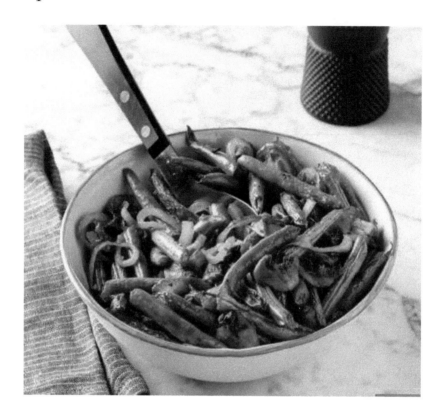

Method:

1. Pre-heat the air fryer at 375 degrees. Merge all of the ingredients in the large-sized bowl by tossing.

2. Assemble the vegetables on the greased air-fryer pot. Cook for 8 -10 minutes until become tender. Redistribute by tossing and cook for 8-10 minutes until they get browned.

69. Air Fried Radishes

Ingredients:

- Quartered Radishes - (about 6 cups)
- Fresh Oregano - 1 tbsp.

- Dried Oregano - 1 tbsp.
- Pepper - 1/8 tsp.
- Salt - 1/4 tsp.
- Olive Oil - 3 tbsp.

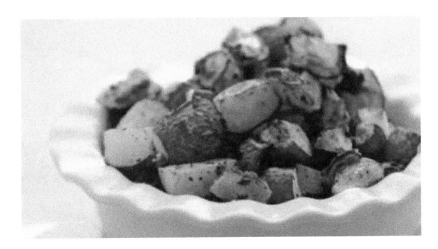

Method:

1. Set the temperature of an air fryer to 375 degrees. Mix the rest of the ingredients with radishes. In an air-fryer pot, put the radishes on greased dish.

2. Cook them for 12-15 minutes until they become crispy & tender with periodically stirring. Take out from the air fryer and serve the radishes in a clean dish.

70. Air Fried Catfish Nuggets

Ingredients

- Catfish fillets (1 inch) - 1 pound
- Seasoned fish fry coating - 3/4 cup
- Cooking oil - to spray

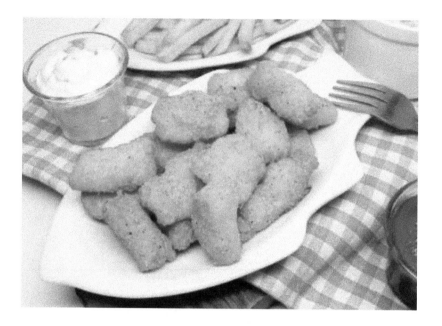

Method

1. Set the temperature of an air fryer to 200C.

2. Coat catfish pieces with seasoned coating mix by proper mixing from all sides.

3. Place nuggets evenly in an oiled air fryer pot. Spray both sides of nuggets with cooking oil. You can work in batches if the size of your air fryer is small.

4. Air fry nuggets for 5-8 minutes. Change sides of nuggets with the help of tongs and cook for more 5 minutes. Shift these delicious nuggets in a clean plate and serve immediately.

CONCLUSION:

This manual served you the easiest, quick, healthy and delicious foods that are made in an air fryer. It is also very necessary to cook food easily and timely without getting so much tired. We've discussed all the 70 easy, short, quick, delicious and healthy foods and dishes. These recipes can be made within few minutes. This manual provides the handiest or helpful cooking recipes for the busy people who are performing their routine tasks. Instead of ordering the costly or unhealthy food from hotels, you will be able to make the easy, tasty and healthy dishes with minimum cost. By reading this the most informative handbook, you can learn, experience or make lots of recipes in an air with great taste because cooking food traditionally on the stove is quite difficult for the professional persons. With the help of an air fryer, you can make various dishes for a single person as well as the entire family timely and effortlessly. We conclude that this cook book will maintain your health and it would also be the source of enjoying dishes without doing great effort in less and budget.

The Healthy Air Fryer Cookbook with Pictures

70+ Fried Tasty Recipes to Kill Hunger, Be Super Energetic and Make Your Day Brighter

By Chef Carlo Leone

Table of Contents:

Introduction

An air fryer is a little kitchen appliance which imitates the outcomes of deep frying foods with the excess grease. As opposed to submerging food in order to fry it, the more food is put within the fryer together with a rather tiny quantity of oil. The food is subsequently "fried" having just hot air cooking. Food is cooked fast Because of the high heat and, because of the small quantity of oil onto the exterior of the meals, the outside will be emptied, like it was fried!

So, here we have discussed 70 best and healthy recipes for you that you can try at home and enjoy cooking using an air fryer.

Chapter 1: Air fryer Basics and 20 Recipes

Type of air fryer:

There're some air fryers that are over $300 and the one I used was less than a hundred. I didn't want you to splurge on the expensive one immediately because I was like what if I don't even use this thing? I want you to know that I'm going to use it first so I bought this for less than $100. This one is perfectly fine. It's big, it cooks a lot and it works just as good if not better than the more expensive models.

I'm going to bring you many air fryer recipes that are super easy. Even though it takes up quite a bit of counter space, it does a good job getting things crispy and delicious. Let's start with four recipes i.e. Bacon, Brussels sprouts, chicken wings and chicken breasts. So, let's get started.

1. Air fryer Bacon Recipe

I'm going to use four slices of bacon and I'm going to cut them in half on the cutting board.

So, here's the air fryer that I have:

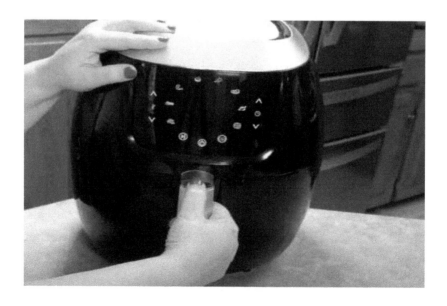

It is a 5.7 quart which is a pretty large air fryer. You take out the drawer and then we're going to lay the bacon inside of the air fryer, as it all fits. You want it to be a single layer so that they get evenly cooked. We're going to put this back in so we set the temperature for 350 degrees and they will cook for about nine minutes. We will also check them a couple of times just to make sure they're not getting too overdone. That's all there is to it, so our air fryer bacon is already and let's pull it out.

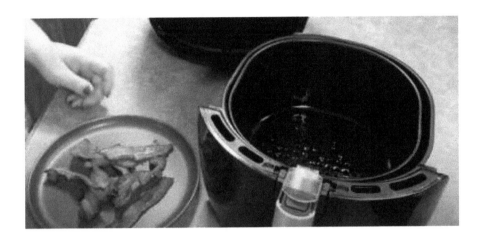

If you wanted it a little crispy, you could leave it in for probably just one more minute but I like it like this.

2. Air Fryer Apple Pie Chips

Let us be honest: If you are craving super-crispy, crunchy apple chips, then baking them in the oven is not good for you. The air fryer, on the other hand, is best.

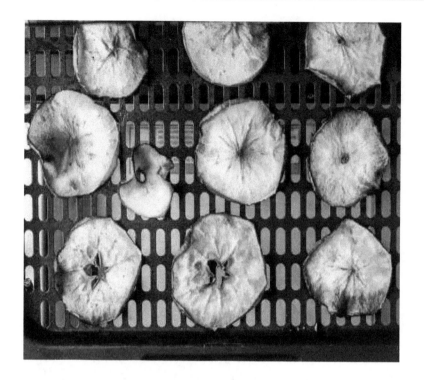

You'll begin by slicing an apple (any variety will probably work, although a red apple generates extra-pretty processors), and in case you've got a mandolin, utilize it as the thinner the slice, the crispier the processor. Toss the pieces with cinnamon and nutmeg, put an even coating into a preheated air fryer, coat with cooking spray, and stir fry until golden. You will have a tasty snack in under 10 minutes. For maximum crunchiness, let cool completely before eating.

Ingredients

- Moderate red apple

- 1/4 tsp ground nutmeg

- 1/2 tsp ground cinnamon

- Cooking spray

Instructions

- ❏ Thinly slice the apple into 1/8-inch-thick slices using a knife or rather on a mandoline.

❏ Toss the apple slices with 1/2 teaspoon ground cinnamon along with 1/4 teaspoon ground nutmeg.

❏ Preheat in an air fryer into 375°F and place for 17 minutes. Coat the fryer basket with cooking spray. Put just one layer of apple pieces into a basket and then spray with cooking spray.

❏ Air fry until golden-brown, rotating the trays halfway through to keep the apples at level, about 7 minutes total.

❏ Allow the chips to cool entirely too crisp.

❏ Repeat with the air fryer for the remaining apple pieces.

3. **Air-fryer Chicken Wings**

We will get started on the chicken wings.

Ingredients:

- 12 Chicken wings

- Salt

- Pepper

Method:

I'm going to put them in the air fryer basket and then I'm going to season them with salt and pepper. I've got these all in a single layer and they're kind of snug in there which is fine because they're going to shrink as they cook.

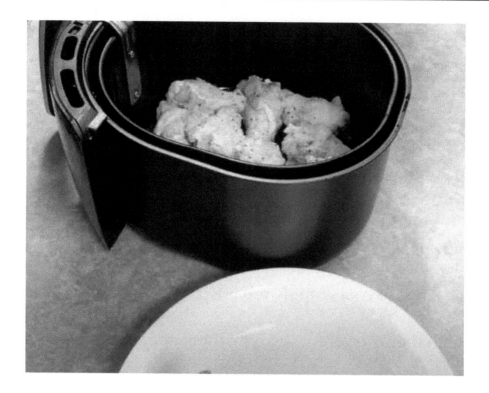

I put in about 12 chicken wings fit in my air fryer basket and now we're going to cook them for 25 minutes at 380 degrees. What that's going to do is it really get them cooked and then we're going to bump up the temperature and we will get them crispy. The first cook on our wings is done and now we are going to put it back in the air fryer at 400 degrees for about three to five minutes to get them nice and crispy. With this recipe and most air fryer recipes, whenever you're cooking things for longer than I would say five minutes, you may want to pull the basket out and shake what's inside. It is to make sure that it gets evenly cooked and I like to do that about every five minutes. Our wings are done. Look at how good they look in there nice and crispy.

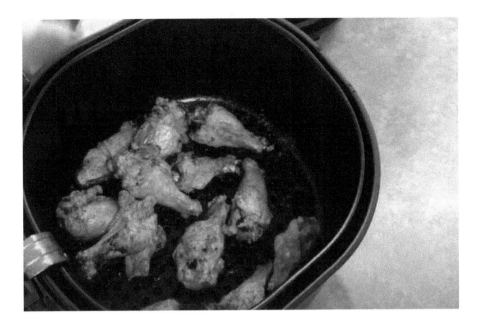

This took about three minutes as I didn't have to do the full five minutes for these.

4. **Air Fryer Mini Breakfast Burritos**

All these air-fried miniature burritos are fantastic to get a catch's go breakfast or perhaps to get a midday snack. Leave the serrano Chile pepper for a spicy version.

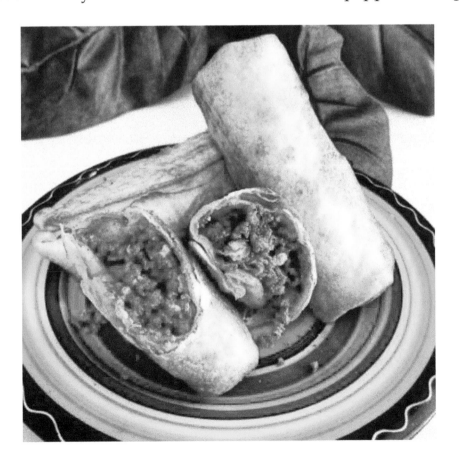

Ingredients

- 1 tablespoon bacon grease

- 1/4 cup Mexican-style chorizo

- 2 tbsp. sliced onion

- 1 serrano pepper, chopped

- salt and ground black pepper to taste

- 4 (8 inch) flour tortillas

- 1/2 cup diced potatoes

- 2 large eggs

- avocado oil cooking spray

Instructions

- ❖ Cook chorizo in an air fryer over medium-high heat, stirring often, until sausage operates into a dark crimson, 6 to 8 minutes.

- ❖ Melt bacon grease in precisely the exact way over medium-high warmth.

- ❖ Add onion and serrano pepper and continue stirring and cooking until berries are fork-tender, onion is translucent, and serrano pepper is tender in 2 to 6 minutes.

- ❖ Add eggs and chorizo; stir fry till cooked and fully integrated into curry mixture in about 5 minutes. Season with pepper and salt.

- ❖ Meanwhile, heat tortillas directly onto the grates of a gasoline stove until pliable and soft.

- ❖ Put 1/3 cup chorizo mixture down the middle of each tortilla.

❖ Fold top and bottom of tortillas over the filling, then roll into a burrito form. Mist with cooking spray and put in the basket of a fryer.

❖ Flip each burrito above, peppermint with cooking spray, and fry until lightly browned, 2 to 4 minutes longer.

5. Herb Chicken Breast

Now let's get to the herb chicken breast.

Ingredients

- Salt

- Pepper

- Chicken Breast

- Smoked Paprika

- Butter

Method:

We've got two chicken breasts. We've got butter, Italian seasoning salt, pepper and smoked paprika. We're going to mix all of that into the butter to give it a quick mix. Now we've got our two chicken breasts here and we're going to spread the mixture over each chicken breast to give it a nice flavorful crust.

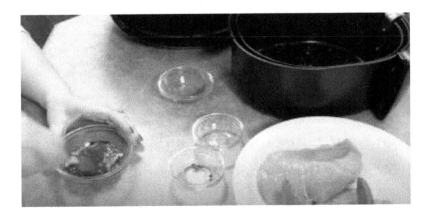

Put these in the air fryer with some tongs. We're ready to cook these in the air fryer.

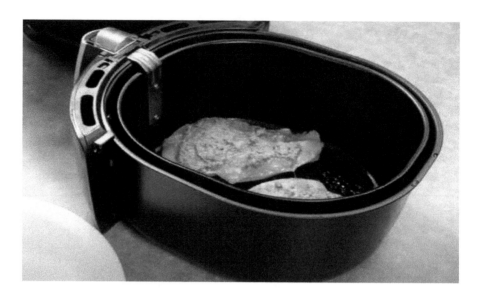

Cook them at 370 degrees for about 10 to 15 minutes and then check it with a meat thermometer to make sure that they're perfectly cooked. Because we don't want them to be overcooked, then they'll be dry and we definitely don't want them to be undercooked.

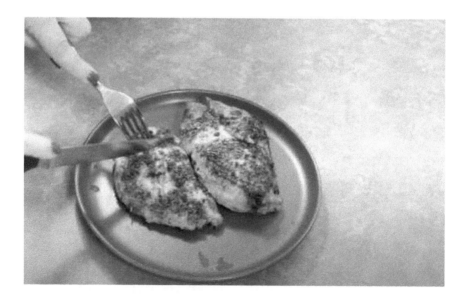

Okay, we pulled our chicken out of the air fryer. We had one chicken breast that was smaller so it came out a little bit earlier and now we have this one that's ready and its right at 165. So, we know that our chickens are not going to be dry. Let's cut into one of these. Those are perfectly cooked and juicy

6. Three Cheese Omelet

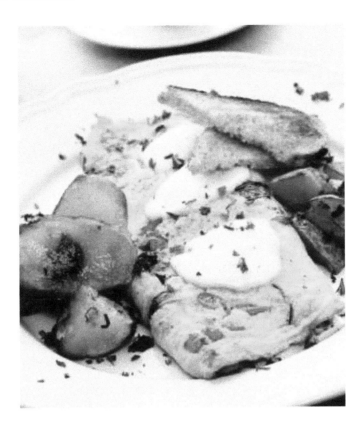

Ingredients

- 3 Tbsp. heavy whipping cream

- ½ tsp salt

- 4 eggs

- ¼ cup cheddar cheese, grated

- ¼ cup provolone cheese

- ¼ tsp ground black pepper

- ¼ cup feta cheese

Method:

❖ Preheat your air fryer to 350 degrees F and line a baking pan using parchment paper. Be sure the pan will fit on your fryer- normally a seven inch round pan will do the job flawlessly.

❖ In a small bowl, whisk together the eggs, cream, pepper and salt

❖ Pour the mixture into the prepared baking pan then place the pan on your preheated air fryer.

❖ Cook for approximately ten minutes or till the eggs are completely set.

❖ Sprinkle the cheeses round the boiled eggs and then return the pan into the air fryer for one more moment to melt the cheese.

7. Patty Pan Frittata

I had a gorgeous patty pan squash sitting on my counter tops and was wondering exactly what to do with this was fresh and yummy for my loved ones. I had not made breakfast however so a summer squash frittata appeared in order! Comparable to zucchini, patty pan squash leant itself well to my fundamental frittata recipe. Serve with your favorite brunch sides or independently. You could also cool and serve cold within 24 hours.

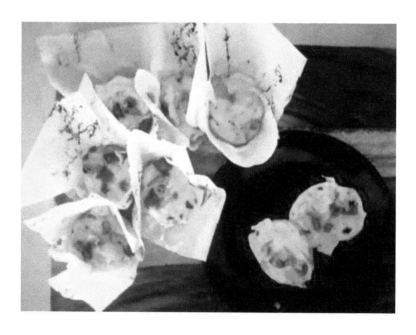

Ingredients

- 1 patty pan squash

- 1 tbsp. unsalted butter

- 4 large eggs

- 1/4 cup crumbled goat cheese

- 1/4 cup grated Parmesan cheese

- salt and ground black pepper to taste

- 1/4 cup

- 2 medium scallions, chopped, green and white parts split

- 1 tsp garlic, minced

- 1 small tomato, seeded and diced

- 1 tsp hot sauce, or to flavor

Instructions

- ❖ Press 5-inch squares of parchment paper to 8 cups of a muffin tin, creasing where essential.

- ❖ Heat butter over moderate heat; stir fry into patty pan, scallion whites, salt, garlic, and pepper. Transfer into a bowl and set aside.

- ❖ Add sausage in the identical way and cook until heated through, about 3 minutes. Add sausage into patty pan mix.

- ❖ Fold in goat milk, Parmesan cheese, and tomato. Add hot sauce and season with pepper and salt. Twist in patty pan-sausage mix. Put frittata mixture to the prepared muffin cups, filling to the peak of every cup and then overfilling only when the parchment paper may encourage the mix.

❖ Put muffin tin in addition to a cookie sheet in the middle of the toaster.

8. Bacon and Cheese Frittata

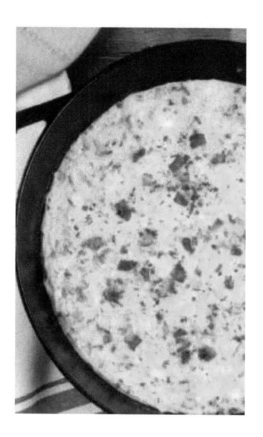

Ingredients

- ½ cup cheddar cheese, grated

- 4 eggs

- ½ cup chopped, cooked bacon

- ½ tsp salt

- 3 Tbsp. heavy whipping cream

- ¼ tsp ground black pepper

Method:

❖ Preheat your air fryer to 350 degrees F and line a baking pan using parchment paper. Be sure the pan will fit on your fryer- normally a seven inch round pan will do the job flawlessly.

❖ In a small bowl, whisk together the eggs, cream, pepper and salt

❖ Stir in the cheese and bacon into the bowl.

❖ Pour the mixture into the prepared baking pan then place the pan on your preheated air fryer.

❖ Cook for approximately 15 minutes or till the eggs are completely set.

9. **Meat Lovers Omelet**

Ingredients:

● ¼ cup cheddar cheese, grated

● ¼ cup cooked, crumbled bacon

● ½ tsp salt

● 4 eggs

● ¼ cup cooked, crumbled sausage

● 3 Tbsp. heavy whipping cream

● ¼ tsp ground black pepper

Method:

❏ Preheat your air fryer to 350 degrees F and line a baking pan using parchment paper. Be sure the pan will fit on your fryer- normally a seven inch round pan will do the job flawlessly.

❑ In a small bowl whisk together the eggs, cream, pepper and salt.

❑ Pour the mixture into the prepared baking pan then place the pan on your preheated air fryer.

❑ Cook for approximately ten minutes or till the eggs are completely set.

❑ Sprinkle the cheeses round the boiled eggs and then return the pan into the fryer for another two minutes to melt the cheese.

10. Crispy Brussels sprouts

Next on our list is air fryer crispy Brussels sprouts.

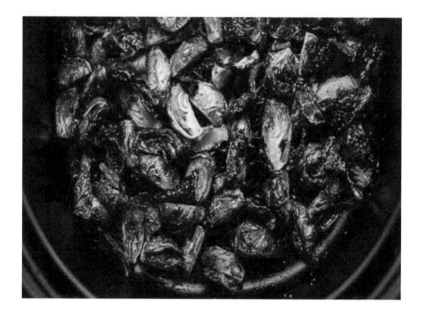

Ingredients:

- Brussels sprouts

- Salt

- Pepper

Method:

Let's get started with these Brussels sprouts. Use fresh Brussels sprouts and we could also use frozen ones. I've got a bag of frozen Brussels sprouts and actually they're still broke. I'm going to season them with some salt and some pepper.

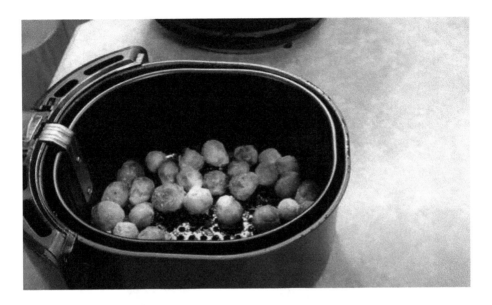

Shake them up and now I'm going to cook them at 400 or I'm going to start with 10 minutes. Let's see how it goes. I think you're going to be surprised because they're crispy. Can you believe that? I think these are better than fresh ones.

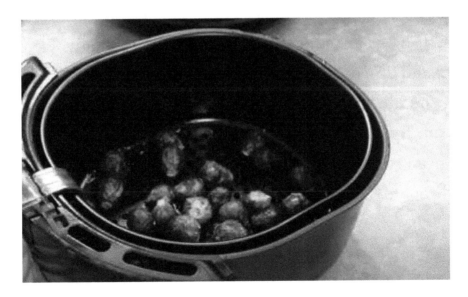

Use frozen if you want to make air fryer Brussels sprouts because the fresh ones take forever to get soft on the inside. You got to cut them into quarters, you've got to trim the leaves off these. They're frozen. I just threw them in the air fryer for 15minutes and they're good to go.

Now what I'm going to show you are actually dessert ideas that you can cook in your air fryer. They come in different sizes and one and a half liter is quite common too, so just check when you buy your own if you do that.

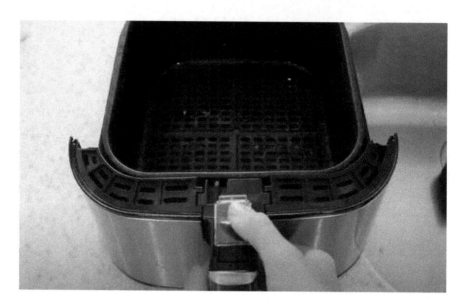

It is a bigger liter air fryer because I promise you, you're going to want to cook everything in this. What I love about this style of air fryer is that it's so simple on the front. You will see that you have got different settings but if you want to cook chips, prawns, fish, steak and muffins as well, it's really easy to adjust the temperature up and down. Also the time up and down as well. Then once you put your tray back in, all you need to do is select your setting and press the play button and the air fryer does everything else for you. It is also really really easy to clean. All you need to do is remove your tray from your air fryer, press the button on at the handle and detach your basket from the tray.

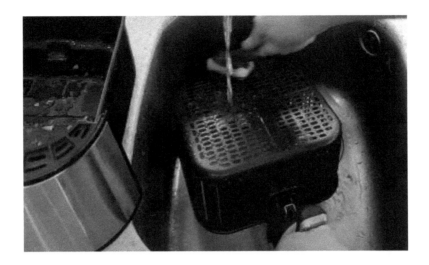

I then use a handheld scrubbing brush which dispenses washing-up liquid and I just go over my basket and my outer tray as well which is where all the fats from your food drip. I just go in with some warm water and my washing up liquid washes it all away. It's got a really nice TEFL coating so everything just wipes off. It's nonstick, then I just leave it on the side, let it dry and then pop it back in my air fryer. At once it is dry, so with all that said I'm just going to jump straight on into the recipes.

11. Hard Boiled Eggs

Ingredients:

- 4 eggs

Method:

➢ Preheat your air fryer to 250 degrees F.

➢ Place a wire rack in the fryer and set the eggs in addition to the rack.

➢ Cook for 17 minutes then remove the eggs and put them into an

➢ Ice water bath to cool and then stop the cooking procedure.

➢ Peel the eggs and love!

1. Spinach Parmesan Baked Eggs

Ingredients:

- 1 Tbsp. frozen, chopped spinach, thawed

- 1 Tbsp. grated parmesan cheese

- 2 eggs

- 1 Tbsp. heavy cream

- ¼ tsp salt

- 1/8 tsp ground black pepper

Method:

❏ Preheat your air fryer to 330 degrees F.

❏ Spray a silicone muffin cup or a little ramekin with cooking spray.

❏ In a small bowl, whisk together all of the components

❏ Pour the eggs into the ready ramekin and bake for 2 minutes.

❏ Enjoy directly from the skillet!

12. Fried hushpuppies.

Inside my home, stuffing is consistently the very popular Thanksgiving dish on the table. Because of this, we create double the amount we all actually need just so we can eat leftovers for a week! And while remaining stuffing alone is yummy, turning it into hushpuppies? Now that is only pure wizardry. Here is the way to use your air fryer to produce near-instant two-ingredient fried hushpuppies.

Ingredients:

- large egg

- cold stuffing

- Cooking spray

Directions:

★ Put 1 large egg in a large bowl and gently beat. Add 3 cups leftover stuffing and stir till blended.

★ Preheat in an air fryer into 355°F and place it for 12 minutes. Put one layer of hushpuppies on the racks and then spray the tops with cooking spray.

★ Repeat with the remaining mixture.

13. Keto Breakfast Pizza

An egg, sausage, and pork rind "crust" holds sauce, cheese, and other savory toppings within this keto-friendly breakfast pizza recipe.

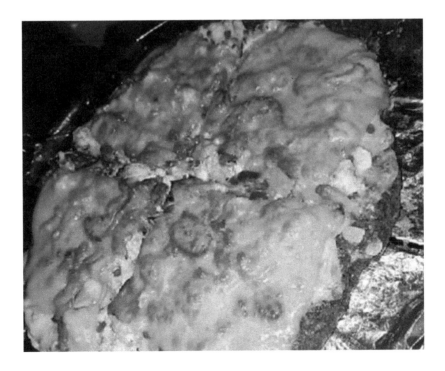

Ingredients

- 3 large eggs, split

- 2 tbsp. Italian seasoning

- 1 cup ready country-style sauce

- 10 tbsp. bacon pieces

- 1 pound bulk breakfast sausage

- cooking spray

- 1/3 cup crushed pork rinds

- 2 tbsp. chopped yellow onion

- 2 tbsp. diced jalapeno pepper

- 1 cup shredded Cheddar cheese

Instructions

★ Grease a rimmed pizza sheet.

★ Spread mixture out on the pizza sheet at a big, thin circle.

★ Meanwhile, spray a large air fryer with cooking spray and heat over medium-high heat. Whisk remaining eggs together in a bowl and then pour into it.

★ Place an oven rack about 6 inches from the heat source and then turn on the oven's broiler.

★ Spread sausage evenly over the beef "crust", sprinkle scrambled eggs. Sprinkle with bacon pieces, onion, and jalapeno.

★ Broil pizza in the preheated oven till cheese is melted, bubbling, and lightly browned, 3 to 5 minutes. Let cool and cut into fourths prior to serving.

14.Mozzarella stick

Ready for the simplest mozzarella stick recipe? These air fryer mozzarella sticks are created completely from pantry and refrigerator staples (cheese sticks and breadcrumbs), which means that you can dig to the crispy-coated, nostalgic bite anytime you would like.

INGREDIENTS:

➤ 1 (12-ounce) bundle mayonnaise

➤ 1 large egg

➤ 1/2 tsp garlic powder

➤ all-purpose flour

➤ 1/2 tsp onion powder

Method:

★ Before frying pan, set the halved cheese sticks onto a rimmed baking sheet lined with parchment paper. Freeze for half an hour. Meanwhile, construct the breading and get outside the air fryer.

★ Whisk the egg and lettuce together in a skillet. Put the flour, breadcrumbs, onion, and garlic powder in a large bowl and whisk to mix.

★ Working in batches of 6, then roll the suspended cheese sticks at the mayo-egg mix to coat, and then in the flour mixture.

★ Pour the coated cheese sticks into the parchment-lined baking sheet. Pour the baking sheet into the freezer for 10 minutes.

★ Heat the fryer to 370°F. Fry 6 the mozzarella sticks for 5 minutes -- it's important not to overcrowd the fryer.

★ Repeat with the rest of the sticks and serve hot with the marinara for dipping.

15. Raspberry Muffins

Ingredients:

- ¼ cup whole milk

- 1 egg

- 1 Tbsp. powdered stevia

- ¼ tsp salt

- ¼ tsp ground cinnamon

- 1 ½ tsp baking powder

- 1 cup almond flour

- ½ cup frozen or fresh raspberries

Steps:

I. Preheat your air fryer to 350 degrees F.

II. In a large bowl, stir together the almond milk, stevia, salt, cinnamon, and baking powder.

III. Add the milk and eggs and then stir well.

IV. Split the muffin batter involving each muffin cup, filling roughly 3/4 of this way complete.

V. Set the muffins to the fryer basket and cook for 14 minutes or till a toothpick comes out when inserted to the middle.

VI.   Eliminate from the fryer and let cool.

16. Sausage Tray Bake

I have just chopped up some new potatoes and then I've got some chipolata sausages so I'm going to make a tray bake.

Ingredients:

- Potatoes

- Chipolata Sausage

- corvette

- Onion

- Garlic

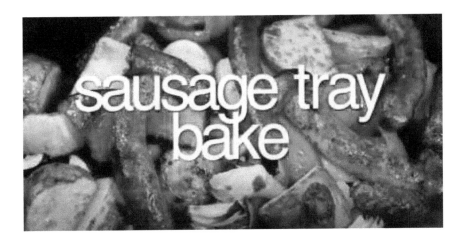

Method:

I would put potato and chipotle sausage into the air fryer for about 20 minutes at first before I add in my other veggies.

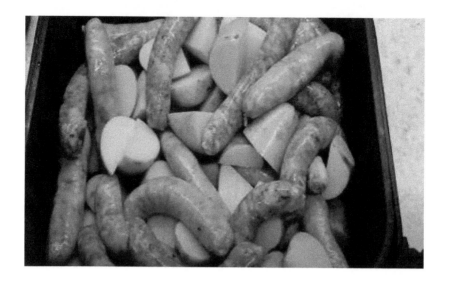

Once these have been in for 20 minutes or so, I will then add in two papers of corvette, an onion and some garlic to go in as well. Cook them for a further 10 minutes and then dinner should be ready.

17. Strawberry Muffins

Ingredients:

- ¼ cup whole milk

- 1 ½ tsp baking powder

- ½ cup chopped strawberries

- 1 egg

- ¼ tsp salt

- ¼ tsp ground cinnamon

- 1 cup almond flour

- 1 Tbsp. powdered stevia

Steps:

1. Preheat your air fryer to 350 degrees F.

2. In a large bowl, stir together the almond milk, stevia, salt, cinnamon, and baking powder.

3. Add the milk and eggs and then stir well.

4. Fold in the berries.

5. Split the muffin batter involving each muffin cup, filling roughly 3/4 of this way complete.

6. Set the muffins to the fryer basket and cook for 14 minutes or till a toothpick comes out when inserted to the middle.

7. Eliminate from the fryer and let cool.

18. Bacon and Eggs for a single

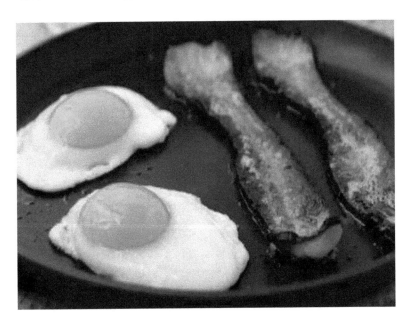

Ingredients:

- 1 Tbsp. heavy cream

- two Tbsp. cooked, crumbled bacon

- 1/4 tsp salt

- 2 eggs

- 1/8 tsp ground black pepper

Directions

❑ Preheat your air fryer to 330 degrees F.

❑ Spray a silicone muffin cup or a little ramekin with cooking spray.

❑ In a small bowl, whisk together all of the components

❑ Pour the eggs into the ready ramekin and bake for 2 minutes.

❑ Enjoy directly from the skillet!

19. **Mini Sausage Pancake Skewers with Spicy Syrup**

These small savory skewers are fantastic for breakfast or a fantastic addition to your brunch buffet. The hot maple syrup garnish kicks up the flavor and adds some zest to sandwiches and sausage.

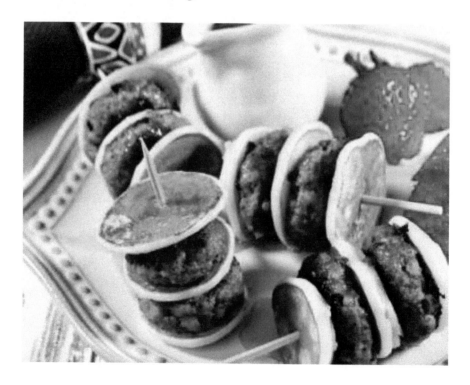

Ingredients

Syrup:

- 4 tbsp. unsalted butter

- 1/2 tsp salt

- 1/2 cup maple syrup

- 1 tsp red pepper flakes, or to taste

Pancake

- 1 cup buttermilk

- 2 tbsp. unsalted butter, melted

- 1 cup all-purpose flour

- 1 large egg

- 1 tbsp. olive oil

- 1 lb. ounce standard pork sausage (like Jimmy Dean®)

- 13 4-inch bamboo skewers

- 2 tablespoons sour cream

- 1/2 tbsp. brown sugar

- 1/4 tsp baking powder

- 1/4 tsp salt

- 2 tsp maple syrup

Instructions

❑ Bring to a boil and cook for 3 to 4 minutes.

❑ Meanwhile, prepare pancakes: whisk flour, sugar, baking powder, and salt in a huge bowl. Whisk buttermilk, egg, sour cream, melted butter and maple syrup together in another bowl. Pour the wet ingredients into the flour mixture. Stir lightly until just blended but slightly lumpy; don't overmix. Let sit for 10 minutes.

❑ Heat in an air fryer over moderate heat. Drop teaspoonfuls of batter onto them to make 1-inch diameter sandwiches.

❑ Cook for approximately 1 to 2 minutes, then reverse, and keep cooking until golden brown, about 1 minute. Transfer cooked pancakes into a plate and repeat with remaining batter.

❑ Heat olive oil at precisely the exact same fryer over moderate heat. Form table-spoonfuls of sausage to 1-inch patties, exactly the exact same size as the miniature pancakes.

❑ Cook until patties are cooked through, about 3 minutes each side. Transfer to a newspaper towel-lined plate.

❑ Blend 3 pancakes and two sausage patties onto each skewer, beginning and end with a pancake.

❑ Repeat to create staying skewers. Serve drizzled with hot syrup.

20. Avocado Baked Eggs

Ingredients:

- 1 Tbsp. heavy cream

- ¼ tsp salt

- ¼ avocado, diced

- 1 Tbsp. grated cheddar cheese

- 2 eggs

- 1/8 tsp ground black pepper

Method:

❏ Preheat your air fryer to 330 degrees F.

❏ Spray a silicone muffin cup or a little ramekin with cooking spray.

❏ In a small bowl, whisk together the eggs, cream, cheddar cheese, salt, and pepper.

❏ Stir in the avocado and pour the eggs into the ready ramekin and bake for 2 minutes.

❏ Enjoy directly from the skillet!

Chapter 2: Air Fryer 50 more Recipes for You!

21. Sausage and Cheese Omelet

Ingredients:

- ¼ cup cheddar cheese, grated

- ½ cup cooked, crumbled sausage

- 4 eggs

- 3 Tbsp. heavy whipping cream

- ½ tsp salt

- ¼ tsp ground black pepper

Method

01. Preheat your air fryer to 320 degrees F and line a baking pan using parchment paper. Be sure the pan will fit on your fryer- normally a seven inch round pan will do the job flawlessly.

02. In a small bowl, whisk together the eggs, cream, pepper and salt.

03. Pour the mixture into the prepared baking pan then place the pan on your preheated air fryer.

04. Cook for approximately ten minutes or till the eggs are completely set.

05. Sprinkle the cheeses round the boiled eggs and then return the pan into the fryer for another two minutes to melt the cheese.

22. Pita bread Pizza

I am making some pita bread pizzas now.

Ingredients:

- Bread

- Tomato puree

- Passat

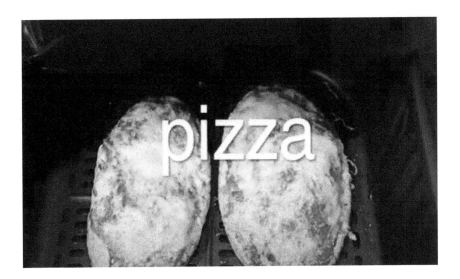

Method:

I usually would make these in the oven and I would put them in there for about 10 to 15 minutes. I'm just going to put some ketchup on top of the pizza bread base.

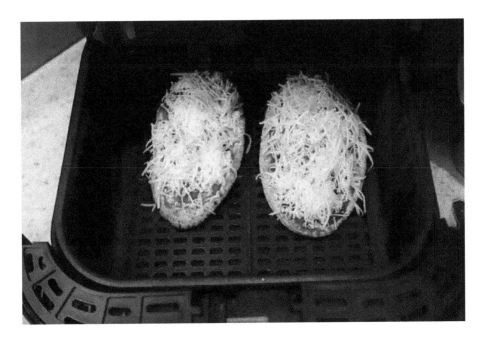

Or you can put tomato puree on there or some pasta whatever you've got. Then I'm just going to put some cheese on really nice and simple. I'm going to pop them on the pizza setting in the air fryer so that's eight minutes when I do my pizzas in the oven the base isn't really nice and crispy. So, I am really pleased with how they've turned out in the air fryer. Pizzas are done, crispy delicious, ready to eat.

23. Air Fryer Hanukkah Latkes

If you have never needed a latke, it is about time we change this. Traditionally served throughout Hanukkah, these crispy fritters -- frequently made with grated potatoes, lettuce, onion, and matzo meal -- are kind of impossible to not love.

Traditionally latkes are fried in oil (or poultry schmaltz!)) , however I wanted to see if I could create them using the popular air fryer. Since the fryer is a high-heat convection oven, the large fan speed and focused warmth yields a crispy potato pancake that is also soft at the middle.

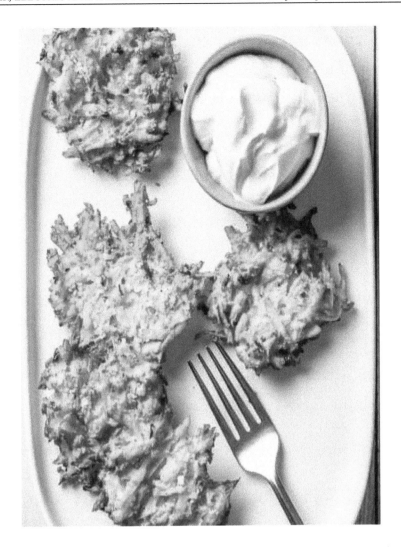

INGREDIENTS

- 1 1/2 Pounds Russet potatoes (2 to 3 tbsp.)

- ½ medium yellow onion

- 1/2 tsp freshly ground black pepper

- Cooking spray

- Two large eggs

- matzo meal

- 2 tsp kosher salt

Description:

❖ Peel 1 1/2 lbs. russet potatoes. Grate the potatoes and 1/2 yellow onion onto the large holes of a box grater. Put with a clean kitchen towel, then pull up the sides of the towel to make a package, and squeeze out excess moisture.

❖ Transfer the curry mixture into a large bowl. Add two large eggs, 1/4 cup matzo meal, two tsp kosher salt, and 1/2 tsp black pepper, and stir to blend.

❖ Preheat the Air Fryer into 375°F and place it for 16 minutes. Coat the air fryer racks together with cooking spray.

❖ Dip the latke mix in 2-tablespoon dollops to the fryer, flattening the shirts to make a patty.

❖ Air fry, rotating the trays halfway through, for 2 minutes total. Repeat with the rest of the latke mix.

24. Salmon Fillet

Now, I'm going to cook some salmon in it.

Ingredients:

- Salmon

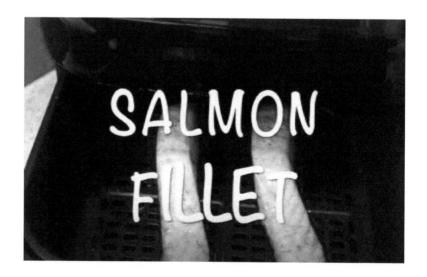

Method:

I put my salmon in, with nothing on top of it, just a salmon filet. I pop it in on the fish sitting for ten minutes and when it comes out it has got the crispy skin ever. The salmon was in for ten minutes and I wanted to show you how crispy the skin is.

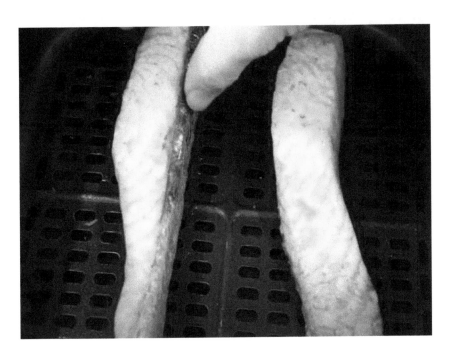

I'm someone who loves eating salmon skin and that is just perfectly done right.

25. Air Fryer Mini Calzones

Among the greatest approaches to utilize an air fryer is a miniature oven that will not heat up your entire kitchen for party snacks. It's possible to turn out batch after batch of wings, mozzarella sticks, and also, yes, miniature calzones which are hot, crispy, and superbly nostalgic by one air fryer.

These mini calzones utilize ready pizza dough to produce delicious pockets full of gooey cheese, piquant tomato sauce, and hot pepperoni that are fantastic for celebrations, after-school snacks, or even for satisfying your craving to get your dessert rolls of your childhood.

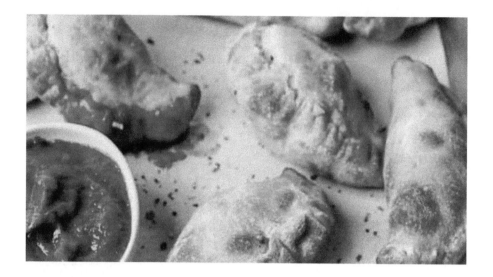

Ingredients:

- All-purpose flour, for rolling the dough out

- Pizza sauce, and more for dipping

- Thinly sliced pepperoni

- miniature pepperoni, chopped

Directions:

- ❖ Utilize a 3-inch round cutter or a large glass to cut 8 to 10 rounds of bread.

- ❖ Transfer the rounds into some parchment paper-lined baking sheet. Gather up the dough scraps, then reroll and replicate cutting rounds out until you've got 16.

- ❖ Top each round with two tsp of sauce, 1 tablespoon of cheese, and one tsp of pepperoni.

- ❖ Working with a single dough around at a time, fold in half an hour, then pinch the edges together to seal. When every calzone is sealed, then use a fork to crimp the borders shut to additional seal.

❖ Heat the air fryer into 375°F. Working in batches of 4, air fry the calzones until golden brown and crispy, about 8 minutes. Serve with extra pizza sauce for dipping, if desired.

26. Fajitas

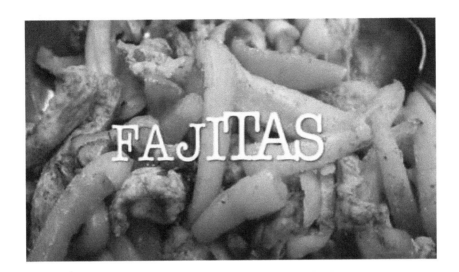

Ingredients:

- Turkey Strips

- Yellow Pepper

- Onion

- Orange Pepper

Method:

It's a night that we are going to be having for heaters. So, here, I've chopped up yellow and orange pepper and also half an onion. I have got some turkey strips.

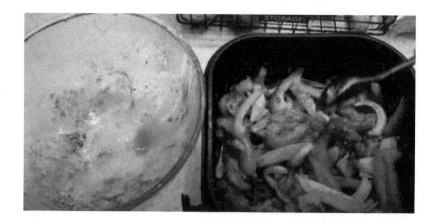

I'll pass it over heat as it makes barbecue flavor onto all of this. So, I'm just going to pop these all into the air fryer together because I think they'll actually cook through at a very similar rate. Then I am going to pop them on the chicken setting and let the air fryer get cooking alright. This is the fajita mix in ten minutes.

I put on the chicken setting which is actually 20 minutes but I was just checking it.

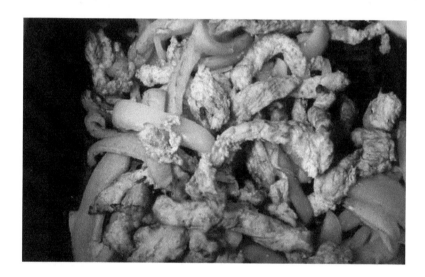

I cut a piece of the turkey and it's perfect all the way through, I cut it like one of the biggest pieces up as well. So, it's absolutely perfect so all this needs is ten minutes in the air fryer and it's done right.

27.Pot Sweet Potato Chips

Replace the humble sweet potato to a freshly-fried bite, and it is sure to be yummy. Sweet potato chips, sweet potato tater tots -- you name it, we will take it.

The comparison between the sweetness of the curry and the saltiness of this bite is really impossible to not love.

These air fryer sweet potato chips provide everything you adore about these deep-fried snacks. That is the great thing about the air fryer that it requires less oil, after all -- you have to bypass the hassle and clutter of heating a massive pot of oil to the stove -- but the "fried" cure comes out evenly as yummy. And unlike a store-bought bag of chips, you have to personalize the seasonings. Here, we are using dried herbs and a pinch of cayenne for an earthy, somewhat spicy beverage.

Ingredients:

- medium sweet potato

- 1 tbsp. canola oil

- 1/2 tsp freshly ground black pepper

- 1/4 tsp paprika

- 1 tsp kosher salt

- 3/4 tsp dried thyme leaves

- Cooking spray

Directions:

❏ Wash 1 sweet potato and dry nicely. Thinly slice 1/8-inch thick using a knife or rather on a mandolin. Set in a bowl, then cover with cool water, and then soak at room temperature for 20 minutes to remove the excess starch.

❏ Drain the pieces and pat very dry with towels. Put into a large bowl, then add 1 tbsp. canola oil, 1 tsp kosher salt, 3/4 tsp dried thyme leaves, 1/2 tsp black pepper, 1/4 tsp paprika, and a pinch cayenne pepper if using, and toss to blend.

❑ Gently coat in an air fryer rotisserie basket with cooking spray.

❑ Air fry in batches: put one layer of sweet potato pieces from the rotisserie basket. Put the rotisserie basket at the fryer and press on.

❑ Preheat the fryer into 340°F and place for 22 minutes, until the sweet potatoes are golden brown and the edges are crispy, 19 to 22 minutes.

❑ Transfer the chips into a newspaper towel-lined plate to cool completely

❑ They will crisp as they cool. Repeat with the remaining sweet potato pieces.

28. Easy Baked Eggs

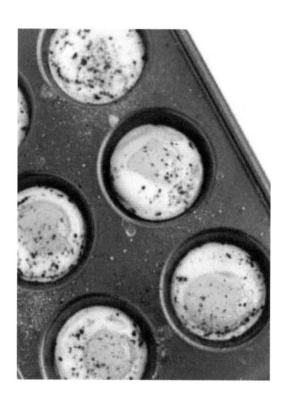

Ingredients:

- 1 Tbsp. heavy cream

- ¼ tsp salt

- 2 eggs

- 1/8 tsp ground black pepper

Method:

➢ Preheat your fryer to 330 degrees F.

➢ Spray a silicone muffin cup or a little ramekin with cooking spray.

➢ In a small bowl, whisk together all of the components

➢ Pour the eggs into the ready ramekin and bake for 6 minutes.

➢ Enjoy directly from the skillet!

29. Air Fryer Buttermilk Fried Chicken

I went to school in the South, so I have had my fair share of crispy, succulent, finger-licking fried chicken. As you might imagine, I had been skeptical about creating a much healthier version from the air fryer.

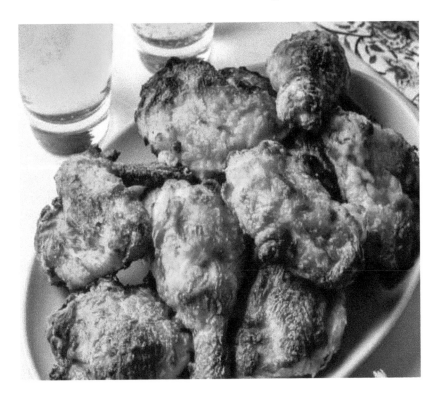

The second I pulled out my first batch, but my worries disappeared. The epidermis was crispy, the coat was cracker-crisp (as it ought to be), and also, above all, the chicken itself was tender and succulent -- the indication of a perfect piece of fried chicken.

Air fryer fried chicken is lighter, quicker, than and not as cluttered as deep-fried chicken. Here is the way to get it done.

Ingredients

- 1 tsp Freshly ground black pepper, divided

- Buttermilk

- 1 tsp Cayenne pepper

- 1 tbsp. Garlic powder

- 2 tbsp. paprika

- 1 tbsp. onion powder

- 1 tsp kosher salt, divided

- all-purpose flour

- 1 tbsp. ground mustard

- Cooking spray

Directions

- ❏ Put all ingredients into a large bowl and season with 1 teaspoon of the kosher salt and 1/2 tsp of honey.

- ❏ Add 2 cups buttermilk and simmer for 1 hour in the fridge. Meanwhile, whisk the remaining 1 tbsp. kosher salt, staying 1/2 tsp black pepper, 2 cups all-purpose flour, 1 tbsp. garlic powder, 2 tbsp. paprika, 1 teaspoon cayenne pepper, 1 tbsp. onion powder, plus one tbsp. ground mustard together into a huge bowl.

❏ Preheat an air fryer into 390°F. Coat the fryer racks together with cooking spray. Remove the chicken in the buttermilk, allowing any excess to drip off. Dredge in the flour mixture, shaking off any excess. Put one layer of chicken in the basket, with distance between the bits. Air fry, turning the chicken hallway through, until an instant-read thermometer registers 165°F from the thickest part

❏ Cook for 18 to 20 minutes, then complete.

30. Keto Chocolate Chip Muffins

Ingredients:

- ¼ tsp salt

- 1 Tbsp. powdered stevia

- ¼ cup whole milk

- 1 egg

- 1 cup almond flour

- 1 ½ tsp baking powder

- ½ cup mini dark chocolate chips (sugar free)

Method:

❖ Preheat your air fryer to 350 degrees F.

❖ In a large bowl, stir together the almond milk, stevia, salt, cinnamon, and baking powder.

❖ Add the milk and eggs and then stir well.

❖ Split the muffin batter involving each muffin cup, filling around 3/4 of this way complete.

❖ Set the muffins to the air fryer basket and cook for 14 minutes or till a toothpick comes out when put to the middle.

❖ Eliminate from the fryer and let cool.

31. Crispy Chickpeas

What, I've got in here are some chickpeas.

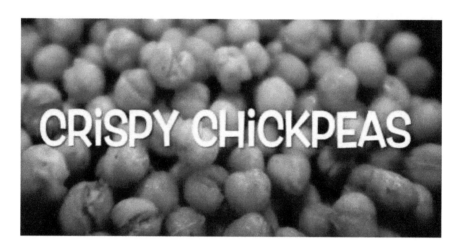

Ingredients:

- Chickpeas

- Olive oil

- Per-peril salt

Method:

I've drained and washed chickpeas and then what I'm going to do is add on some olive oil and then also the periphery salt. The reason I put some olive oil on is because it just helps the pair of results stick to the chickpeas.

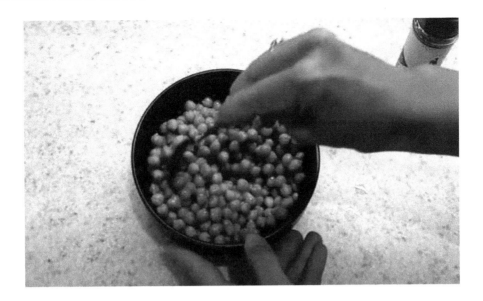

Then I'm just going to mix everything in together and pop them into the air fryer for about 15 minutes. On the chip setting these are great little snacks to make like pre dinner snacks. Instead of having crisps or if you're watching a movie, instead of having popcorn these are good little things. Also, if you are having a salad they're really nice to go in your salad as well.

32.Keto Blueberry Muffins

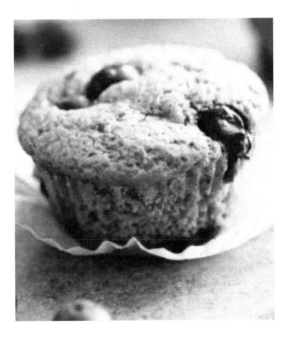

Ingredients:

- 1 egg

- ¼ tsp salt

- 1 cup almond flour

- 1 Tbsp. powdered stevia

- 1 ½ tsp baking powder

- ¼ cup whole milk

- ¼ tsp ground cinnamon

- ½ cup frozen or fresh blueberries

Steps:

1) Preheat your air fryer to 350 degrees F.

2) In a large bowl, stir together the almond milk, stevia, salt, cinnamon, and baking powder.

3) Add the milk and eggs and then stir well.

4) Split the muffin batter involving each muffin cup, filling roughly 3/4 of this way complete.

5) Set the muffins to the air fryer basket and cook for 14 minutes or till a toothpick comes out when put to the middle.

6) Eliminate from the fryer and let cool.

33. Air Fryer Donuts

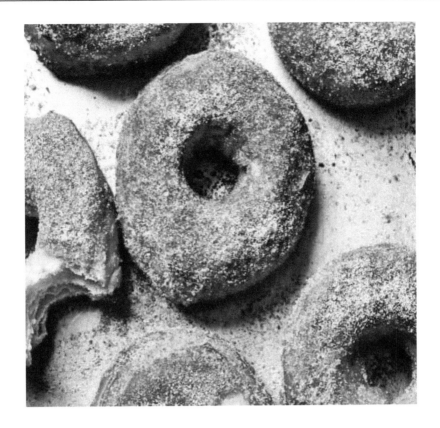

Ingredients

- ground cinnamon

- granulated sugar

- Flaky large snacks,

- Jojoba oil spray or coconut oil spray

Instructions

★ Combine sugar and cinnamon in a shallow bowl; place aside.

★ Remove the cookies from the tin, separate them and set them onto the baking sheet.

★ Utilize a 1-inch round biscuit cutter (or similarly-sized jar cap) to cut holes from the middle of each biscuit.

★ Lightly coat an air fryer basket using coconut or olive oil spray (don't use nonstick cooking spray like Pam, which may damage the coating onto the basket)

★ Put 3 to 4 donuts in one layer in the air fryer (that they shouldn't be touching). Close to the air fryer and place to 350°F. Transfer donuts into the baking sheet.

★ Repeat with the rest of the biscuits. You can also cook the donut holes they will take approximately 3 minutes total

★ Brush both sides of this hot donut with melted butter, put in the cinnamon sugar, and then turn to coat both sides.

34. Sausage and Spinach Omelet

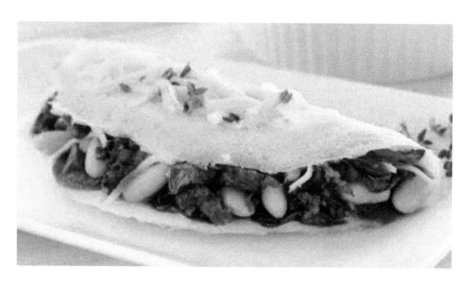

Ingredients:

½ cup baby spinach

4 eggs

¼ cup cheddar cheese, grated

½ cup cooked, crumbled sausage

3 Tbsp. heavy whipping cream

½ tsp salt

¼ tsp ground black pepper

Directions

I.   Preheat the air fryer at around 330 F.

II.   In a small bowl, whisk together the eggs, cream, pepper and salt.

III.   Fold in the cooked sausage and sausage.

IV.   Pour the mixture into the prepared baking pan then place the pan on your

V.   Cook for approximately ten minutes or till the eggs are completely set.

VI.   Sprinkle the cheeses round the boiled eggs and then return the pan into the fryer

VII.   Fryer for another two minutes to melt the cheese.

35.Air Fryer Potato Wedges

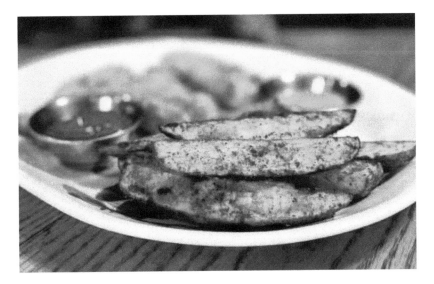

Perfectly crisp and seasoned potato wedges directly from your air fryer. It will not get any simpler than this!

Ingredients

→ 2 medium Russet potatoes, cut into wedges

→ 1/2 tsp sea salt

→ 1 1/2 tsp olive oil

→ 1/2 tsp chili powder

→ ⅛ teaspoon ground black pepper

→ 1/2 tsp paprika

→ 1/2 tsp parsley flakes

Instructions

❖ Place potato wedges in a large bowl.

❖ Put 8 wedges at the jar of the air fryer and cook for 10 minutes.

❖ Flip wedges with tongs and cook for another five minutes.

36. Chocolate Chip Cookies in Air fryer

They are my day pick-me-up, my after-dinner treat, also, sometimes, a part of my breakfast. I keep either frozen cookies or baked biscuits in my freezer -- true my friends know and have come to appreciate when they come around for dinner or even a glass of wine.

The kind of chocolate chip cookie I enjoy all, depends upon my mood. Sometimes I need them super doughy, and sometimes challenging and crisp. If you're searching for one someplace in between -- gooey on the inside and crunchy on the outside -- I have discovered the foolproof way of you. It entails cooking them on your air fryer.

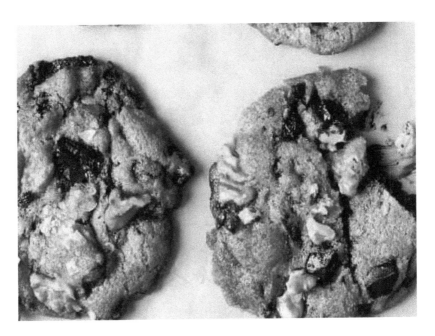

When using your fryer to create biscuits, be certain that you always line its base with foil to aid with simple cleanup. You will also need to line the basket or racks using parchment paper. Buy paper which has holes in it, cut some slits to the newspaper, or make sure you leave space around it which will allow for even cooking and flow of the air. With these suggestions, you're on your way to cookie victory!

Ingredients:

- Granulated sugar

- vanilla extract

- dark brown sugar

- 1 tsp kosher salt

- 2 large eggs

- 3/4 cup chopped walnuts

- 1 tsp baking soda

- Flaky sea salt, for garnish (optional)

- all-purpose flour

- Cooking spray

INSTRUCTIONS

❖ Put 2 sticks unsalted butter in the bowl of a stand mixer, fitted with the paddle attachment and also let it sit till softened. Insert 3/4 cup granulated sugar and 3/4 cup packed dark brown sugar and beat it on medium speed till blended and fluffy within 3 to 4 minutes. Add 1 tablespoon lemon extract, 2 big eggs, and 1 tsp kosher salt, and beat until just blended. After that, add 1 tea-spoon baking soda plus 2 1/3 cups all-purpose flour in increments, mixing until just blended.

❖ Add 2 cups chocolate balls and 3/4 cup chopped peppers and stir with a rubber spatula until just blended.

❖ Preheat in an air fryer, at 350ºF and set to 5 minutes. Line the fryer racks with parchment paper, make sure you leave space on all sides for air to leak.

❖ Reduce 2-tablespoon scoops of this dough on the racks, setting them 1-inch apart. Gently flatten each spade marginally to earn a cookie form.

❖ Sprinkle with flaky sea salt, if using. Bake until golden brown, about 5 minutes. Remove the racks out of the fryer and let it cool for 3 to 5 minutes to place. Repeat with the remaining dough.

37. Crispy Coated Veggies

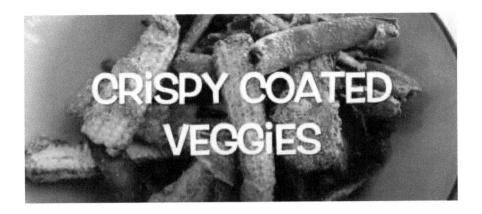

Ingredients:

- Vegetables

- Egg

- Paprika

- Salt & Pepper

Method:

I'm making some crispy coating of vegetables in this bowl. I have got one egg beaten up. This is actually almond flour but you can use normal flour and then I popped in some paprika. I've also put in some salt and pepper here too. Then I'm going to dip my veggies into my egg and then I'll put them into the flour mixture, then into the air fryer for probably about eight minutes.

38. Ranch Pork Chops in Air fryer

Ingredients

- 4 boneless, center-cut pork chops, 1-inch thick

- aluminum foil

- cooking spray

- 2 Tsp dry ranch salad dressing mix

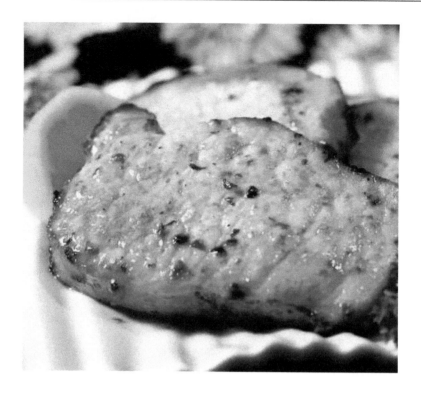

Directions

★ Put pork chops on a plate and then gently spray both sides with cooking spray. Sprinkle both sides with ranch seasoning mixture and let them sit at room temperature for 10 minutes.

★ Spray the basket of an air fryer with cooking spray and preheat at 390 degrees F (200 degrees C).

★ Place chops in the preheated air fryer, working in batches if needed, to guarantee the fryer isn't overcrowded.

★ Flip chops and cook for 5 minutes longer. Let rest on a foil-covered plate for 5 minutes prior to serving.

39.Quesadillas

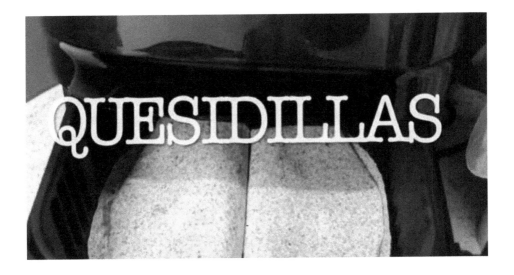

Ingredients:

- Refried Beans

- Cheese

- Peppers

- Chicken

Method:

I'm going to be using the El Paso refried beans in the tin. I will spread that onto the wrap and then I'm just going to sprinkle some cheese on top.

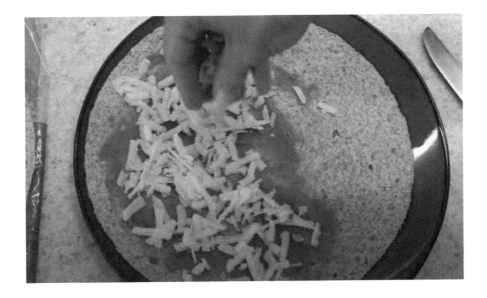

This is a really basic wrap so usually when we have routes we'll add some like peppers in here as well and loads of other bits like chicken. I just wanted to show you how well they cook in the air fryer. You pop them in on the pizza setting and in 8 to10 minutes they are done. Really crispy and ready to eat.

40. Pecan Crusted Pork Chops at the Air Fryer

The air-fryer makes simple work of those yummy pork chops. The chops make good leftovers too, since the pecan crust does not get soggy!

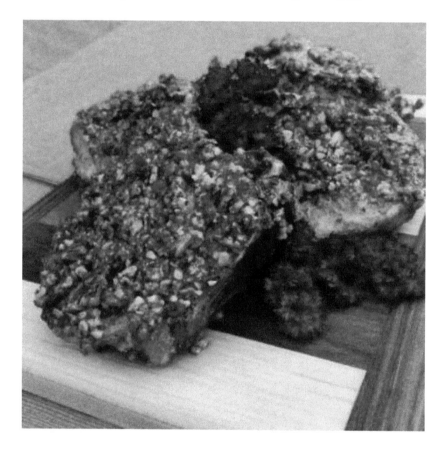

Ingredients:

- Egg

- Pork

- Pecans

- Simmer

Instructions

➢ Add egg and simmer until all ingredients are well blended. Place pecans onto a plate.

➢ Dip each pork dip in the egg mix, then put onto the plate together with the pecans

➢ Press pecans firmly onto either side until coated. Spray the chops on both sides with cooking spray and set from the fryer basket.

➢ Cook at the fryer for 6 minutes. Turn chops closely with tongs, and fry until pork is no longer pink in the middle, about 6 minutes more.

41. Crispy Chicken Thighs

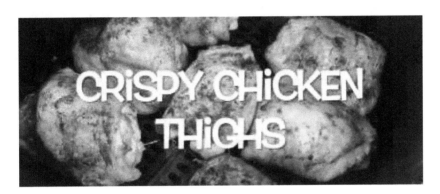

Ingredients

- Chicken thighs

- Pepper

- Olive oil

- Paprika

- Salt

Method:

I've got some chicken thighs. These have got bone-in and skinned on so what I've done is just put some olive oil on top of them with some paprika and some salt and pepper. Then I just rubbed everything into the chicken skin so I'm going to pop these into my air fryer. Press the chicken button and let the air fryer just do its thing.

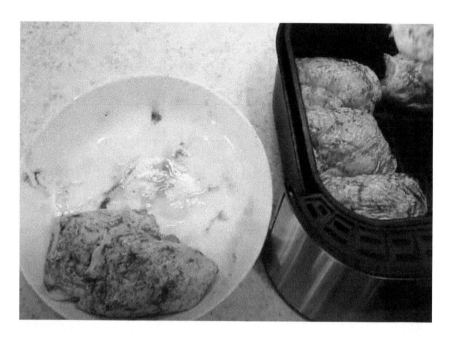

This skin is super crispy that is perfectly done and it's been in there for 20 minutes. I just wanted to show you all the fat that came out of that chicken so here are all the oils that came off.

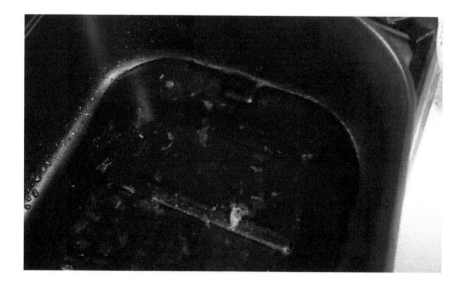

So those are what your chicken would be sitting in but instead it's all just tripped underneath the air fryer.

42. Bacon-Wrapped Scallops with Sirach Mayo

This yummy appetizer is ready quickly and easily in the air fryer and served with a hot Sirach mayo skillet. I use the smaller bay scallops because of this. If you're using jumbo scallops, it'll require a longer cooking time and more bits of bacon.

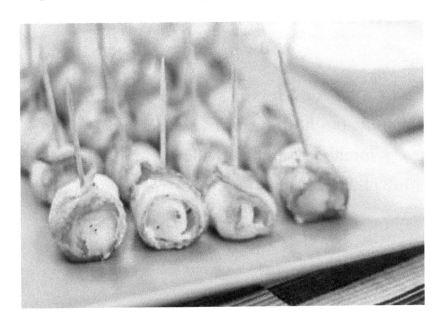

Ingredients

- 1/2 cup mayonnaise

- 1 pinch coarse salt

- 2 tbsp. Sirach sauce

- 1 pound bay scallops (about 36 small scallops)

- 1 pinch freshly cracked black pepper

- 12 slices bacon, cut into thirds

- 1 serving olive oil cooking spray

Instructions

★ Mix mayonnaise and Sirach sauce together in a little bowl.

★ Preheat the air fryer to 390 degrees F (200 degrees C).

★ Season with pepper and salt. Wrap each scallop with 1/3 piece of bacon and fasten with a toothpick.

★ Spray the air fryer basket with cooking spray. Put bacon-wrapped scallops from the basket in one layer; divide into two batches if needed.

★ Cook at the air fryer for 7 minutes. Check for doneness; scallops should be wheat and opaque ought to be crispy. Cook 1 to 2 minutes more, if needed, checking every moment. Remove scallops carefully with tongs and put on a newspaper towel-lined plate to absorb extra oil out of the bacon.

43. Homemade Chips

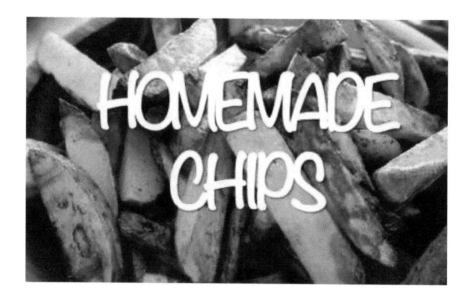

Ingredients

- Chip

- Olive oil

- Paprika

- Salt

Method:

Now I'm going to do some chips. I've just cut up some potatoes into chip shapes and then I am going to put some olive oil on top. Some paprika and some salt and the main reason I'm putting olive oil on top is basically for the paprika and the salt to stick to the surface of the chips. I'll just pop these in and then I'll put them onto the chip setting and let them cook away for about 18 minutes. I will be staring these halfway through because I'm doing quite a few chips as well. I will probably have to put these on for another 10 minutes after the 18 minutes is done.

44.Easy Air Fryer Pork Chops

Boneless pork chops cooked to perfection with the help of an air fryer. This recipe is super easy and you could not ask for a more tender and succulent chop.

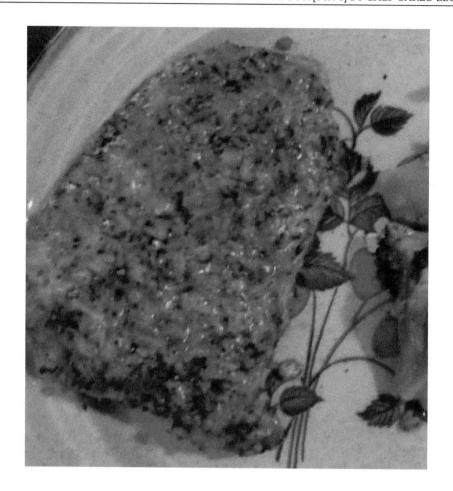

Ingredients

- 1/2 cup grated Parmesan cheese

- 1 tsp kosher salt

- 4 (5 oz.) center-cut pork chops

- 2 tbsp. extra virgin olive oil

- 1 tsp dried parsley

- 1 tsp paprika

- 1 tsp garlic powder

- 1/2 teaspoon ground black pepper

Instructions

❏ Preheat the fryer to 390 degrees F.

❏ Combine Parmesan cheese, paprika, garlic powder, salt, parsley, and pepper in a level shallow dish; combine well.

❏ Stir every pork chop with olive oil. Dredge both sides of each dip from the Parmesan mixture and put on a plate.

❏ Put 2 chops from the basket of the fryer and cook for 10 minutes; turning halfway through cook time.

45. Corn on the Cob

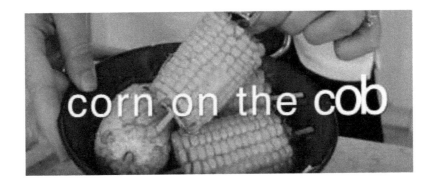

Ingredients:

- Corn

- Butter

- Salt

Method:

We're going to do some corn on the cob. What I'm going to do is just pop them into my air fryer but not put anything on top of them. I'm going to put them in on the prawn settings.

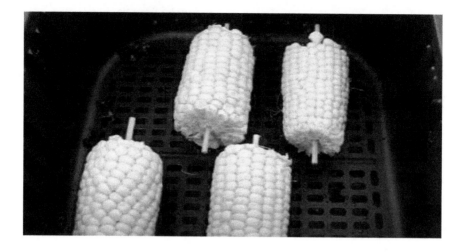

It's just eight minutes, after ten minutes like I said, I will then add some butter on top and a little bit of salt. They're ready to eat.

46. Air Fryer Broiled Grapefruit

This hot and warm grapefruit with a buttery candy topping is the best accompaniment for your Sunday brunch and makes a lovely snack or dessert. I love to add a pinch of sea salt in the end to actually bring out the tastes.

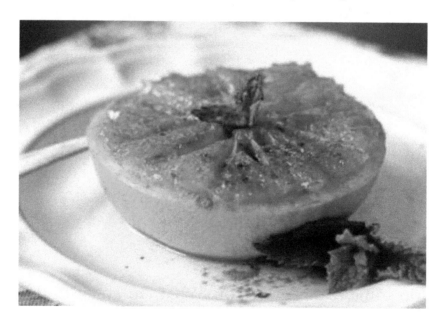

Ingredients

- 1 red grapefruit, refrigerated

- aluminum foil

- 1 tbsp. brown sugar

- 1/2 teaspoon ground cinnamon

- 1 tbsp. softened butter

- 2 tsp sugar

Instructions

➢ Cut grapefruit in half crosswise and slice off a thin sliver away from the base of every half, when the fruit is not sitting at level. Use a sharp paring knife to cut around the outer edge of this grapefruit and involve every section to generate the fruit easier to consume after cooking.

➢ Combine softened butter 1 tbsp. brown sugar in a small bowl. Spread mix over each grapefruit in half. Sprinkle with remaining brown sugar levels.

➢ Cut aluminum foil into two 5-inch squares and put each grapefruit half one square; fold the edges up to catch any juices. Place in the air fryer basket.

➢ Broil in the fryer until the sugar mixture is bubbling, 6 to 7 minutes.

47.Kale Crisps

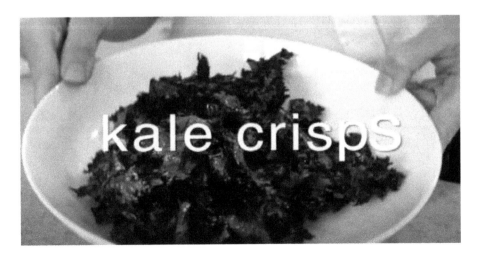

Ingredients:

- Kale

- Olive oil

- Salt

Method:

I'm going to make some kale crisps now. So, the first thing we're going to do list, get my kale and chop off the thick stocky bits. Once I've chopped that out, I will then just dice my kale up into kind of chunks and then I'll pop them into a bowl. Put some olive oil on top and some salts give everything a mix around.

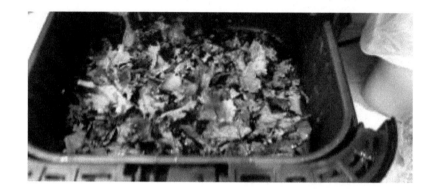

I'll pop them into my air fryer and on the prong setting. The reason I put them on the prong setting is because that's just a quick eight minute setting and that's the perfect amount of time that these kale crisps take to cook. When they come out, they are super nice and crunchy and they taste delicious.

48. Air Fryer Brown Sugar and Pecan Roasted Apples

A sweet and nutty topping made with brown sugar and pecans adds amazing flavor to apples since they cook to tender perfection at the air fryer.

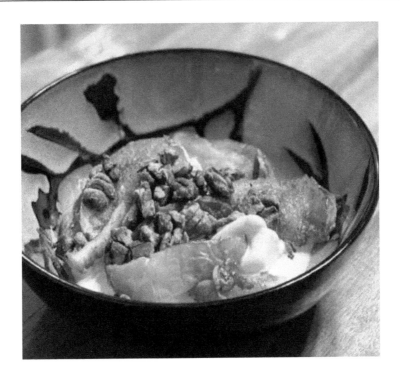

Ingredients

- 1/4 tsp apple pie spice

- 2 tbsp. coarsely chopped pecans

- 1 tbsp. brown sugar

- 1 tbsp. butter, melted

- 1 tsp all-purpose flour

- 2 medium apples, cored and cut into wedges

Instructions

→ Preheat the air fryer to 350 degrees F

→ Put apple wedges in a skillet drizzle with butter and toss to coat. Arrange apples in one layer in the air fryer basket and then sprinkle with pecan mixture.

→ Cook in the preheated air fryer until apples are tender, 10 to 15 minutes.

49. Sausage Rolls

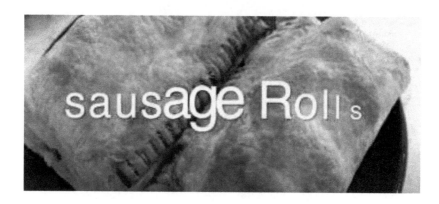

Ingredients:

- Sausage

- Puff pastry

- Cheese

- Chutney

- Milk

Methods:

Today we're going to make some really easy sausage rolls. So, I've just got some puff pastry and some sausages. What I'll do is I'll cut the puff pastry into four pieces. I'll then lay a sausage into each one of the pieces along with some grated cheese.

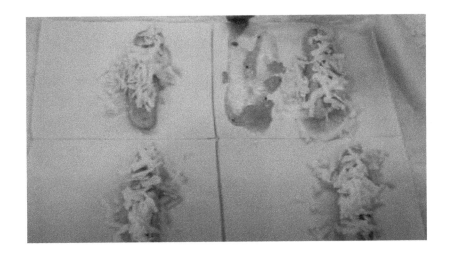

I like to have some chutney in the house as well. I'll just fold over the pastry and then secure it with a fork at the edges. So, it doesn't open up. I then just also get a bit of milk as well or you can use a beaten egg and just brush it over the top so it goes nice and golden brown. I'll pop it into my air fryer on the chip setting because they do need a good18 minutes in there to make sure the sausages are nice and cooked.

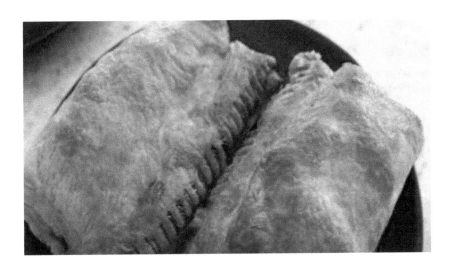

After the 18 minutes they're ready to eat.

50. Air Fryer French Fries

It will not get more classic than French fries; the normally accepted technique is fairly, dare I say, air tight, but I really do have one additional trick in shop! Last, dip them in honey mustard, hot ketchup, garlic aioli, or all 3 blended together, such as I did

Ingredients

- 1 lb. russet potatoes, peeled

- 1/2 tsp kosher salt

- 2 tsp vegetable oil

- 1 pinch cayenne pepper

Instructions

- ❖ Slice segments into sticks too around 3/8 inch-wide.

- ❖ Cover potatoes with water and let boil for 5 minutes to discharge excess starches.

- ❖ Drain and cover with boiling water with several inches (or put in a bowl of boiling water). Let sit for 10 minutes.

- ❖ Drain potatoes and move onto several paper towels. Transfer to a mixing bowl drizzle with oil, season with cayenne, and toss to coat.

- ❖ Stack potatoes in a dual layer in the fryer basket. Slide out basket and throw fries; keep frying until golden brown, about 10 minutes longer. Toss chips with salt in a mixing bowl.

51.Cheese on Toast

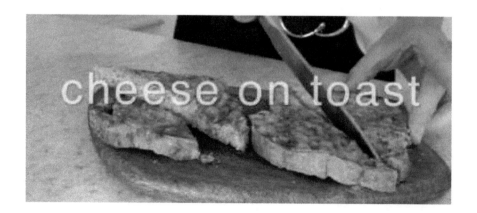

Ingredients:

- Bread

- Garlic butter

- cayenne pepper

Method:

I'm going to show you how to make a really quick and easy cheese on toast. How I make my cheese on toast is I get the bread and I put garlic butter on each side of the bread.

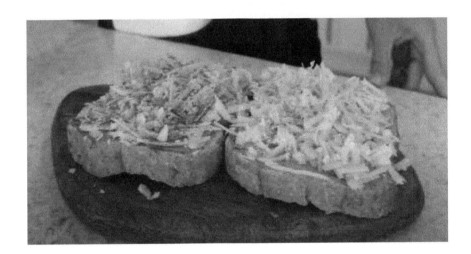

For me this is a very important step. I then grate quite a generous amount of cheese and then sprinkle it over the top. I will also add a little dash of cayenne pepper on top. Pop into my air fryer on the pizza button so that is for eight minutes at 160 degrees. Once the time is up, it comes out perfect every single time with a real nice crunchy piece of toast.

52. Tomato Pork Chops

It is a rather quick and easy recipe.

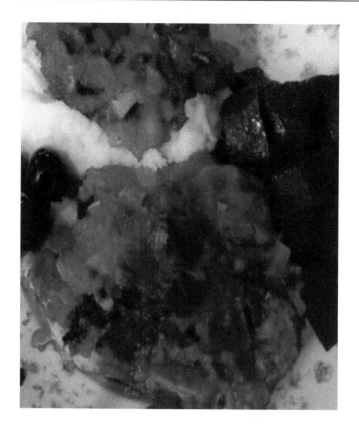

Ingredients

- 1 bell pepper - sliced, your color option

- 1 (15 oz.) can tomato sauce

- garlic powder to flavor

- 4 pork chops

- 1 tsp, sliced

- pepper and salt to taste

Directions

- ❖ Dredge the pork chops in flour, add to the pan and brown well on both sides.

❖ Add the onion and bell pepper, stir and cook for 5 minutes in the air fryer, or until nearly tender. Return pork chops to skillet and pour into the sauce. Permit the sauce to begin bubbling and reduce heat.

❖ Simmer for half an hour and season with garlic powder, pepper and salt to taste.

53. Veggie Egg Bread

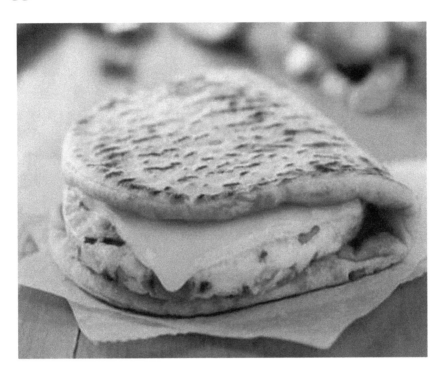

Ingredients:

- 1 tsp salt

- ½ pound cream cheese

- 10 eggs

- 4 cups grated zucchini

- 1 cup grated cheddar cheese

- ½ cup chopped tomatoes

- ½ tsp ground black pepper

- ½ cup sliced mushrooms, cooked

- ½ cup almond flour

- 2 tsp baking powder

Directions

❖ Be sure the pan will fit on your air fryer- normally a seven inch round pan will do the job flawlessly.

❖ Stir together the almond milk, pepper, salt and baking powder.

❖ In another bowl, beat the cream cheese until its smooth and nice afterward insert the eggs. Beat until well blended.

❖ Add the zucchini into the cream cheese mixture and stir until incorporated.

❖ Add the dry mix to the cream cheese jar and then stir well.

❖ Pour into the prepared pan and then cook at the fryer for 45 minutes

54. Easy Muffins

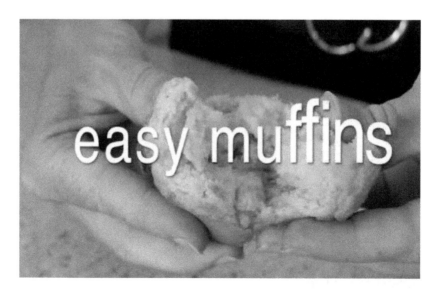

Ingredients:

- Sugar

- Butter

- Flour

- Eggs

- Milk

- Salt

Method:

We're going to make cupcakes. I have got a hundred grams of sugar, 250 grams of butter, 250 grams of flour, 4 eggs, a splash of milk and a dash of salt. We're just going to whisk this all up. I have got some of these cupcake holders. They're silicon ones. I'm going to add it to those and then we'll put them into the air fryer on the cupcake setting and let them cook away.

55. Almond Flour Pancake

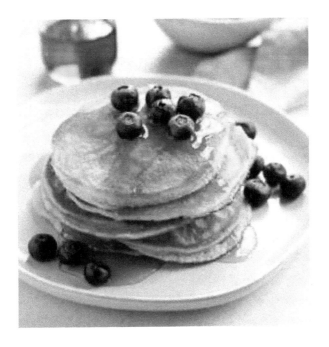

Ingredients:

- 1 teaspoon vanilla extract

- 1 1/4 cup almond milk

- two Tbsp. granulated erythritol

- 1 teaspoon baking powder

- 2 eggs

- 1/2 cup whole milk

- 2 Tbsp. butter, melted

- 1/8 tsp salt

Directions

- ❖ Be sure the pan will fit on your air fryer- normally a seven inch round pan will do the job flawlessly.

- ❖ Put the eggs, butter, milk and vanilla extract in a blender and puree for around thirty minutes.

- ❖ Add the remaining ingredients into the blender and puree until smooth.

- ❖ Pour the pancake batter to the prepared pan and set from the fryer.

- ❖ Cook for 2 minutes or until the pancake is puffed and the top is gold brown.

- ❖ Slice and serve with keto sugar free!

56. Zucchini and Bacon Egg Bread

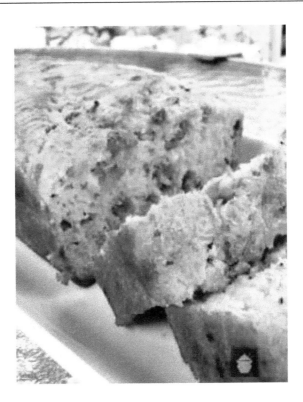

Ingredients:

- ½ cup almond flour

- 1 tsp salt

- ½ pound cream cheese

- 10 eggs

- 2 tsp baking powder

- ½ tsp ground black pepper

- 1 pound bacon cooked and crumbled

- 4 cups grated zucchini

- 1 cup grated cheddar cheese

Directions

❖ Be sure the pan will fit on your air fryer- normally a seven inch round pan will do the job flawlessly.

❖ Stir together the almond milk, pepper, salt and baking powder.

❖ In another bowl, beat the cream cheese until its smooth and nice afterward insert the eggs. Beat until well blended.

❖ Add the zucchini into the cream cheese mixture and stir until incorporated.

❖ Add the dry mix to the cream cheese jar and then stir well.

❖ Pour into the prepared pan and then cook at the fryer for 45 minutes

57. Raspberry Almond Pancake

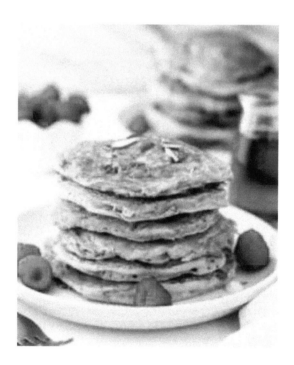

Ingredients:

- 1/2 cup whole milk

- 2 Tbsp. butter, melted

- 1 teaspoon almond extract

- 2 eggs

- two Tbsp. granulated erythritol

- 1 teaspoon baking powder

- 1/8 tsp salt

- 1 1/4 cup almond milk

- 1/4 cup frozen or fresh desserts

Directions

I.   Preheat your air fryer to 420 degrees F and line a baking pan using parchment paper. Be sure the pan will fit on your air fryer- normally a seven inch round pan will do the job flawlessly.

II.   Put the eggs, butter, milk and almond extract in a blender and puree for around thirty minutes.

III. Add the remaining ingredients into the blender and puree until smooth.

IV.   Pour the pancake batter to the pan and stir in the raspberries

V.   Lightly.

VI.   Put in the fryer.

VII. Slice and serve with keto sugar free!

58. Maple Brussel Sprout Chips

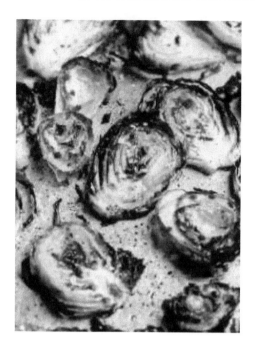

Ingredients:

- 2 Tbsp. olive oil

- 1 tsp sea salt

- 1 Pound Brussel Sprouts, ends removed

- 1 tsp maple extract

Method:

➤ Preheat your air fryer to 2400 degrees F and line the fryer tray with parchment paper.

➤ Peel the Brussels sprouts leaf at a time, putting the leaves in a massive bowl as you pare them.

➤ Toss the leaves using the olive oil, maple extract and salt then disperse onto the prepared tray.

➤ Bake for 15 minutes at the fryer, tossing halfway through to cook evenly.

➤ Serve warm or wrap in an airtight container after chilled.

59. Sweet and Tangy Apple Pork Chops

That is a recipe that I made using the thought that apples and pork go beautifully together! The seasonings provide the pork a pleasant and slightly spicy flavor. The apple cider increases the sweetness, while still bringing an exceptional tartness, since it's absorbed into the meat. Serve with applesauce, if wanted. Hope you like it!

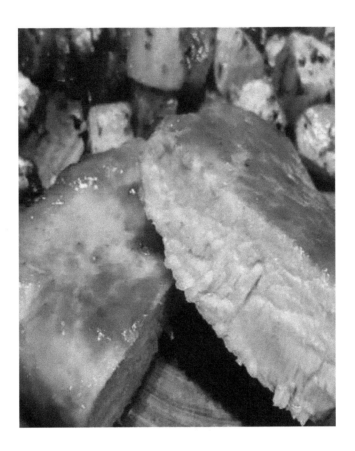

Ingredients:

- 3 tbsp. brown sugar

- 1/2 tsp garlic powder

- 2 tbsp. honey mustard

- 1 tsp mustard powder

- 1/2 teaspoon ground cumin

- 1 lb. pork chops

- 2 tbsp. butter

- 1/2 tsp cayenne pepper (Optional)

- 3/4 cup apple cider

Instructions

❏ Mix brown sugar, honey mustard, mustard powder, cumin, cayenne pepper, and garlic powder together in a small bowl. Rub pork chops and let sit on a plate for flavors to split into pork chops, about 10 minutes.

❏ Melt butter in a large skillet over moderate heat; include apple cider. Organize coated pork chops from the skillet;

❏ Cook until pork chops are browned, 5 to 7 minutes each side.

60. Maple Brussel Sprout Chips

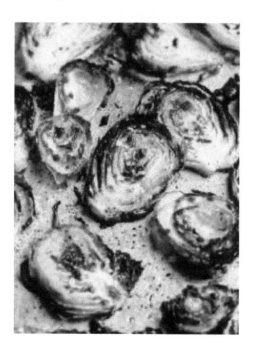

Ingredients:

- 2 Tbsp. olive oil

- 1 tsp sea salt

- 1 Pound Brussel Sprouts, ends removed

- 1 tsp maple extract

Method:

➤ Preheat your air fryer to 2400 degrees F and line the fryer tray with parchment paper.

➤ Peel the Brussels sprouts leaf at a time, putting the leaves in a massive bowl as you pare them.

➤ Toss the leaves using the olive oil, maple extract and salt then disperse onto the prepared tray.

➤ Bake for 15 minutes at the fryer, tossing halfway through to cook evenly.

➤ Serve warm or wrap in an airtight container after chilled.

61.Blueberry Pancake

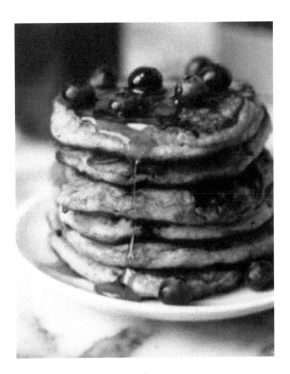

Ingredients:

- 2 Tbsp. butter, melted

- 1 teaspoon vanilla extract

- 1 1/4 cup almond milk

- 2 eggs

- 1 teaspoon baking powder

- 1/8 tsp salt

- 1/4 cup frozen or fresh blueberries

- 1/2 cup whole milk

- Two Tbsp. granulated erythritol

Directions

1. Preheat your air fryer to 400 degrees F and line a baking pan using parchment paper. Be sure the pan will fit on your fryer- normally a seven inch round pan will do the job flawlessly.

2. Put the eggs, butter, milk and vanilla extract in a blender and puree for around thirty minutes.

3. Add the remaining ingredients into the blender and puree until smooth.

4. Pour the pancake batter to the pan and stir in the blueberries

5. Put in the fryer.

6. Slice and serve with keto sugar free!

62. Chocolate Croissants

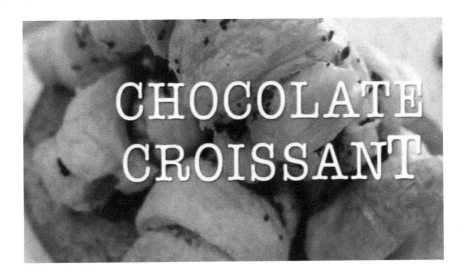

Ingredients

- Puff pastry

- Flake chocolate

Method:

I wanted to show you how to make some chocolate croissants in your air fryer as well. So, what I have got here is one roll of puff pastry and then to go on top to make it chocolatey, I have got some flake chocolate. What I'm going to do is roll out my puff pastry and then I'm going to crumble some flake chocolates all over the pastry.

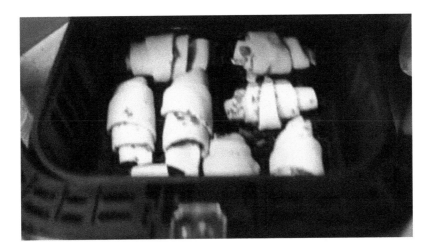

I'm then going to cut my pastry into eight. I'm going to cut them into fours and then I'll cut each four diagonally and then I'll roll them up into a croissant shape. Pop them into my air fryer, cook them on the muffin button which is a twelve minutes setting and then when they come out they are really really nice, chocolatey and delicious.

63. Strawberry Pancake

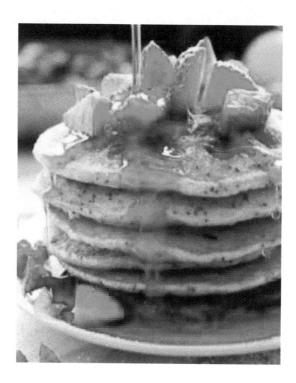

Ingredients:

- 1 teaspoon baking powder

- 1/8 tsp salt

- 1/4 cup fresh chopped tomatoes

- 2 eggs

- 1 teaspoon vanilla extract

- 1 1/4 cup almond milk

Directions

I.   Pre-heat the air fryer for around 15 minutes.

II.   Put the eggs, butter, milk and vanilla extract in a blender and simmer for about half an hour.

III.   Add the remaining ingredients into the blender and puree until smooth.

IV.   Pour the pancake batter to the pan and stir in the berries gently.

V.   Put in the fryer.

VI.   Slice and serve with keto sugar free!

64. Cheesy Zucchini Bake

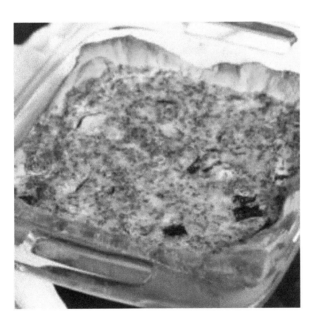

Ingredients:

- 2 tsp baking powder

- ½ tsp ground black pepper

- 1 tsp salt

- ½ cup almond flour

- 4 cups grated zucchini

- ½ pound cream cheese

- 10 eggs

- 1 cup grated cheddar cheese

Method:

1. Be sure the pan will fit on your air fryer- normally a seven inch round pan will do the job flawlessly. If it's possible to fit a bigger pan, then do so!

2. Stir together the almond milk, pepper, salt and baking powder.

3. In another bowl beat the cream cheese until its smooth and nice afterward insert the eggs. Beat until well blended.

4. Add the zucchini into the cream cheese mixture and stir until incorporated.

5. Add the dry mix to the cream cheese jar and then stir well.

6. Pour into the prepared pan and then cook at the fryer for 45 minutes.

65. Basil-Garlic Grilled Pork Chops

I had been tired of the exact same old agendas, and opted to try out something new... WOW! These chops are excellent!! They're fantastic for casual entertaining or family dinner. Together with the fresh basil and grated garlic, the taste is quite refreshing! Everybody will adore these!

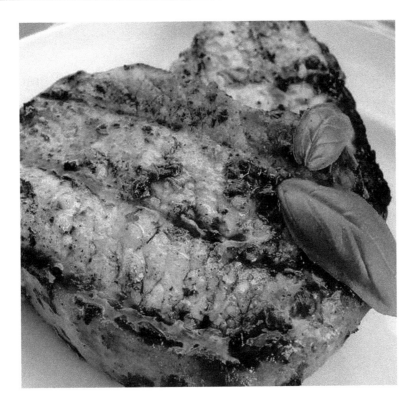

Ingredients

- 4 (8 ounce) pork chops

- 4 cloves garlic, minced

- ¼ cup chopped fresh basil

- 1 lime, juiced

- salt and black pepper to taste

Instructions

- ❖ Toss the pork chops with all the carrot juice in a bowl until evenly coated. Toss with ginger and garlic. Season the chops to taste with pepper and salt. Set aside to marinate for half an hour.

- ❖ Cook the pork chops on the fryer till no longer pink at the middle, 5 to 10 minutes each side.

66. Full English breakfast

Full English breakfast is one that my family really really likes. We have lived in England for a while so my kids really look forward to Saturday morning so that we make full English breakfast. However today I'm going to be showing you a special way to make it stress free.

I'm going to be starting off with the hash browns.

Ingredients:

- Potatoes

- Cheese

- Egg

- Salt

- Pepper

- Chili Flakes

- Sausage

Method:

So, the hash brownies are going to be composed of potatoes. I'm going to be using two, then I'm also going to be using cheese. This is shredded cheese and this is like the equivalent of one and a half cups of cheese. We are also going to be using one egg, this is one raw egg and some all-purpose flour, and this is the equivalent of two huge teaspoons of flour. We will be using some pepper along with chili flakes and finally of course some salt to taste. Right, so these are the ingredients that I'm going to be using for the hash browns.

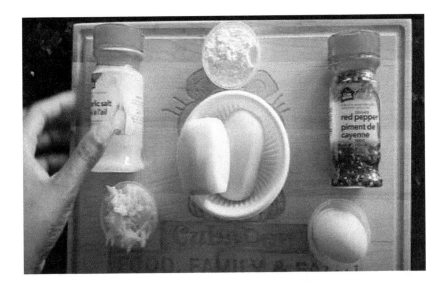

Before we start off with hash browns let's move on to all the other ingredients or condiments that are going to make up the English breakfast so part of the traditional ones we also use would be the eggs so this will make up we're going to make sunny side up eggs I'm going to be using some tomatoes some sausage, so this is not this is not the same way you have a traditional English breakfast.

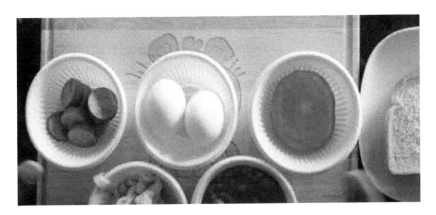

This isn't the same kind of way the sausage is or the way to slice but this is fine. Then we're going to be including baked beans right. So, this is a shop bought and actually there's still one more ingredient I'm going to be using: bacon. This is raw thinly sliced bacon and we have two slices of bread right. So, that's all the components or the condiments are going to go into the full English breakfast.

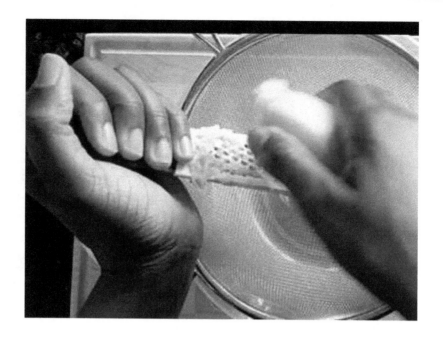

Let's start off straight away with the hash browns because all these other things are pretty much ready to go. Let's start with the preparation of the hash browns. So the first thing I'm going to be doing to grate the potatoes. With grated you can use any size. I want to use the really thin size because I want it more or less almost if it's already mashed or boiled. Because I'm going to be putting it in an array, I want it to take as little time as possible in order to get the potatoes done. If you've had English breakfast before let me know what you include or what you remove. I know people have different types of English breakfast at different times. Yeah, I know there's the black pudding, if you're a traditional English person you probably like black pudding instead.

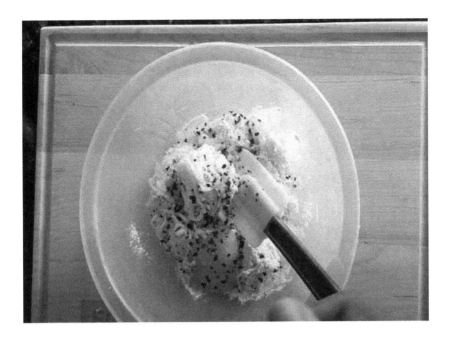

We're done with the grating of the potatoes and I've rinsed it out in sense that I've put some water in. I'm giving it a good squeeze to make sure all the water is gone. This helps to remove the majority of the starch in the potatoes. So it's completely up to you, if you want to skip this process in the sense that you want to rinse out some of the water from the potatoes. Okay so that done, the next thing we're going to move on to the mixing. I'm going to put in my flour. This is two teaspoons but it seems like I'm going to use only one. Then I remember eggs, had a full raw egg for my potato to make the hash browns. I also have some cheese, add some salt to taste and some chili flakes. I like something hot and spicy and yeah that's why I add that. So, I give this a really good mix for hash browns, people usually sometimes add butter so it's completely up to you what you want to include in your own hash browns. I'm just keeping my own soft shots sweet and simple. You can add or subtract as much as you want.

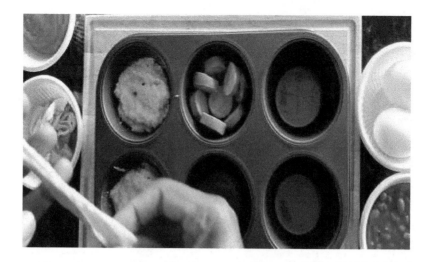

I'm going to give my tray a spray just to oil it, because what I'm going to do guys, this is something different. I'm going to start off with the hash browns. I'm putting everything and it's going to come out like a cup sort of like a cupcake, because my cans are a bit deep. I'm going to spread it into two sections right because I want it to cook all the way through so the potatoes are going to come out, sort of like a cupcake or potato cups. I'm also going to give this another spray right now, this is different.

I'm going to put in oops my sausages right, to line them all in here. As I'm using the air fryer for everything stress less so hopefully this should work for a bachelor or spencer or a small family or just making breakfast for somebody for just one person in the family. This works pretty good. I'm going to put them in first so the next thing that is going to be included in the air fryer all three of them are going in now is the bacon. I'm going to put the bacon this way, alternatively, I could have chopped up the bacon and put them in one of these sections. Maybe I would actually just do that so that you have a look-see at its rest of the bacon. I'm just going to cut this one in here.

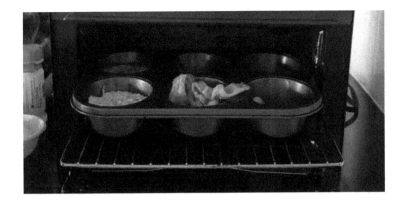

Throw it into the extra bit there again, I'm not going to be bothered about these bacon, because you know they're going to come up with their own oil. It's going to go into the air fryer oven. Put it in the air fryer oven and let it fry just turning the timer to one hour. It's an air fryer oven and the specific degree setting should be up on your screen and yeah so once this is ready again, like I said it's halfway into the cooking of the sausages of the hash browns and the bacon.

I'm now going to include the baked beans and the eggs because those ones will actually take less time compared to what you've got in the oven. I've had these in the air fryer and I can see that my bacon is coming out nicely.

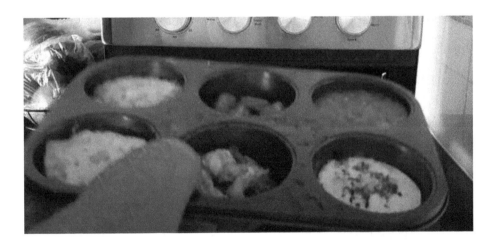

You see that so it depends on you if this is how you like your bacons this is the point in which you take them out. So, I'm just going to chuck the monotone section of the cupcake bits. What I'm going to do is to put the ones that are under done on the top and the ones that are already getting as crisp, I'm going to put them at the bottom. Now I'm just trying to get my stuff together. I'm scooping out all the sausages tone section so that I have two sections free for me to put my eggs and my baked beans. I'm going to have the egg sunny side up, I'm not going to spray the container again because all the bacon oil is in the egg, is in the cupcake holder. I'm just going to break two eggs and putting two into one section and then add some salt and some chili flakes. Our egg begins to cool, then I'm also going to put in the baked beans right in the final section. We are all good to go so I just want to show you guys what it looks like.

We've got the eggs we've got the baked beans we've got everything in the section in the containers. I'm going to have the the tomatoes, I'm just going to line them on top here and yeah voila. I know for some people it's a lot of work but this is really stress less. The only bit where you have lots of work to do is with the grating of the potatoes and that's pretty much it. We're going to allow these now to cook all the way through by the time the egg is done and the baked paint is ready, the entire dish should be ready. We're about 30 minutes into the entire thing and it's looking really really good. I just want to bring this and mix up the sausages a bit, yeah and put this back because you need a couple of minutes to go. You can see the egg, you can see the bacon everything is looking wonderful. I'm going to move this all the way back because I want to put my tomatoes just to give it a little bit of somehow grilled max and then my bread right just to heat it up.

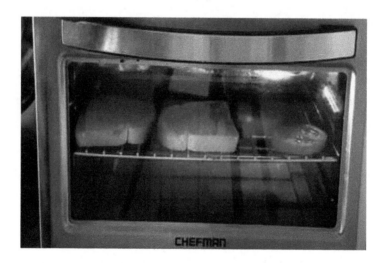

Let it give me somewhat like a mini toast. I'm going to shut this down now its done 30 minutes and it's done right. I'm not looking to get toasted bread but I just want this really warm. It's not toasted but it's warm and really crispy. I'm going to get the bread out of the way and the same thing with the tomatoes. So they're just warm so that when the breakfast is being eaten it's really nice and warm and fuzzy. Let's get onto plating it okay we are all ready, can you see that looks really good so and this is every single thing in one place right. So, our potatoes looks properly cooked a bit hot, our hash browns potatoes looks good and you can see our sausages. It did really really well cooked properly right and the same thing with the bacon so you can see all crispy or crunchy. I was able to achieve breakfast.

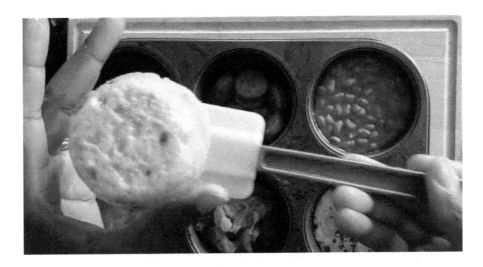

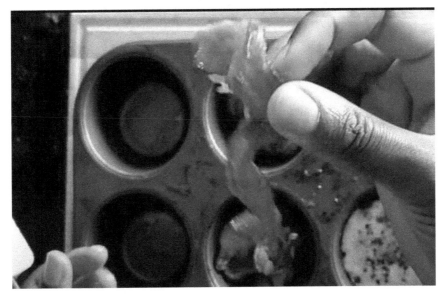

It took me about 30 minutes to make the entire dish so you can see my eggs yummy yummy yummy. I'm just going to dish this out and yeah so you can see the entire dish all presented for you. This is our English breakfast right you have the bread, we've got the bacon, I'm going to put in the sausages. This is a wonderful breakfast. All I really did was just to check it up at various times and baked beans is ready. This could actually is pretty decent meal and I think can it's perfect for more than one person. We have got egg there's not mushroom, there is no black pudding but this is completely fine the way it is right. So, this is what our full English breakfast looks like on some days and I've got the eggs, I've got the bacon, I still have some bacon there in the tray because I did make a lot so, still have some eggs.

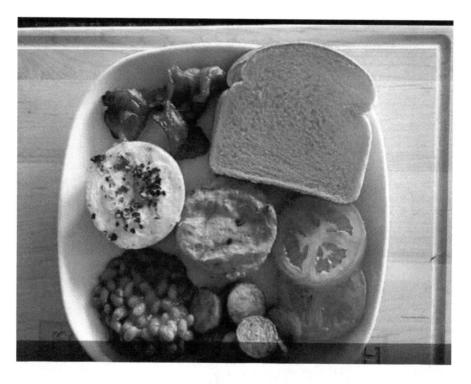

I have got some bacon some bread, yeah with a glass of milk or a cup of coffee you're good to go.

67. Garlic Brussel Sprout Chips

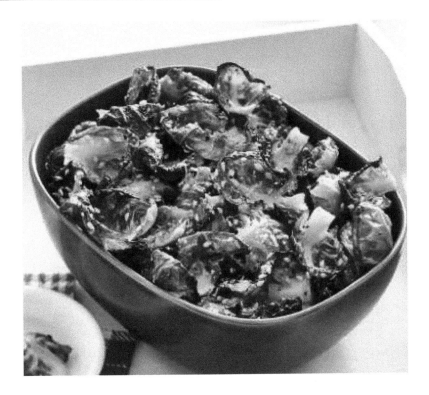

Ingredients:

- 1 tsp sea salt

- 1 Pound Brussel Sprouts, ends removed

- 2 Tbsp. olive oil

- 1 tsp garlic powder

Method:

❖ Preheat your air fryer to 2400 degrees F and line the fryer tray with parchment paper.

❖ Peel the Brussels sprouts leaf at a time, putting the leaves in a massive bowl as you pare them.

❖ Toss the leaves together with olive oil, garlic powder and salt then disperse onto the prepared tray.

❖ Bake for 15 minutes at the fryer, tossing halfway through to cook evenly.

68. Home and Asparagus

Ingredients:

- 1/4 teaspoon ground black pepper

- 1/4 tsp salt

- 1 lb. asparagus spears

Directions

❏ Preheat your air fryer to 400 degrees F and line your fryer tray using a

❏ Set the cod filets onto the parchment and sprinkle with the pepper and salt and rub the spices to the fish.

❏ Top the fish with the remaining components then wrap the parchment paper around the fish filets, surrounding them entirely.

❏ Put the tray in the fryer and bake for 20 minutes.

69. Herbed Parmesan Crackers

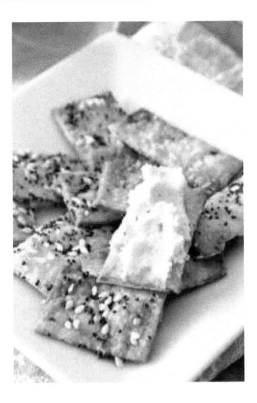

Ingredients:

- 2 Tbsp. Italian seasoning

- ½ cup chia seeds

- 1 ½ cups sunflower seeds

- 1 egg

- 2 Tbsp. butter, melted

- Salt

- ½ tsp garlic powder

- ½ tsp baking powder

- ¾ cup parmesan cheese, grated

Method:

❑ Set the sunflower seeds and chia seeds in a food processor until finely mixed to a powder. Put into a large bowl.

❑ Add the cheese, Italian seasoning, garlic powder and baking powder to the bowl and combine well.

❑ Add the melted butter and egg and stir till a wonderful dough forms.

❑ Put the dough onto a sheet of parchment and then put the following slice of parchment on top.

❑ Roll the dough into a thin sheet around 1/8 inch thick.

❑ Remove the top piece of parchment and lift the dough with the underside parchment and set onto a sheet tray which can fit in the air fryer.

❑ Score the cracker dough to your desired shape and bake for 40-45cminutes.

❑ Break the crackers aside and enjoy!

70. Salmon and Asparagus

Ingredients:

- ¼ tsp ground black pepper

- 1 ¾ pound salmon fillets

- ¼ tsp salt

- 1 pound asparagus spears

- 1 Tbsp. lemon juice

- 1 Tbsp. fresh chopped parsley

- 3 Tbsp. olive oil

Method

→ Preheat your air fryer to 400 degrees F and line your fryer tray using a long piece of parchment paper.

→ Set the salmon filets onto the parchment and sprinkle with the salt and pepper and rub the spices to the fish.

→ Top the fish with the rest of the ingredients then wrap the parchment paper around the fish filets, surrounding them completely.

→ Put the tray in the fryer and bake for 20 minutes.

71.Super Seed Parmesan Crackers

Ingredients:

- ½ tsp baking powder

- 1 egg

- 2 Tbsp. butter, melted

- 1 cups sunflower seeds

- ¾ cup parmesan cheese, grated

- 2 Tbsp. Italian seasoning

- ½ cup chia seeds

- ½ cup hulled hemp seeds

- ½ tsp garlic powder

- Salt

Method:

★ Preheat your air fryer to 300 degrees F.

★ Put into a large bowl.

★ Add the cheese, Italian seasoning, garlic powder and baking powder to the bowl and combine well.

★ Add the melted butter and egg and stir till a wonderful dough forms.

★ Put the dough onto a sheet of parchment and then put the following slice of parchment on top.

★ Roll the dough into a thin sheet around 1/8 inch thick.

★ Remove the top piece of parchment and lift the dough with the underside parchment and set onto a sheet tray which will fit from the air fryer.

★ Score the cracker dough to your desired shape and bake for 40-45 minutes.

★ Break the crackers aside and enjoy!

Conclusion

We have included 70 best recipes for you in this book. So, just try it out and then give us feedback with images of cooking.

Wood Pellet Smoker Grill Cookbook

Discover Tens of Succulent Recipes and Learn 9+1 Beginners Tricks to Make Your First Grills with No Pressure

By

Chef Carlo Leone

Table of Contents

Introduction

The hottest trend in the BBQ and grilling community have been pellet grills. Since technology has not really improved much in the industry in the last three decades or so, individuals are enthusiastic about the amazing functionality and comfort that pellet grills are bringing to the sector. However, it's crucial to learn how they function in order to fully appreciate what they have to deliver. So, if you're new to grilling or smoking pellets and you're thinking about how pellet grills operate, then you've come to the right place.

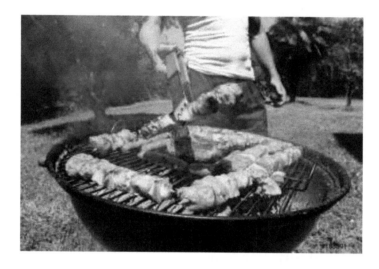

Barbecuing is the oldest form of cooking worldwide. Low-and-slow smoking and cooking over indirect heat is the standard concept of barbecuing. There is little question regarding the findings obtained from barbecuing utilizing haze, indirect fire, sauces, rubs, and natural meat juices. Among grilling and barbecuing, there is a big distinction, but many people are ignorant because they use all words loosely.

Smoker-grills with wood pellets is ideal units for barbecuing.

In this book, you will get to know each and everything you need to learn about the know-how of a Wood Pellet Smoker Grill.

This book provides you with various tips and tricks that you need to know in order to enjoy the process of barbequing and making it a deliciously funny activity.

Also, various basic recipes are provided for you to start with your grilling with ease in the comfort of your home.

Chapter 1- Wood Pellet Smoker Grills

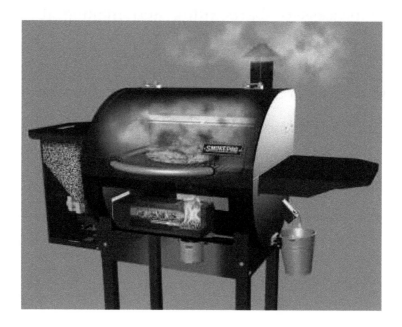

1.1 What is a Pellet Smoker Grill?

A barbecue pit using compressed hardwood sawdust such as apple, plum, hickory, pine, oak, mesquite, and other wood pellets to roast, grill, smoke and bake is the clinical concept of a wood pellet smoker-grill. The smoker-grill wood pellet provides you with taste profiles and moisture that can only be obtained through hardwood cooking. Grill temperatures on certain versions vary from 150 °F to well over 600 °F, depending on the maker and platform.

Wood pellet smoker-grills are succulent, cosy and clean, unparalleled by gas grills and charcoal. The smoke composition is milder than you may be accustomed to from other cigarettes. They produce the flexibility and advantages of a convection oven due to their architecture. Smoker-grills with wood pellets is safe and easy to work.

In short outdoor cookers that incorporate components from smokers, kitchen ovens, charcoal smokers, and gas grills are pellet grills. They use 100% of natural hardwood pellets, the fuel supply that enables direct or indirect heat to be generated by Pellet Grills.

Fueled by wood pellets, utilizing an electronic control panel, they will smoke and grill and bake to automatically feed fuel pellets to the flames, regulate the ventilation of the grill, and maintain constant cooking temperatures.

1.2 Working of a Pellet Smoker Grill

Wood pellets are placed into a hopper-called storage container. An auger that is operated by electricity then feeds the pellets into a cooking chamber. The wood pellets ignite by combustion, warming the cooking chamber. After that, the air is pulled in by intake fans. Across the boiling area, flame and smoke are then emitted.

Rather like an oven, pellet grills provide you digitally or with a knob with reliable temperature regulation, typically varying from 180 ° F to 500 ° F. So, "low and slow" or searing hot both can be cooked by you.

In order to check the core temperature of the beef, most pellet grills do have a meat probe that can link with the control board. There is a proprietary Sear Zone plate for grills that requires implicit or explicit heat and eight separate cooking methods.

1.3   Basic Components of a Wood Pellet Smoker

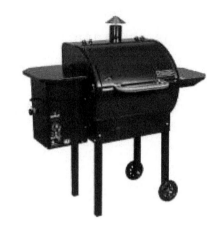

The following provided are the basic components of a wood pellet smoker grill: -

1. Hopper

This is where they store the wood pellets. Be sure you hold a good quantity of pellets based on the cook's range, the cook's temperature, and the capability of the hopper.

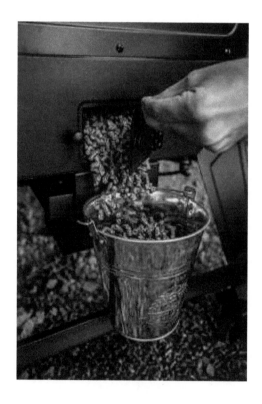

2. Firepot

This is where the fire and burn the wood pellets that ignite the barbecue. For the pellet shaft, which holds the auger, the wide hole in the firepot is; the bottom center gap below it is for the igniter tube, and the other holes are for the ventilation of the fan. After a few cooks, it is a good idea to empty or vacuum out the ashes in order to enable the igniter to function more effectively.

3. Auger

The pellets are then loaded via the auger, the feed system that provides the fire pot with the pellets.

4. Fan

As it ensures a constant and/or steady airflow, the fan is very critical, maintaining the pellets trying to burn in the firepot and culminating in cooking convection.

5. Igniter Rod

The wood pellets are ignited in the firepot by this rod. The ignitor rod and the pellet feed tube that is required by the auger to supply pellets to the firepot can be seen with the firepot away.

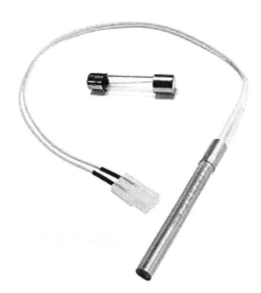

6. Hear Deflector

A specially crafted plate covering the firepot is the heat deflector. The goal is to absorb the heat and distribute it uniformly under the grease/drip plate, converting the wood pellet smoker-grill into a wood-fired convection oven effectively.

7. Resistive Temperature Detector (RTD) / Thermocouple

The thermal sensor that supplies the input loop to the controller is the RTD or thermocouple. For better heat readings, deep clean the thermocouple regularly.

8. Flame Zone Pan

For clear, high-temperature grilling, it is used in tandem with searing grates and attachments for the griddle.

9. Drip Pan

In indirect frying, smoking, baking and roasting, the oiled pan is used. It routes the grease generated to the grease bucket during cooking. It is recommended to scrape off an appropriate caked-on residue from cooks. Also, substitute the foil per few cooks if utilizing foil.

10. Grease Bucket

Runoff fat and oil from cooking activities are extracted from the grease bucket. Accumulation of grease relies on how often you want to cut from beef and poultry fat caps and extra fat. Lining the foil grease bowl tends you clear up.

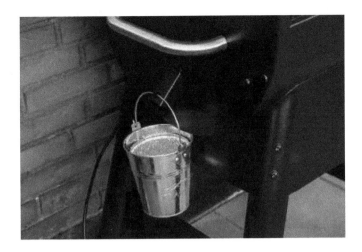

1.Controller

To preserve the set-point temperature, the controller, which normally comes in several types, regulates the air and pellet movement.

1.4   Using your Wood Pellet Smoker Grill

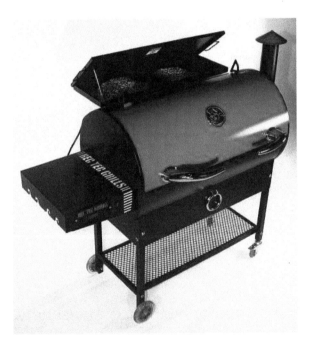

1. Assembly

If a nearby distributor assembles your product for you or you order your unit from a big box retailer, you will need to install your wood pellet smoker-grill. Whether you order the product directly from the vendor or via an online distributor, the unit would also be shipped on a pallet by a ground carrier. But don't dread; assembly isn't as rough as it seems or as complicated as you would imagine.

Only set out all of the bits, and yes, before you begin assembly, make sure you read the directions. Tech help and assistance are just a phone call away, and several suppliers have excellent customer care.

You'll find the design and directions will help you to create your smoker-grill wood pellet easily in an hour or less. In most units, the foundation and legs are often mounted. You will have your device full of wood pellets and ready for the initial burn-in in no time. Be sure you have someone to support you if and where the directions ask for two persons. By choosing to do things yourself, do not harm yourself.

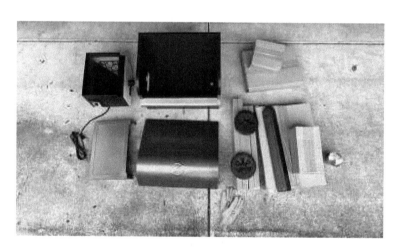

2. Ignition

Wood pellet smoker-grills require standard household 120 VAC or 12 VDC outlets. For powering the ignition and service, wood pellet smoker-grills require regular household 120 VAC or 12 VDC outlets. For, e.g., certain devices, such as the Davy Crockett tailgate device from Green Mountain Grills, are built to use 12 VDC from a car battery or a deep-cycle battery. They also have a 120 VAC AC/DC converter for usage. The power requirements are actually very limited for wood pellet smoker-grills and are used for four items: fan, auger, controller and igniter rod.

Smoker-grills with wood pellets are very safe and easy to work. Inside the fire pot, the fire/flames are limited and completely protected by the oil pan, which gives indirect cooking and avoids flare-ups. Typically, based on the maker, one of two factors can arise when you turn on your device. Your pit either goes through a particular power-up series, or a typical scenario follows it.

The controller is flipped on, the igniter rod is triggered (it will glow red hot), the auger feeds a certain volume of pellets into the firepot, and the fan feeds air into the firepot through numerous tiny holes to start and sustain the fire. The igniter rod is either switched off after a fixed period (4 minutes or longer) or when the pit exceeds a set temperature, depending on your controller. To stop flame-outs, PID controllers can switch the igniter rod back on when the temperature falls below a fixed temperature.

3. Initial Burn-In

To burn out all oils and chemicals used in the processing phase, the burn-in technique is used.

With hardwood barbecue-grade wood pellets, fill the hopper. Because the transmission of the first pellets to the firepot can take ten or more minutes for the auger, put half a handful of pellets in the firepot. Attach the device into a 120 VAC electrical socket with grounding. Just turn on your grill. Place temperature between 350 ° F and 450 ° F if you have a digital controller, and allow the grill to operate at temperature for 30 to 60 minutes (check your owner's manual for precise temperature settings and time). Convert the temperature setting to strong if your grill has an LMH controller.

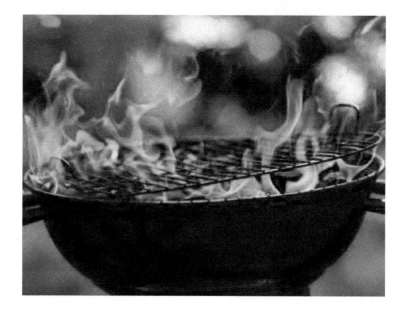

4. Testing for Hot Spots on Your Wood Pellet Smoker-Grill

Not all wood pellet smoker-grills are identical, but I promise that you will be able to smoke and prepare some of the best food your family and friends will ever experience by knowing about your barbecue! To have a working knowledge of the barbecue, it just takes a few cooks to train.

You'll want to monitor the temperature of the grill surface for uniform heat and hotspots. The biscuit test is one simple way to do this.

In the corners, front, back, and middle of the barbecue pick up a box of refrigerator biscuits and position them. As per the instructions on the box, cook the biscuits. You can discover where the hotter and colder places are in your device with this exercise.

Place your food and prepare it according to the data you've gained.

The use of a remote temperature probe to measure the temperatures at the same positions as the biscuit test is needed for a more technical process. At each biscuit spot, put a remote temperature probe, check the temperature, contrast it to the fixed point on your controller and, if any, record the temperature variations. No matter how nice your grill controller is, regardless of the position of the RTD/thermocouple, you'll notice discrepancies. To attain the temperatures you like, just change your grill's fixed temperatures accordingly.

Cleaning Your Wood Pellet Smoker-Grill

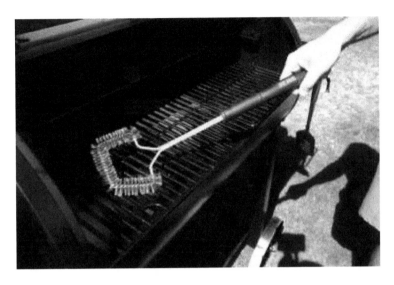

It is highly recommended that you keep your smoker-grill with wood pellets as clean as possible. It only takes a couple of minutes to keep the pit clean before you cook. Cleanliness ensures that your cooks are always penetrated with fresh and clean smoke. For the best results, after every hard cook or after every two to four short cooks, replace the foil on the grease drop pan. If you choose not to use foil, then make sure that the caked residue is often scraped off from your drip pan. There is nothing other than the gases burning off at elevated temperatures from rancid old grease. Using a barbecue wire brush to scrub and hold them clean after each cooker, when the grill grates are still hot. Wipe down both sides of the grates using paper towels. When handling the grates and cleaning your pit, I strongly suggest you wear disposable rubber gloves.

Once your pit fully cools down, remove the drip pan and regularly remove any ash from the firepot and the body of the pit using a shop vacuum cleaner.

Although smoker-grills with wood pellets are incredibly effective, you will still accumulate some ash.

Large quantities of ash in the firepot will decrease the unit's efficiency and might not cause the igniter rod to ignite pellets properly at star-tup. During a roast, an ash accumulation in the body of the pit has a chance to be blown around and collected on the beef.

Chapter 2-Tricks and Techniques

2.1 Quality Meat and Seasonings

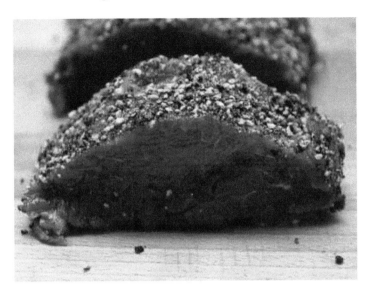

For excellent and personalized cuts of meats, sausages and poultry, and as well as wonderful rubs, seasonings, and barbecue sauces, don't forget your friendly neighbourhood butcher shop.

Low-and-slow cooking, grilling, smoking, frying, roasting, etc., are always worth the seasoning.

It is strongly suggested that you go out and visit the nearest butcher shops and meat markets to see if you can even locate the jewel in the rough that will create an excellent crowd of your next chef.

FTC-In order to redistribute the juices into the product, this significant acronym stands for "Foil-Towel-Cooler" and is a popular process used for retaining and/or resting cooked meats, such as pork butts, turkey and brisket. It provides a final product that is juicy and tender. For example, to accomplish these effects, pit masters, professionals, caterers, and restaurants utilize industrial units such as a Cambro. The FTC is lovingly referred to as the Cambro of the unfortunate guy.

To hold the juices contained, double-wrap the cooked meat in heavy-duty aluminium foil. Before you put it in a cooler, cover the foiled meat in a wide towel. Minimize air room if needed by covering the majority of the cooler with towels to help prevent the heat from dissipating. Depending on the meat and/or the period available before serving, FTC pork butts and briskets are processed in a locked cooler for a minimum of 2 hours and up to 4 to 6 hours. When processing meat, take care, since it may always be too hot to handle even after resting for hours.

2.2 USDA Minimum Internal Temperatures

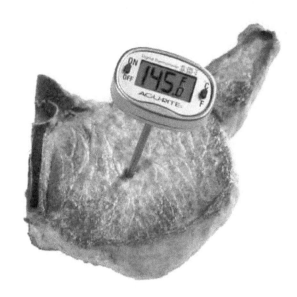

As determined with an automated food thermometer, cook all food at these required internal temperatures before extracting it from the heat source. For purposes of personal choice, you can choose to cook at higher temperatures.

1. Indirect and Direct Grill Setup

Both smoker-grills with wood pellets are built mainly for indirect cooking. To cook more slowly and uniformly, indirect cooking utilizes deflected fire. The heat deflector is a stainless-steel plate that sits above the fire pot, as described before. It collects the heat from the fire and radiates it out like a convection oven does, ensuring that the heat is spread around it, giving a cook that is more uniform. Direct cooking uses direct, high heat to cook, much as the name suggests. It's a quicker time to cook, which doesn't make for many infusions of smoke, but it does give you the iconic grill marks. More producers are now starting to provide the versatility of a direct cooking setup, and a limited number have a built-in hybrid design that both offers indirect and direct cooking power without needing to alter any configuration.

- **Indirect Setup**

You'll be using an indirect rig for several wood pellet smoker-grill recipes. Per your manufacturer's user manual, mount your grease pan. In order for the grease fat to fall out, the Grease pan is built to slant in the path of the grease bucket. Otherwise, at higher temperatures, the grease would collect on the pan, which might become a flare-up safety problem.

- **Direct Setup**

You will need to swap your indirect pan with a direct pan because your machine has built-in direct cooking capabilities. To customize it for direct cooking, you can need to detach one or more cover plates in certain units or slip the top part of a combination pan. To close or expose the gaps, you slip the cover in one direction or the other. Shuttered holes are for indirect cooking, whereas direct cooking is for open holes. Searing gratings are not obligatory. They can have greater results when grilling and cooking directly since they are built to sear and sizzle foods easier by focusing the fire.

2. Ingredients

Feel free to replace, delete, and incorporate some ingredients dependent on your tastes, taste buds, and ingredients on hand, depending on how relaxed you are in the kitchen or with the grill. Strict adherence to the list of ingredients can deliver impressive results, but do not be afraid to tweak it here and there.

3. Prepping for the Grill

Before taking the food to the barbecue, the prep portion is all the preparation you do. Planning ahead is the number one goal in the prep period. Offer yourself plenty of time, read the recipe, and examine every move or process in which you can have concerns. To allow the seasonings, rubs, marinades and brines to do their magic, recipes can call for refrigeration overnight or for hours after making preparations. Before beginning your preparation, gather all required ingredients and cooking equipment. Before starting, make sure the proteins are safely thawed in the refrigerator if you do not use fresh beef, poultry, or seafood. Be vigilant to have good sanitary facilities, above all.

There may be occasions when the processes of planning and guidance can occur concurrently. You may opt to preheat before finishing the cooking, based on the length of time your wood pellet smoker-grill needs to preheat, much as in a conventional indoor oven.

4. On the Wood Pellet Smoker Grill

Unless otherwise stated, it is strongly recommended to start with a complete pellet hopper and a clean wood pellet smoker-grill configured for indirect fire. If required, prior to putting the meat on the plate, insert the grill meat probe(s) or remote meat probe(s) into the thickest part of the protein. Bear in mind that each smoker grill for wood pellets is different, and so the time to create various recipes may vary accordingly. Depend on internal temperatures at all times. Just to find out that it's undercooked, you won't believe how scrumptious a piece of meat might look.

You can soon discover when you grow confident with your wood pellet smoker-grill that cooking directions can be adjustable as long as the correct internal temperature is met by your finished product.

2.3 General Information and Tips

1. Preheating

According to factory start-up procedures, times for heating up your wood pellet smoker-grill can differ. The trick is to run a few experiments to grasp your barbecue.

2. Thawing Food

Always thaw food in the refrigerator to be healthy to avoid illness; immerse it in freezing water, adjust the water every 30 minutes and ensure that the food remains submerged; or use the freezer to defrost the food. On the countertop, do not thaw the frozen food.

3. Internal Temperature

Often use a wireless instant-read thermometer such as a Thermapen or an analogous device to cook at internal temperatures. Before putting the protein on the grill, probe thermometers should be inserted and put in the thickest section of the beef, not reaching the bone.

4. Tenting

Until slicing or eating, many recipes ask for resting the meat under a foil tent. Tenting is a simple process.

In the middle, fold sheets of aluminium foil, fan it opens into a tent form and position it loosely over the food. Instead of placing them on the serving tray, tenting tends to preserve heat as the food redistributes the natural juices. By tenting, crispy skin texture on poultry and crisp on meats may be affected.

5. The Stall

A natural part of the cooking process is the stall, also known as the plateau or zone. Large cuts of meat reach a point when cooked at low temperatures, where the core temperature stops rising for a period of time. After the collagen melts, most cuts of meat tenderize, and the fibres begin to separate. The stall will experience every big chunk of meat, such as a pork butt (shoulder) or beef brisket. It can last minutes or as long as three hours and normally occurs from 155 ° F to 170 ° F at internal meat temperatures. It's not a question of whether, but when, the stall is going to happen. In your wood pellet smoker-grill, you may be tempted to turn the heat up, but practice patience; just ride it out so as not to affect the meat being cooked.

6. The Texas Crutch

A technique is commonly known as the "Texas crutch" will decrease your cooking time and bypass the stall for those who cannot wait out the stall. The most preferred version of the Texas crutch is to consider removing the meat from the stall before it reaches its full size. When the internal temperature reaches 160 °F, remove the meat, then double wrap it in heavy-duty aluminium foil, ensuring that any meat probes are inserted into the meat. Wrap the foil around the probe until it attains your desired internal temperature, and return the meat to the grill.

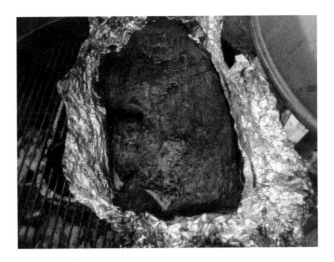

7. Carving Meat

Always carve meat across the grain, not with it, to get the most tender outcomes. Searching for the simultaneous lines running down the meat identifies the direction that the grain is running. Slice the muscle fibre lines perpendicular to them.

8. Protect your Skin

While handling raw meat and spicy peppers like jalapeños, wear food-grade latex-free nitric gloves.

9. Keep your Prep Surface Clean

It is highly recommended that plastic food wrap and/or heavy-duty aluminium foil line your prep area. When dealing with raw meat, this simplifies clean-up and is also more hygienic.

10. Curing Salt

Curing salt contains salt and nitrite, which is used in some low-and-slow recipes and should not be used to season food at the table or during the cooking process. Significant quantities can be lethal, but when curing meat, it is harmless in small quantities.

11.Smoke Issues

The higher the temperature, the lower smoke is produced by a wood pellet smoker-grill. No noticeable smoke above 300°F will be produced by most units. Therefore, when a recipe initially calls for extremely high temperatures, use any pellets of your choice, as the pellets will not influence the flavour.

2.4 Simple tricks for beginners

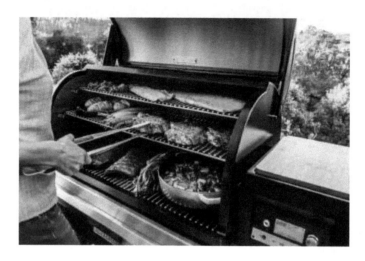

1. Allow yourself some time to get acquainted with your new grill/smoker

Allow yourself time to familiarize yourself with your new grill/smoker. We know you're going to be anxious to give it a try, but don't be overly ambitious. Start with chicken, salmon steaks or fillets, pork loin tenderloin, Cornish hens, blade steaks, or other fairly affordable cuts that can be completed in 2 hours or less, instead of a whole brisket that might take 15 hours or more, or a budget-busting prime rib roast.

2. Don't let your meat come to room temperature before cooking

Whichever meat you select, put it straight from the refrigerator on the preheated grill/smoker. Do not allow it to reach room temperature before cooking, as many recipes suggest.

3. Take advantage of your pellet grill's searing capabilities

Many pellet grills feature searing capabilities, which means that temperatures above 500 °C can be reached. Again, for information on your particular model, check your owner's manual.

4. Use the reverse sear method

Don't think about smoking the meat at a lower temperature and then finishing it at a high temperature. This two-step approach is particularly useful for smoking crisp (not rubbery) skin chicken, or the "reverse sear technique" often used for thicker steaks or prime ribs.

5. Use your pellet grill just like an oven

Just like an oven, your smoker/pellet grill can be used, capable of baking, roasting, braising, etc. But the inclusion of wood smoke gives much more fascinating flavours to food.

6. Experiment with pellet flavours

Experiment with the flavours of pellets. Certain pellet labels are somewhat subtle.

7. Position your grill at least 6 feet away from your home

At least six feet from any buildings, overhangs, bushes, etc., place your barbecue.

8. Always store pellets in a dry place

Pellets can always be kept in a dry spot. Otherwise, it'll transform to sawdust, and if it's an augur, to anything like a stone!

9. Use the upper rack of your grill for cooking something that's prone to drying out

Convection and radiant heat are also generated by your pellet grill. Place them on the upper rack to shield them from the heat radiating from the bottom while you are frying anything that is vulnerable to drying out, such as thin fish fillets or chicken breasts. You can balance a wire rack on fire bricks or buy after-market racks if your machine doesn't come with an upper rack. To produce moisture, you may also place a pan of water or other liquid on the grill grate.

10. Season your new pellet grill

Season your new pellet grill according to directions from the manufacturer. This burns off the production process of any residual oils.

11. Identify any hot spots — most grills have them

As directed by the owner's manual, preheat your grill to medium-high, then lay slices of cheap white bread shoulder to shoulder across the grater. Watch carefully, then after a couple of minutes, flip. Take a photo of the findings. The darkest bread will show where the temperature could be warmer

12. Invest in a good meat thermometer

At grill level, a laser-type thermometer will give you a more precise temperature reading than an integrated dome thermometer. Determine your grill model's temperature range from lowest to highest.

13. Use lower temperatures to generate more smoke

At lower temperatures, especially in the "low and slow" range between 225 and 275, you will generate more smoke.

14. Never allow the pellets in the pellet hopper to run out

Never allow it to run out of the pellets in the pellet hopper. If this occurs, before relighting the barbecue, check the owner's manual. To reassure yourself to top off the pellets, set a timer if you have to.

15. Invest in a smoking tube to supplement the smoke generated by your grill

If you want to complement your pellet grill with the smoke produced, or even cold smoke, engage in a smoking tube.

16. Clean your grill frequently

To prevent the build-up of ash or oil, clean your grill regularly. Much like a sharp-bladed spatula or putty knife, a shop-type vacuum is a must. Don't neglect to sweep the exhaust or chimney.

17. Use heavy-duty foil for easier clean-up

To protect the oil tray and to line the grease bucket, use high-duty foil. (Also, hollow containers may be used as bucket liners, such as coffee or tomato cans.)

18. Remove the grease bucket after each cook

Take the grease bucket off the side of the grill after each cooker and hide it in a secure position to keep it out of the hands of pets, coyotes or other hungry creatures.

19. Smoke vegetables and side dishes on your new grill

Using the new grill to smoke or roast vegetables or side dishes.

Chapter 3-Appetizers Recipes

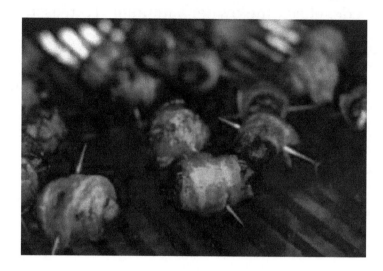

3.1 Atomic Buffalo Turds

Ready in about 2 hours and 50 minutes | Servings-6 to 10 | Difficulty-Hard

Ingredients

- 3/4 cup of shredded Monterey Jack and cheddar cheese blend

- Half teaspoon of red pepper flakes

- Eight ounces of regular cream cheese

- Ten medium jalapeño peppers

- One teaspoon of garlic powder

- Ten thinly sliced bacon strips, cut in half

- One teaspoon of smoked paprika

- Twenty Little Smokies sausages

- Half teaspoon of cayenne pepper

Instructions

1. Firstly, if you use your food service gloves, we need to ready the grill for that. Clean the jalapeño peppers and slice them lengthwise. Carefully extract the seeds

and veins using a spoon or paring knife, and dispose of them. On a vegetable grilling tray, put the jalapeños and set them aside.

2. Mix the cream cheese, shredded cheese, paprika, cayenne pepper, garlic powder, and red pepper flakes in a small cup, if using, until they are thoroughly absorbed.

3. With the cream cheese mixture, cover the hollowed jalapeño pepper pieces.

4. On top of each half of the packed jalapeño pepper, put a Little Smokies sausage.

5. Wrap each half of the jalapeño pepper with half a slice of thin bacon.

6. To secure the bacon to the sausage, use a toothpick, making sure not to pierce the pepper. On a grilling tray or skillet, position the ABTs.

7. For indirect cooking, set up your wood pellet smoker-grill and preheat it to 250°F using hickory pellets or a mix.

8. Smoke the jalapeño peppers for one and a half to 2 hours at 250 ° F before the bacon is fried and crunchy.

9. Remove the ABTs from the grill and leave to rest before serving for 5 minutes.

3.2 Garlic Parmesan Wedges
Ready in about 45 minutes | Servings-3 | Difficulty-Moderate

Ingredients

- A quarter cup of extra-virgin olive oil

- 3/4 teaspoon of black pepper

- 3/4 cup of grated Parmesan cheese

- Three tablespoons of chopped fresh cilantro

- Three large russet potatoes

- One and a half teaspoons of salt

- Two teaspoons of garlic powder

- Half cup of blue cheese or ranch dressing per serving, for dipping (optional)

Instructions

1. Using a vegetable brush to gently clean the potatoes with cold water and allow the potatoes to dry.

2. Lengthwise, cut the potatoes in half and then split both halves into thirds.

3. To clean away all the humidity that is emitted as you cut the potatoes, use a paper towel. Moisture prevents the wedges from being crispy.

4. In a wide cup, put the potato wedges, pepper, salt, olive oil, and garlic powder and toss gently with your hands to ensure that the oil and spices are equally spread.

5. Arrange the wedges on a non-stick grilling tray/pan/basket on a single sheet.

6. For indirect cooking, set up your wood pellet smoker-grill and preheat it to 425 ° F using any form of wood pellet.

7. Place your preheated smoker-grill on the grilling tray and roast the potato wedges for Fifteen minutes before turning. Roast the potato wedges until the potatoes are fork-tender on the inside and crunchy golden brown on the outside, for an extra 15 to 20 minutes.

8. Sprinkle with Parmesan cheese on the potato wedges and garnish with, if needed, cilantro or parsley. If needed, serve with ranch dressing blue cheese for dipping.

3.3 Bacon-Wrapped Asparagus
Ready in about 45 minutes | Servings-4 to 6 | Difficulty-Hard

Ingredients

- Extra-virgin olive oil

- One pound of thick fresh asparagus

- Five slices of thinly sliced bacon

- One teaspoon of Pete's Western Rub

Salt and pepper as per taste

Instructions

. Snap and trim the woody ends of the asparagus so that they are both around the same weight.

. Divide the asparagus into three-spear packets and spray it with olive oil. With one slice of bacon, seal each package and then sprinkle with the seasoning or salt and pepper to taste.

. Configure your indirect cooking wood pellet smoker-grill, putting Teflon-coated fiberglass mats on top of the grates. Using some kind of pellets, preheat to 400°F. It is possible to preheat the grill when heating the asparagus.

. For 25 to 30 minutes, grill the bacon-wrapped asparagus until the asparagus is soft and the bacon is fried and crispy.

3.4 Bourbon BBQ Smoked Chicken Wings
Ready in about 2 hours and 50 minutes | Servings-6 | Difficulty-Hard

Ingredients

Wings

• Sweet and smoky chicken rub or your favorite store-bought rub

Four pounds of chicken wings

Two tablespoons of vegetable oil

Bourbon BBQ Sauce

• Five finely minced cloves of garlic

Half finely minced medium sweet yellow onion

• Half cup of bourbon

• A quarter cup of tomato paste

- Two cups of ketchup
- Half cup of packed light brown sugar
- 1/3 cup apple cider vinegar
- A quarter cup of Worcestershire sauce
- Two tablespoons of liquid smoke
- Half tablespoon of kosher salt
- Half teaspoon of black pepper
- A quarter teaspoon of cayenne pepper
- A few dashes of hot sauce (optional)

Instructions

For sauce

1. Over medium heat, add a drizzle of olive oil to a saucepan. Add the garlic and onion and cook for about 5 minutes. Add the bourbon and continue cooking for approximately 3 minutes.

2. To break it up, add tomato paste and whisk. Add all the remaining components of the sauce and whisk to combine. Increase the heat and bring it to a boil. Simmer for about 15-20 minutes and reduce the heat to medium-low or low.

3. When you like a smooth, glossy sauce, pour sauce through a fine-mesh sieve to strain out pieces of onion and garlic. Set aside to cool. Store the leftover BBQ sauce for 2-3 weeks in the refrigerator in an airtight container.

For wings

1. Pat dry chicken wings with a clean paper towel. In a large mixing bowl, add the wings and toss with the vegetable oil. Ensure that each wing is coated; add rub and massage into the wings.

2. Add pellets of hickory wood to the hopper. Turn on the smoker, open the lid and set the setting for the smoke. Smoke-free heat, lid open, 5-10 minutes, until very smoky. Set the smoker to 250 F degrees by adding chicken wings to the oiled grill grates. Close the smoker's lid and smoke for 2 hours and 30 minutes, or until the internal temperature of the chicken wings reaches 165 degrees F. To ensure precise cooking temperatures, use an instant reading meat thermometer.

3. With bourbon BBQ sauce, change the smoker setting to high and braise chicken wings on both sides. Cook the wings on the other side for 5 minutes, then flip them over and cook for 3-5 minutes.

4. To remove chicken wings from a foil or parchment coated plate or baking sheet, select Shut down on smoker. Allow 5-10 minutes to rest. Turn it off and unplug the smoker.

5. Eat the wings as they are, or brush them with extra BBQ sauce. Dip in the blue cheese or ranch dressing for a traditional experience and serve with celery and carrots.

3.5   Brisket Baked Beans

Ready in about 2 hours and 30 minutes | Servings-10 to 12 | Difficulty-Hard

Ingredients

- Two tablespoons of extra-virgin olive oil
- One large diced yellow onion,
- One medium diced green bell pepper
- One medium diced red bell pepper
- Two to six diced jalapeño peppers
- Three cups of chopped Texas-Style Brisket Flat
- One (28-ounce) can of baked beans, like Bush's Country Style Baked Beans

- One (28-ounce) can of pork and beans

- One (14-ounce) can of rinsed and drained red kidney beans

- One cup of barbecue sauce

- Half cup of packed brown sugar

- Three chopped garlic cloves

- Two teaspoons of ground mustard

- Half teaspoon of kosher salt

- Half teaspoon of black pepper

Instructions

1. Heat the olive oil in a skillet over medium heat, and then add the diced onion, peppers and jalapeños. Cook for about 8 to 10 minutes, occasionally stirring, until the onions are translucent.

2. Combine the chopped brisket, pork, baked beans and beans, cooked onion, kidney beans and peppers, barbecue sauce, brown sugar, ground mustard, garlic, black pepper and salt in a 4-quart casserole dish.

3. Use the pellets of choice to install your wood pellet smoker-grill for indirect cooking and preheat it to 325 ° F. Cook the uncovered brisket of baked beans for one and a half to 2 hours until the beans are dense and bubbly. Allow 15 minutes to rest before serving.

3.6   Crabmeat-Stuffed Mushrooms

Ready in about 50 minutes | Servings-4 to 6 | Difficulty-Moderate

Ingredients

- Extra-virgin olive oil

- Six medium portobello mushrooms

- 1/3 cup of grated Parmesan cheese

For the crabmeat stuffing

Two tablespoons of extra-virgin olive oil

Eight ounces of fresh crabmeat, or canned or imitation crab meat

1/3 cup of chopped celery

1/3 cup of chopped red bell pepper

Half cup of chopped green onion

Half cup of Italian bread crumbs

Half cup of mayonnaise8 ounces cream cheese, at room temperature

Half teaspoon of minced garlic

One tablespoon of dried parsley

Half cup of grated Parmesan cheese

A quarter teaspoon of Old Bay seasoning

A quarter teaspoon of kosher salt

A quarter teaspoon of black pepper

Instructions

1. Using a damp paper towel, clean the mushroom caps. Cut and set aside the stems.

2. With a spoon, extract the brown gills from the undersides of the mushroom caps and dispose of them.

3. Get the crabmeat stuffing ready. Drain, rinse and remove any shell bits when using canned crabmeat.

4. Heat olive oil over medium-high heat in a skillet. Add the celery, green onion and bell pepper, and sauté for 5 minutes. Set to cool aside.

5. In a large bowl, mix the cooled sautéed vegetables gently with the rest of the ingredients.

6. Cover the crabmeat stuffing and refrigerate it until ready to use.

7. Fill the crab mixture with each mushroom cap, creating a mound in the center.

8. Sprinkle with extra-virgin olive oil and sprinkle the Parmesan cheese with each stuffed mushroom cap. In a 10 x, 15-inch baking dish, put the stuffed mushrooms.

9. Install your wood pellet smoker-grill for indirect heat and use any pellets to preheat to 375 ° F.

10. Bake for 30 to 45 minutes until the stuffing is hot and the mushrooms are beginning to release their juices (165 °F measured with an instant-read digital thermometer).

3.7 Hickory-Smoked Moink Ball Skewers

Ready in about 1 hour and 50 minutes | Servings-6 to 9 | Difficulty-Hard

Ingredients

- Half pound ground pork sausage

- Half pound ground beef

- One large egg

- Half cup of Italian bread crumbs

- Half cup of minced red onions

- Half cup of grated Parmesan cheese

- A quarter cup of finely chopped parsley

- A quarter cup of whole milk

- Two minced garlic cloves

- One teaspoon of oregano

- Half teaspoon of kosher salt

- Half teaspoon of black pepper

- Half pound thinly sliced bacon, cut in half

- A quarter cup of barbecue sauce

Instructions

. Combine the ground pork sausage, ground beef, egg, onion, parmesan cheese, bread crumbs, parsley, milk, salt, garlic, oregano, and pepper in a large bowl. Don't overwork the flesh.

. Form one and a half-ounce meatball, roughly 1 inch in diameter, and place them on a fiberglass mat coated with Teflon.

. Wrap half a slice of thin bacon with each meatball. On six skewers, spear the moink balls (3 balls per skewer)

. For indirect cooking, configure your wood pellet smoker-grill.

. Using hickory pellets, preheat your wood pellet smoker-grill to 225°F.

. For 30 minutes, smoke the Moink Ball Skewers.

. Raise the pit temperature to 350 ° F until the internal temperature of the meatballs reaches 175 ° F, and the bacon is crunchy (approximately 40 to 45 minutes).

. During the last 5 minutes, brush the moink balls with your favourite barbecuing sauce.

3.8   Smashed Potato Casserole

Ready in about 1 hour and 55 minutes | Servings-8 | Difficulty-Hard

Ingredients

- A quarter cup of (Half stick) salted butter
- Ten bacon slices
- One small thinly sliced red onion
- One small thinly green sliced bell pepper
- One small thinly sliced red bell pepper
- One small thinly sliced yellow bell pepper
- Three cups of mashed potatoes

- 3/4 cup of sour cream

- One and a half teaspoons of Texas Barbecue Rub

- Four cups of frozen hash brown potatoes

- Three cups of shredded sharp cheddar cheese

Instructions

1. Over medium heat, cook the bacon in a large skillet until crisp, about 5 minutes on each side. Set aside the bacon.

2. To a glass container, transfer the rendered bacon grease.

3. Warm the butter or bacon grease in the same large skillet, over medium heat, and sauté the red onion and bell peppers until al dente. Just set aside.

4. Spray non-stick cooking spray on a 9 to 11-inch casserole dish and spread the mashed potatoes on the bottom of the dish.

5. Layer the sour cream and season with Texas Barbecue Rub over the mashed potatoes.

6. On top of the potatoes, layer the sautéed vegetables and keep the butter or bacon grease in the pan.

7. Sprinkle with half a cup of sharp cheddar cheese, followed by brown potatoes with frozen hash.

8. Spoon over the hash browns with the residual butter or bacon fat from the sautéed vegetables and top with crumbled bacon.

9. Top with one and a half of the remaining cups of sharp cheddar cheese and cover with a lid or aluminium foil over the casserole dish.

10. Use the pellets of choice to customize your wood pellet smoker-grill for indirect cooking and preheat it to 350 ° F.

11. For 45 to 60 minutes, bake the mashed potato casserole until the cheese is bubbling.

2. Before serving, let it rest for 10 minutes.

3.9 Roasted Vegetables

Ready in about 1 hour | Servings-4 | Difficulty-Moderate

Ingredients

One cup of small halved mushrooms

One medium sliced and halved yellow squash

One small chopped red onion

Six medium stemmed asparagus spears

A quarter cup of roasted garlic–flavoured extra-virgin olive oil

Three minced garlic cloves

One teaspoon of dried oregano

Half teaspoon of black pepper

One cup of cauliflower florets

One medium sliced and halved zucchini

One medium chopped red bell pepper

- Six ounces of small baby carrots

One cup of cherry or grape tomatoes

Two tablespoons of balsamic vinegar

- One teaspoon of dried thyme

- One teaspoon of garlic salt

Instructions

1. Place in a large bowl the florets of cauliflower, mushrooms, yellow squash, red bell pepper, zucchini, carrots and red onions, tomatoes and asparagus.

2. Stir in the vegetables with olive oil, garlic, balsamic vinegar, thyme, oregano, black pepper and garlic salt

3. Toss the vegetables gently with your hand until they are fully encased with olive oil, herbs, and spices.

4. Spread the seasoned vegetables evenly on a non-stick grilling tray/pan/basket

5. For indirect cooking, set up your wood pellet smoker-grill and preheat it to 425 ° F using any form of wood pellet.

6. To the preheated smoker-grill, transfer the grilling tray and roast the vegetables for 20 to 40 minutes, or until the veggies are al dente. Immediately serve.

3.10 Applewood-Smoked Cheese

Ready in about 3 hours |Servings-Many| Difficulty-Hard

Ingredients

One-to-two and a half-pound block of the following suggested cheeses like

- Sharp cheddar
- Gouda
- Extra-sharp 3-year cheddar
- Pepper Jack Swiss
- Monterey Jack

Instructions

1. Break the cheese blocks into compact sizes to maximize smoke penetration based on the form of the cheese blocks.

2. To allow a very thin skin or crust to develop that serves as a barrier to heat but enables the smoke to enter, let the cheese sit uncovered on the counter for 1 hour.

3. Mount a cold-smoke package to customize your wood pellet smoker-grill for indirect fire and plan for cold-smoking.

4. Ensure that the louver vents of the smoker box are completely open to allow the box to avoid moisture.

5. Preheat your smoker-grill wood pellet to 180 ° F, or if you have one, use the smoke mode, using apple pellets for a milder smoke taste.

6. Put the cheese on non-stick grill mats of Teflon-coated fiberglass and cold-smoke for 2 hours.

7. Take the smoked cheese and use a cooling rack to allow it to cool on the counter for an hour.

8. Vacuum-seal and mark your smoked cheeses for a minimum of 2 weeks before refrigerating to enable the smoke to absorb and mellow the cheese's taste.

3.11 Bacon Cheddar Sliders

Ready in 45 minutes | Servings-6 to 10 | Difficulty-Moderate

Ingredients

- Half teaspoon of garlic salt
- Half teaspoon of garlic powder
- Half teaspoon of black pepper
- Half cup of mayonnaise
- Six (1-ounce) slices of sharp cheddar cheese, cut in half
- One and a half pounds ground beef
- Half teaspoon of seasoned salt
- Half teaspoon of onion powder
- Six bacon slices, cut in half
- Two teaspoons of creamy horseradish

- Half small red onion, thinly sliced
- Ketchup
- Half cup of sliced kosher dill pickles12 mini buns

Instructions

1. In a medium dish, blend together the ground beef, seasoned salt, garlic salt, garlic powder, black pepper and onion powder

2. Divide the meat mixture into 12 equal portions and form them into small, thin, circular patties and set aside (approximately 2 ounces each).

3. Over medium pressure, cook the bacon in a medium skillet until crisp, around 5 to 8 minutes. Only put back.

4. Mix the mayonnaise and horseradish, if used, in a wide bowl to render the sauce. In order to use a griddle accessory, customize your wood pellet smoker-grill for direct cooking. Check with your supplier

5. And see if they have a griddle accessory that fits your special smoker-grill for wood pellets.

6. For better non-stick results, coat the griddle's cooking surface with cooking spray.

7. Using the pellets of your choosing, preheat your wood pellet smoker-grill to 350°F. Your griddle's surface should be around 400°F.

8. Grill the patties on either side for 3 to 4 minutes before they are cooked to an internal temperature of 160°F.

9. If needed, put on each patty a slice of sharp cheddar cheese while the patty is still on the griddle or after the patty has been removed from the griddle. On the bottom half of each roll, put a dollop of the mayonnaise mixture, a red slice of onion, and a burger patty. Pickle slices, sausage, and ketchup on top.

3.12   Teriyaki Steak Bites

Ready in 1 hour and 45 minutes | Servings-4 | Difficulty-Moderate

Ingredients

Teriyaki Marinade

One tablespoon of light brown sugar packed

One teaspoon of garlic salt

Two pounds of top sirloin steak

A quarter cup of teriyaki sauce

One teaspoon of garlic powder

One tablespoon of soy sauce

Half teaspoon of pepper

One tablespoon of apple cider vinegar

Instructions

1. Mix all of the marinade components together in a tiny mixing bowl.

2. Trim the steak and split it into 2-inch bits. Place in the Ziploc bag and add in the steak top marinade. Squeeze out as much air as you can and lock the jar. Put in the fridge for a period of 8 hours or overnight.

3. The steak bites are prepared to be smoked to 225 degrees according to the instructions of the maker until ready to smoke.

4. Place it on the smoker grates or on a rack right away. Remove the leftover marinade. Smoke for 1 hour and 30 minutes or until 135-140 degrees F is the internal temperature. Remove from the smoker and quickly serve.

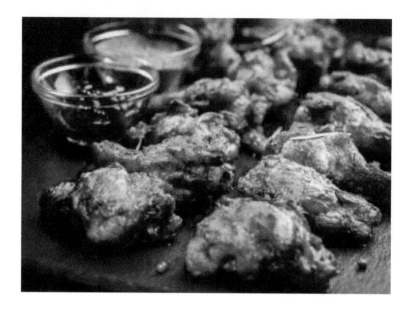

Chapter 4-Lunch Recipes

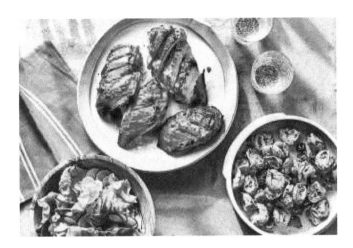

4.1   Jan's Grilled Quarters

Ready in about 2 hours and 15 minutes (marination time excluded) |Servings-4| Difficulty-Hard

Ingredients

- Four fresh or thawed frozen chicken quarters
- Four tablespoons of Jan's Original Dry Rub
- Four to Six tablespoons of extra-virgin olive oil

Instructions

1. Trim any extra skin and fat off the chicken parts. Peel the chicken skin gently and rub the olive oil on and under each quarter of the chicken skin.

2. Season with Jan's Initial Dry Rub on and below the skins and on the backs of the chicken parts.

3. To allow the flavors time to absorb, seal the seasoned chicken pieces in plastic wrap and refrigerate for 2 to 4 hours.

4. Customize your wood pellet smoker-grill for indirect cooking and use some pellets to preheat to 325 ° F.

5. On the barbecue, position the chicken quarters and cook at 325 ° F for 1 hour.

6. To finish the chicken quarters and crisp the skins, lift the pit temperature to 400 ° F after an hour.

7. When the interior temperature, at the thickest areas of the thighs and legs, exceeds 180 ° F, take the crispy chicken quarters off the grill, and the juices flow out.

8. Until eating, rest the grilled spicy chicken quarters under a loose foil tent for 15 minutes.

4.2 Cajun Spatchcock Chicken

Ready in about 3 hours 20 minutes (marination time excluded) |Servings-4| Difficulty-Hard

Ingredients

- Four to five-pound fresh or thawed frozen young chicken
- Four tablespoons of Cajun Spice Rub
- Four to Six tablespoons of extra-virgin olive oil

Instructions

1. Set the breast-side chicken down on a cutting board.

2. In order to extract it, cut down both sides of the backbone using kitchen or poultry shears.

3. To flatten it, turn the chicken over and push tightly down on the breast. Loosen the skin of the breast, thigh, and drumstick gently and peel it down.

4. Apply the olive oil liberally under and on the skin. Season the chicken under the skin on both sides and directly over the flesh.

5. To allow the flavors time to absorb, cover the chicken in plastic wrap and let it sit for 3 hours in the refrigerator.

. For indirect cooking, customize your wood pellet smoker-grill and preheat it to 225°F using hickory, pecan pellets, or a mix.

. For an hour and a half, smoke the chicken.

. Increase the pit temperature to 375 ° F after one and a half hours at 225 ° F, and roast until the internal temperature at the thickest section of the breast exceeds 170 ° F and the thighs are at least 180 ° F.

. Until slicing, rest the chicken under a loose foil tent for 15 minutes.

4.3   Smoked Pork Tenderloins

Ready in about 2 hours (marination time excluded) | Servings-6 | Difficulty-Hard

Ingredients

Two pork tenderloins (one and a half to two pounds)

A quarter cup of Jan's Original Dry Rub or Pork Dry Rub

A quarter cup of roasted garlic–flavored extra-virgin olive oil

Instructions

1. Trim all of the meat's extra fat and silver skin.

2. Apply with olive oil and dust both sides of the tenderloins with the rub.3. For 2 to 4 hours, seal the seasoned tenderloins in plastic wrap and refrigerate.

3. For indirect cooking, set up your wood pellet smoker-grill and preheat it to 230°F utilizing hickory or apple pellets.

4. Take off the plastic wrap from the meat and place the smoker-grill probes of your wood pellet or a remote meat probe into the thickest section of each tenderloin. If your grill does not have meat probe capability or if you do not have a remote meat probe, use a wireless instant-read thermometer for internal temperature readings during the cooker.

5. Set the tenderloins directly on the grill and smoke them at 230 ° F for 45 minutes.

6. Increase the temperature of the pit to 350 ° F and finish cooking the tenderloins for around 45 more minutes until the interior temperature exceeds 145 ° F at the thickest stage.

7. Until cooking, rest the pork tenderloins under a thin foil tent for 10 minutes.

4.4   Pellet Grill Smokehouse Burger

Ready in about 1 hour 30 minutes | Servings-6 | Difficulty-Hard

Ingredients

- Two pounds of ground chuck

- One tablespoon of paprika

- One and a half teaspoons of kosher salt

- Six thick-cut bacon slices

- One tablespoon of soy sauce

- One medium-sized red onion

- Six Kaiser rolls

- Six tablespoons ketchup

- A quarter cup of Dijon mustard

- Two teaspoons of onion powder

- One and a half teaspoons of black pepper

- A quarter cup of unsalted butter

- One tablespoon of Worcestershire sauce

- Six sharp Cheddar cheese slices

- ¾ cup mayonnaise

- Hickory hardwood pellets

Instructions

1. In compliance with the manufacturer's guidance, fill a pellet jar with hardwood pellets into an electronic pellet grill. Set the temperature of the pellet grill to 415 °F, close the lid and preheat for 10 to 15 minutes.

2. In a big tub, blend the beef, paprika, mustard, garlic powder, onion powder, pepper and salt together. Form into six patties (4-inch-wide).

3. In a broad cast-iron or another heat-resistant pan, place the bacon and place it on the grill grate. Close the lid and grill for 25 to 30 minutes until the bacon is mostly crisp and most of the fat is made. Take the bacon out of the pan and drain it on paper towels. Drain skillet drippings; do not wipe clean skillet.

4. Melt the butter on the grill in a pan. To the skillet, add soy sauce and Worcestershire sauce, then mix to blend. Attach the onions to the skillet and position them on one side of the grill. Place the patties and shut the cover on the other side. Grill before a meat thermometer is placed from 130 ° F to 135 ° F in patty registers, 7 1/2 to 10 minutes per hand. Top the patties with slices of cheese, cover, and barbecue for 1 to 2 minutes before the cheese is melted. Put the buns on the grill, cut side down, and grill for around 1 minute until toasted.

5. Uniformly distributed mayonnaise and ketchup on sliced sides of buns. Place bun bottoms with patties, bacon, and onions; cover with tops, and serve immediately.

4.5 Roasted Leg of Lamb

Ready in about 2 hours 30 minutes (marination time excluded) |Servings-8| Difficulty-Hard

Ingredients

- Half cup of roasted garlic–flavored extra-virgin olive oil

- Three minced garlic cloves

- Two tablespoons of dried oregano

- Half teaspoon of black pepper

- One (Four pounds) boneless leg of lamb

- A quarter cup of dried parsley

- Two tablespoons of fresh-squeezed lemon juice or one tablespoon of lemon zest

- One tablespoon of dried rosemary

Instructions

1. Remove some netting from the lamb's leg. Trim off any wide bits of gristle, fat, and silver skin.

2. Mix the olive oil, garlic, parsley, lemon juice or zest, rosemary, oregano and pepper in a shallow dish.

3. On the inner and outer surfaces of the boneless leg of the lamb, add a spice rub.

4. To protect the boneless leg of lamb, use silicone food-grade cooking bands or butcher's twine. To build and retain the simple shape of the lamb, use bands or twine.

5. Cover the lamb loosely with plastic wrap and chill overnight to allow the meat to penetrate the seasonings.

6. Take the lamb from the fridge and let it stand for an hour at room temperature.

7. Use the pellets of choice to rig your wood pellet smoker-grill for indirect cooking and preheat it to 400 ° F.

8. Break the lamb's plastic wrap.

9. Insert the thickest portion of the lamb with your wood pellet smoker-grill meat probe or a remote meat probe. If your grill does not have meat probe capability or if you do not have a remote meat probe, use a wireless instant-read thermometer for internal temperature readings during the cooker. At 400 °F, roast the lamb until the internal temperature exceeds the ideal doneness at the thickest section.

10. Until cutting against the grain and cooking, rest the lamb under a loose foil tent for 10 minutes.

4.6   Teriyaki Smoked Drumsticks

Ready in about 2 hours 30 minutes (marination time excluded) |Servings-4| Difficulty-Hard

Ingredients

Three teaspoons of Poultry Seasoning

- Ten chicken drumsticks

- Three cups of teriyaki marinade and cooking sauce

  One teaspoon of garlic powder

Instructions

1. Mix the cooking sauce and marinade with the poultry seasoning and garlic powder in a medium bowl.

2. To facilitate marinade penetration, peel back the skin on the drumsticks.3. Place the drumsticks in a marinating pan or 1-gallon sealable plastic bag and pour over the drumsticks the marinade mixture. Overnight, refrigerate.

3. Rotate the morning chicken drumsticks.

4. Configure the indirect cooking of your wood pellet smoker grill.

5. To drain on a cooking sheet on your counter while the grill is preheating, replace the skin over the drumsticks and hang the drumsticks on a poultry leg-and-wing rack. If you don't own a poultry leg-and-wing rack, you can use paper towels to lightly pat the drumsticks dry.

6. Using hickory or maple pellets, preheat your wood pellet smoker-grill to 180°F.

7. Marinated chicken drumsticks should be smoked for 1 hour.

8. Increase the pit temperature to 350 ° F after an hour and cook the drumsticks for a further 30 to 45 minutes before the interior temperature of the thickest section of the drumsticks exceeds 180 ° F.

9. Before serving, rest the chicken drumsticks under a loose foil tent for 15 minutes.

4.7   Applewood Walnut-Crusted Rack of Lamb

Ready in about 2 hours (marination time excluded) |Servings-4| Difficulty-Hard

Ingredients

- Two minced garlic cloves
- Half teaspoon of kosher salt
- Half teaspoon of rosemary
- One cup of crushed walnuts
- Three tablespoons of Dijon mustard
- Half teaspoon of garlic powder
- Half teaspoon of black pepper
- One rack of lamb (one to two pounds)

Instructions

1. In a small bowl, combine the garlic, mustard, garlic powder, pepper, salt, and rosemary together.

2. Spread evenly on all sides of the lamb with the seasoning mix and sprinkle with the crushed walnuts. To stick the nuts to the meat, press the walnuts lightly with your hand.

3. Wrap the walnut-crusted lamb rack loosely with plastic wrap and cool overnight to allow the meat to penetrate the seasonings.

4. To allow it to reach room temperature, remove the walnut-crusted rack of lamb from the refrigerator and let it relax for 30 minutes.

. For indirect cooking, configure your wood pellet smoker-grill and preheat it to 225 ° F using apple pellets.

. Put the bone-side lamb rack down directly on the grill.

. Smoke at 225 ° F until the thickest part of the lamb rack, measured with a digital instant-read thermometer, reaches the desired internal temperature as you are near the times listed in the chart.

. Before serving, rest the lamb under a loose foil tent for 5 minutes.

4.8   Hot-Smoked Teriyaki Tuna

Ready in about 9 hours 10 minutes | Servings-4 | Difficulty-Hard

Ingredients

Two cups of Mr. Yoshida's Traditional Teriyaki Marinade and Cooking Sauce

Two (10-ounce) fresh tuna steaks

Instructions

. Slice the tuna into slices that are uniformly thick, about 2 inches thick.

2. Place the tuna slices along with the marinade in a 1-gallon sealable plastic bag and place it in a shallow baking dish in case of a leak. Let the tuna rotate every hour and sit in the refrigerator for 3 hours.

3. Remove the tuna from the marinade after 3 hours and lightly pat it dry with a paper towel.

4. Enable the tuna to air-dry for 2 to 4 hours in the refrigerator, uncovered, until pellicles form.

5. For indirect cooking, configure your wood pellet smoker-grill and preheat it to 180 ° F using alder pellets.

6. On a Teflon-coated fiberglass mat or directly on the grill grates, place the tuna pieces, and smoke the tuna for an hour.

7. Increase the temperature of the pit to 250°F after 1 hour. Cook for another 1 hour until the internal temperature reaches 145 degrees F.

8. Remove the tuna from the grill and leave to rest before serving for 10 minutes.

4.9   Baked Fresh Wild Sockeye Salmon

Ready in about 40 minutes | Servings-6 | Difficulty-Moderate

Ingredients

- Two fresh wild sockeye salmon fillets
- 3/4 teaspoon of Old Bay seasoning
- Two teaspoons of Seafood Seasoning

Instructions

1. Rinse the salmon fillets with cool water and wipe them dry with a paper towel.

2. Lightly brush the fillets with the seasonings.

3. Customize your wood pellet smoker-grill for indirect cooking and preheat to 400°F using some pellets.

4. Lay the skin-side down of salmon on a Teflon-coated fiberglass mat or directly on the grill grates.

5. Bake the salmon for 15 to 20 minutes before the internal temperature exceeds 140°F, and/or the meat flakes easily with a fork.

6. Rest the salmon for 5 minutes before eating.

4.10   Bacon Cordon Bleu

Ready in about 3 hours 15 minutes | Servings-6 | Difficulty-Hard

Ingredients

- Three large skinless and butterflied boneless chicken breasts
- Three tablespoons of Jan's Original Dry Rub or Poultry Seasoning

Twelve slices of provolone cheese

Twenty-four bacon slices

Three tablespoons of roasted garlic–flavored extra-virgin olive oil

Twelve slices of black forest ham

Instructions

. Weave four bacon slices closely together, leaving extra room at the ends. Alternate bacon slices are interlocked by the bacon weave and used to wind around the chicken cordon bleu.

. Spritz or brush two thin chicken breast fillets on both sides with olive oil.

. With the seasoning, clean all sides of the chicken breast fillets.

. On the bacon weave, plate one seasoned chicken fillet and finish with one slice of each ham and Provolone cheese.

. Using another chicken fillet, ham, and cheese, repeat the operation. Fold in half the chicken, ham and cheese.

. To cover the chicken cordon blue fully, overlap the bacon strips from opposite ends.

. To keep the bacon strips in place, use silicone food-grade cooking bands, butcher's twine, or toothpicks.

. For the leftover chicken breasts and ingredients, repeat the procedure.

. Configure your wood pellet smoker-grill with apple or cherry pellets for indirect cooking and preheating for smoking (180 ° F to 200 ° F).

10. For 1 hour, smoke the bacon cordon bleu.

11. Increase the pit temperature to 350°F after smoking for an hour.

12. If the internal temperature exceeds 165 ° F and the bacon is crisp, the bacon cordon bleu is cooked.

13. Until eating, rest under a loose foil tent for 15 minutes.

4.11 Pulled Hickory-smoked Pork Butts

Ready in about 11 hours (marination time excluded) |Servings-20 or more| Difficulty-Hard

Ingredients

- Two (10-pound) boneless pork butts, vacuum-packed or fresh
- 3/4 cup of Pork Dry Rub, Jan's Original Dry Rub or your favorite pork rub
- One cup of roasted garlic–flavored extra-virgin olive oil

Instructions

1. If you see fit, take off the fat cap and any readily accessible broad portions of surplus fat from each pork ass. Some tend to reduce the fat cap to a quarter of an inch or keep the whole fat cap on because they assume that when they roast, the melting fat bastes the butts. In areas protected by fat, this process prevents the development of bark.

2. Break each butt of pork in half. To keep the meat intact through cooking and handling, use silicone food-grade cooking bands or butcher's twine.

3. Rub the oil over all the sides of each pork ass. Sprinkle a liberal sum of the rub with each pork butt and pat it with your fist.

4. The seasoned boneless pork butts are individually double-wrapped in plastic wrap and refrigerated overnight.

5. For indirect cooking, set up your wood pellet smoker-grill and preheat it to 225 ° F utilizing hickory pellets.

6. Takedown the pork butts from the refrigerator and, when preheating your wood pellet smoker-grill, remove the plastic wrap.

7. There's no need for pork butts to totally hit room temperature. In the thickest section of one or more pork butts, place your wood pellet smoker-grill meat

probes or a remote meat probe. If your grill does not have meat probe capability or you do not possess a remote meat probe, for internal temperature measurements, use an instant-read wireless thermometer during the cook.3. Smoke the butts of pork for 3 hours.

8. Increase the pit temperature to 350 °F after 3 hours and cook before the butts' internal temperature exceeds 160 °F.

9. Take the butts of pork from the barbecue and cover each one in heavy-duty aluminum foil twice. Take caution to ensure that when you double-wrap them, you hold the meat probes in the butts.

10. To your 350°F pellet smoker-grill, return the wrapped pork butts.

11. Until the internal temperature of the pork butts exceeds 200 ° to 205 ° F, continue cooking the foil-wrapped pork butts.

12. Prior to pulling and cooking, remove the pork butts and FTC for 3 to 4 hours.

13. Using your preferred pulling tool, pull the smoked pork butts into little succulent shreds.

14. Mix the pulled pork butts with any remaining liquid if you'd like. On a fresh-baked roll topped with coleslaw, serve the pulled pork with barbecue sauce or serve the pulled pork with condiments such as lettuce, tomato, red onion, mayo, horseradish and cheese.

4.12   Pellet Grill Pork Loin with Salsa Verde

Ready in about 1 hour 15 minutes | Servings-8 | Difficulty-Hard

Ingredients

Salsa Verde

- Half cup of finely chopped shallots
- ⅓ cup chopped fresh cilantro

- One tablespoon of chopped capers
- One teaspoon of grated garlic
- One teaspoon of kosher salt
- Four chopped anchovy fillets
- One cup of olive oil
- ⅓ cup of chopped fresh flat-leaf parsley
- A quarter cup of chopped fresh dill
- One teaspoon of grated lemon zest
- One teaspoon of grated fresh ginger
- ¾ teaspoon crushed red pepper

Pork Loin

- Two teaspoons of kosher salt
- Three tablespoons of fresh lemon juice
- Three and a half pounds boneless
- One teaspoon of black pepper

Instructions

1. Prepare Salsa Verde: In a medium dish, stir together all the ingredients. Just set aside.

2. Prepare the Pork Loin: Fill a pellet jar with hardwood pellets on an electric pellet grill as instructed by the maker. Set the temperature of the pellet grill to 350 °F, close the lid and preheat for 10 to 15 minutes. Sprinkle the pork with salt and pepper all around.

3. Place the pork on the grill, close the lid, and grill on both sides until lightly browned, about 7 1/2 minutes per side. Spin the pork up with the fat cap if necessary, and finish with half the Salsa Verde. Cover the lid and barbecue for 25

to 30 minutes before a meat thermometer inserted into the thickest part registers 140 ° F.

. Take the pork off the grill and let it sit for 15 minutes before slicing. Mix the lemon juice and the remaining Salsa Verde together, and spoon over the sliced pork.

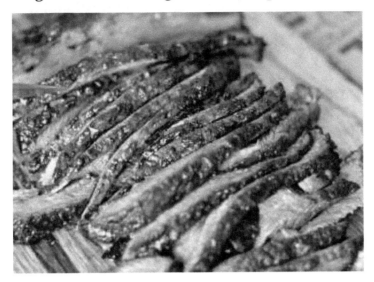

Chapter 5-Dinner Recipes

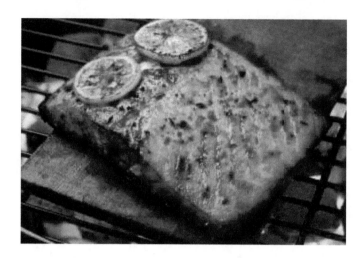

5.1   Roasted Tuscan Thighs

Ready in about 1 hour and 45 minutes (marination time excluded) | Servings-4 | Difficulty-Hard

Ingredients

- Eight chicken thighs
- Three teaspoons of Tuscan Seasoning or any Tuscan seasoning, per thigh
- Three tablespoons of roasted garlic–flavored extra-virgin olive oil

Instructions

1. Trim any extra skin from the chicken thighs to prepare for shrinkage, preserving a quarter of an inch.

2. Peel back the skin gently to clear any large fat deposits under the skin and on the back of the leg.

3. Apply the olive oil gently on and under the skin and back of the thighs. Season with Tuscan seasoning on and below the surface and back of the thighs.

4. To allow the flavors time to absorb before roasting, seal the chicken thighs in plastic wrap and refrigerate for 1 to 2 hours.

. Configure your wood pellet smoker-grill for indirect cooking and use some pellets to preheat to 375 ° F.

. Roast the chicken thighs for 40 to 60 minutes, depending on your wood pellet smoker-grill, before the internal temperature at the thickest section of the thighs exceeds 180 ° F. Until eating, rest the roasted Tuscan thighs under a loose foil tent for 15 minutes.

5.2   Smoked Bone-In Turkey Breast

Ready in about 5 hours | Servings-6 to 8 | Difficulty-Hard

Ingredients

One (eight to ten pound) bone-in turkey breast

Five tablespoons of Jan's Original Dry Rub or Poultry Seasoning
Six tablespoons of extra-virgin olive oil

Instructions

1. Trim away some extra turkey breast fat and skin.

2. Separate the skin from the breast cautiously, keeping the skin preserved. Within the breast hollow, under the skin and on the skin, apply the olive oil.

3. Season the breast cavity generously with rub or seasoning, under the surface, and on the skin.

4. Place the turkey breast, breast-side up, in a V-rack for better handling or directly on the grill grates.

5. Enable the turkey breast on your kitchen countertop to rest at room temperature when preheating your wood pellet smoker barbecue.

6. For indirect cooking, set your wood pellet smoker-grill and preheat it to 225°F utilizing hickory or pecan pellets.

7. For 2 hours, smoke the bone-in turkey breast at 225 °F on the V-rack or directly on the grill grates.

8. Elevate the temperature of the pit to 325 ° F after 2 hours of hickory smoke. Roast until an internal temperature of 170 ° F hits the thickest section of the turkey breast, and the juices run clear.

9. Before cutting against the grain, rest the hickory-smoked turkey breast under a loose foil tent for 20 minutes.

5.3   Crab-Stuffed Lemon Cornish Hens

Ready in about 2 hours 15 minutes (marination time excluded) |Servings-2 to 4| Difficulty-Hard

Ingredients

- Two Cornish hens
- Four tablespoons of Pete's Western Rub or any poultry rub
- One halved lemon
- Two cups of Crabmeat Stuffing

Instructions

1. Rinse the hens inside and out vigorously and pat off. Loosen the breast and leg skin cautiously. Under and on the skin and inside the cavity, rub the lemon. Rub the Western Pete's Rub under and on the skin of the breast and thigh. Return the skin to its original location cautiously.

2. To allow the flavors time to mature, seal the Cornish hens in plastic wrap and refrigerate for 2 to 3 hours.

3. Prepare according to the guidelines for the Crabmeat Stuffing. Before stuffing the hens, make sure it has cooled absolutely. Stuff each hen cavity loosely with the crab stuffing.

. To hold the stuffing in, bind the Cornish hen legs together with butcher's twine.

. Set your wood pellet smoker-grill with some pellets for indirect cooking and preheat to 375 ° F.

. Place the stuffed hens inside a baking dish on a shelf. If you don't have a rack small enough to match, you may also directly position the hens in the baking bowl.

. The hens are roasted at 375 ° F until the internal temperature exceeds 170 ° F at the thickest section of the breast, the thighs exceed 180 ° F, and the juices run clear.

. To see if it has hit a temperature of 165°F, measure the crabmeat stuffing.

. Until eating, rest the roasted hens under a loose foil tent for 15 minutes.

5.4   Double-Smoked Ham

Ready in about 2 hours | Servings-8 to 12 | Difficulty-Hard

Ingredients

One (ten pounds) applewood-smoked, boneless, fully cooked, ready-to-eat ham or bone-in smoked ham

Instructions

1. Take the ham from its wrapping and allow to rest for 30 minutes at room temperature.

2. Depending on what kind of wood was used for the initial smoking, customize your wood pellet smoker-grill for indirect cooking and preheat it to 180°F using apple or hickory pellets.

3. Directly put the ham on the grill grates and smoke the ham at 180°F for 1 hour.

4. Elevate the pit temperature to 350 ° F after an hour.

5. Cook the ham for around one and a half to 2 more hours before the internal temperature exceeds 140 ° F.

6. Until cutting against the grain, cut the ham and cover it in foil for 15 minutes.

5.5   Easy No-Fail Pellet Smoker Ribs

Ready in about 6 hours | Servings-4 | Difficulty-Hard

Ingredients

- Two racks of Baby Back or Spare Ribs
- BBQ Rib Rub

Instructions

1. Begin preheating your pellet smoker at 225 degrees F as you are prepping the ribs. Following the directions and start-up procedure of your pellet smoker brand is critical.

2. Ribs normally come on the underside of the rack with a thin coat of rough muscle. This is known as the silver skin, and it has to be extracted so that the meat can penetrate the seasonings.

3. On a sheet tray, put the ribs and apply around 2-3 tablespoons of rib rub each hand. You don't want to coat them fully to make any of the meat peek in.

4. You may position the rack (or two racks) directly on the grates until the smoker is preheated and let them burn. Leave them for at least 4 hours alone. The shorter you open your barbecue, the shorter your cooking period would be. You ought to keep an eye on the temperature of the smoker to ensure it remains where it is placed.

5. It will take 4 or 5 hours for a rack of baby back ribs to cook, and it will take 6 to 7 hours for spare ribs.

6. Pick up the ribs with tongs at the end of the cooking time, and if the bark splits and the ribs are nearly cut in two, they are cooked. Keep on smoking if not.

7. Add sauce to the BBQ. You should cover them with a thin film of your preferred BBQ sauce when the ribs are about to come out of the smoker (they passed the bending test). For 30 more minutes, keep them on the smoker at 225 degrees F so that the sauce will caramelize.

5.6 Texas-Style Brisket Flat

Ready in about 10 hours 45 minutes | Servings-8 to 10 | Difficulty-Hard

Ingredients

- Six and a Half pound beef brisket flat
- Half cup of Texas-Style Brisket Rub or your favorite brisket rub
- Half cup of roasted garlic–flavored extra-virgin olive oil

Instructions

1. Trim the brisket's fat cap off and extract any silver skin.2. Rub the trimmed meat with olive oil on both ends.

2. Apply the rub on both sides of the brisket, making sure that the rub is thoroughly coated.

3. Double-cover the brisket in plastic wrap and refrigerate overnight to reach the beef with the rub, or you can quickly sear the brisket if you choose.

4. Take the brisket from the fridge and put the smoker-grill wood pellet or a remote meat probe into the thickest portion of the meat. If you don't have a meat probe, capabilities or a remote meat probe on your barbecue, then use an instant-read optical thermometer for internal temperature readings during the cooker.

5. For indirect cooking, set up your wood pellet smoker-grill and preheat it to 250 ° F using mesquite or oak pellets.

6. At 250°F, smoke the brisket before the inner temperature exceeds 160°F (about 4 hours).

7. Remove the grill from the brisket, double-wrap it in heavy-duty aluminum foil, make sure the meat probe is left in place, and add it to the grill for smokers.

8. Increase the temperature of the pit to 325 ° F, then cook the brisket for another 2 hours before the internal temperature exceeds 205 ° F.

9. The foiled brisket is cut, wrapped in a cloth, and put in a cooler. Let sit 2 to 4 hours in the cooler before slicing against the grain and serving.

5.7   Hickory-Smoked Prime Rib of Pork

Ready in about 4 hours 15 minutes (marination time excluded) | Servings-6 | Difficulty-Hard

Ingredients

- One (Five pounds) rack of pork, about six ribs
- Six tablespoons of Jan's Original Dry Rub, Pork Dry Rub or your favorite pork roast rub
- A quarter cup of roasted garlic–flavored extra-virgin olive oil

Instructions

1. Trim the fat cap and silver skin off the pork rack. A rack of pork has a membrane on the bones, much like a slice of ribs. Using a spoon handle under the bone membrane to loosen the membrane from the bones so you can reach the membrane with a paper towel to take it off.

2. On both sides of the beef, rub the olive oil liberally. Season with the seasoning, coating the beef on both sides. 3. The seasoned rack of pork is double covered in plastic wrap and refrigerated for 2 to 4 hours or overnight.

3. Take the seasoned pork rack from the refrigerator and let it rest for 30 minutes before cooking at room temperature.

. For indirect cooking, set up your wood pellet smoker-grill and preheat it to 225 ° F utilizing hickory pellets.

. Insert into the thickest portion of the rack of pork the wood pellet smoker-grill meat probe or a remote meat probe. Using an instant-read wireless thermometer while cooking for internal temperature readings if your grill does not have meat probe capability or you do not have a remote meat probe.

. Set the rib-side of the rack down directly on the grill grates.

. For 3 to 3 and a half hours, smoke the pork rack before the internal temperature exceeds 140 ° F.

. Remove from the smoker's meat and let it rest 15 minutes before being carved under a loose foil tent.

5.8   Meaty Chuck Short Ribs

Ready in about 6 hours 35 minutes | Servings- 2 to 4 | Difficulty-Hard

Ingredients

English-cut 4-bone slab beef chuck short ribs

Three to five tablespoons of Pete's Western Rub

Three to four tablespoons of yellow mustard or extra-virgin olive oil

Instructions

1. Remove some silver skin by trimming the fat cap off the ribs, leaving a quarter of an inch of fat.

2. To season the meat correctly by working a spoon handle under the membrane to get a slice raised, separate the membrane from the bones. To catch the membrane, use a paper towel to take it off the bones.

3. Slather both sides of the short rib slab with mustard or olive oil. With the rub, season liberally on both edges.

4. Using mesquite or hickory pellets, set up your wood pellet smoker-grill for indirect heat and preheat to 225 ° F.

5. In the thickest section of the slab of ribs, place your wood pellet smoker-grill or a remote meat probe. If your grill does not have meat probe capability or you do not have a remote meat probe, then for internal temperature measurements, use an instant-read optical thermometer during the cooker.

6. On the grill, put the short ribs bone-side down and smoke for 5 hours at 225 ° F.

7. If the ribs have not achieved an internal temperature of at least 195 ° F after 5 hours, so the pit temperature can rise to 250 ° F before the inner temperature exceeds 195 °F to 205 ° F.

8. Until eating, rest the smoked short ribs under a loose foil tent for 15 minutes.

5.9 Roasted Duck à l' Orange

Ready in about 3 hours and 50 minutes | Servings-3 to 4 | Difficulty-Hard

Ingredients

- One (Five to six-pound) frozen Long Island, Peking, or Canadian duck

- One large orange, cut into wedges

- Half small red onion, quartered

- Three tablespoons of Pete's Western Rub or Poultry Seasoning, divided

- Three celery stalks, chopped into large chunks

For the sauce

- Two cups of orange juice

- Two tablespoons of orange marmalade

- Three teaspoons of grated fresh ginger

- Two tablespoons of soy sauce

- Two tablespoons of honey

Instructions

1. Remove any giblets from the duck's cavity and neck and keep or dispose of them for some purpose. With a paper towel, clean the duck and pat it off.

2. From the tail, spine, and cavity section, trim any extra fat. Using the tip of a sharp paring knife to poke the duck skin all over to make sure that it does not reach the duck meat to promote the removal of the fat layer under the flesh.

3. With one tablespoon of rub or seasoning, season the interior of the cavity.

4. With the remaining rub or seasoning, season the outside of the duck.

5. Stuff the space with orange wedges, celery, and onion. To aid hold the stuffing in, bind the duck legs together with butcher's twine. On a small rack in a shallow roasting pan, put the duck breast-side up.

6. Mix the ingredients in a saucepan over low heat to create the sauce and boil until the sauce thickens and is syrupy.

7. Enable to cool and put aside.

8. Set up your wood pellet smoker-grill for indirect cooking and use some pellets to preheat it to 350 ° F.

9. Roast the duck for 2 hours at 350°F.

10. Brush the duck liberally with the orange sauce after 2 hours.

11. Roast the orange-glazed duck for another 30 minutes and check that the internal temperature exceeds 165 °F at the thickest section of the legs.

12. Until cooking, rest the duck under a loose foil tent for 20 minutes.

13. Throw out the orange wedges, onion and celery. Quarter the duck with shears of poultry and serve.

5.10   Peteizza Meatloaf

Ready in about 3 hours 30 minutes | Servings-8 | Difficulty-Hard

Ingredients

For meatloaf

- Two large eggs
- One cup of Italian bread crumbs
- Half teaspoon of seasoned salt
- One pound pork sausage
- One pound ground beef
- Half teaspoon of garlic salt
- Half teaspoon of ground pepper
- Half teaspoon of granulated garlic
- Half cup of pizza sauce, plus an additional half cup for serving

For stuffing

- Two tablespoons of extra-virgin olive oil
- 2/3 cup of sliced green bell pepper
- A pinch of salt and black pepper
- Three ounces of sliced pepperoni sausage
- One cup of sliced portobello mushrooms
- 2/3 cup of sliced red onion
- Half cup of sliced red bell pepper
- Two cups of shredded mozzarella cheese
- Two cups of shredded cheddar or Jack cheese

Instructions

1. Combine the meatloaf components thoroughly with your hands in a wide bowl to achieve maximum performance.

. Heat the olive oil over medium-high heat in a medium skillet and sauté the mushrooms, green bell pepper, red onion and red bell pepper until the vegetables are al dente for about 2 minutes. With a pinch of salt and black pepper, season the vegetables. Then set it aside.

. Flatten the meatloaf into a 3/8-inch-thick rectangle on parchment paper. Range the sautéed vegetables thinly over the meat. Cover the mozzarella with the veggies, accompanied by the cheddar or Jack. Cover the pepperoni with the cheese.

. Using the parchment paper to roll the meatloaf, ensuring the ends and all seams are covered.

. Set up your wood pellet-smoker grill for indirect heat and use oak pellets or a mix to preheat it to 225 ° F.

. Smoke a meatloaf with stuffed pizza for 1 hour.

. Increase the pit temperature to 350 °F after an hour, and cook until the stuffed pizza meatloaf's internal temperature exceeds 170 °F.

. Cover the meatloaf with the leftover half cup of pizza sauce and allow to stand for 15 minutes under a loose foiled tent before eating.

5.11   Shrimp-Stuffed Tilapia

Ready in about 1 hour 10 minutes | Servings-5 | Difficulty-Moderate

Ingredients

- Two tablespoons of extra-virgin olive oil

- One and a half teaspoons of Seafood Seasoning or Old Bay seasoning

- Five (four to six-ounce) fresh farmed tilapia fillets

- One and a half teaspoons of smoked paprika

For the shrimp Stuffing

- One tablespoon of salted butter

- One cup of Italian bread crumbs

- One large egg, beaten

- One and a half teaspoons of Fagundes Famous Seasoning or salt and pepper

- One pound of cooked, peeled, deveined, tail-off shrimp

- One cup of finely diced red onion

- Half cup of mayonnaise

- Two teaspoons of fresh chopped parsley or dried parsley

Instructions

1. Get the shrimp stuffing packed. To cut the shrimp finely, use a food processor, salsa maker, or knife.

2. Melt the butter and sauté the red onion in a small skillet over medium-high heat until it is translucent around 3 minutes. Put aside to let the room temperature cool.

3. In a wide cup, mix the shrimp, the cooled sautéed onion and the remaining ingredients.

4. Cover the shrimp stuffing and refrigerate it before ready to use. Shrimp stuffing can be used within two days.

5. With olive oil, rub all sides of the fillets.

6. On the backside of each filet, spoon 1/3 cup of the stuffing. Reddish stripping is on the backside of the tilapia fillet.

7. On the lower half of the fillet, flatten out the stuffing. Fold the tilapia in half and make careful to keep the fish in place with two or more toothpicks.

8. With the smoked paprika and seafood seasoning or Old Bay seasoning, dust each fillet.

9. Configure your wood pellet smoker-grill for indirect cooking and use any pellets to preheat it to 400 °F.

10. On a nonstick grilling tray, position the stuffed fillets.

11. Bake the tilapia for 30 to 45 minutes, or until the fish quickly flakes and hits an internal temperature of 145°F.

12. Rest the fish for 5 minutes before serving.

5.12 Easy Smoked Chicken Breasts

Ready in about 45 minutes | Servings-4 | Difficulty-Moderate

Ingredients

- One tablespoon of Olive Oil

- Two tablespoons of Turbinado Sugar

- Two tablespoons of Paprika

- One teaspoon of Black Pepper

- Two tablespoons of garlic powder

- Four Skinless Chicken Breasts Large Boneless

- Two tablespoons of Brown sugar

- One teaspoon of Celery Seed

- Two tablespoons of Kosher salt

- One teaspoon of Cayenne Pepper

- Two tablespoons onion powder

Instructions

1. Mix all the dried ingredients together in a tub.

2. On both sides, pat the chicken breasts to dry and drizzle each side with a little olive oil.

3. Sprinkle the rub liberally on top of the chicken breasts. Enable 15 minutes, or up to 30 minutes, to sit in the fridge (place plastic wrap over the top if over 15 minutes of rest time.)

4. Hot a cigarette smoker (use the super smoke on Traeger) with the lid opened for 5 minutes. Increase the heat to 350 degrees and, as it warms up, shut the cover for 15 minutes.

5. Place the chicken on the grill, spiced side down, and season the underside of the chicken liberally. Cook with the lid closed for 12-13 minutes.

6. Switch over the chicken and cook at 165-170 degrees for another 10-12 minutes or until finished.

7. Take the chicken from the grill and lay a cutting board with foil over the end. Prior to slicing, let the chicken rest for 3-5 minutes.

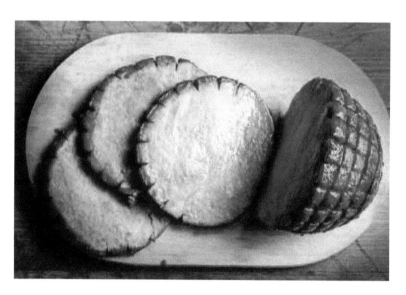

Conclusion

To conclude, the wood pellet smoker grill is scrumptious, pleasant and clean, unmatched by barbecue or gas grills. The smoke composition is milder than you may be accustomed to from other cigarettes. They produce the flexibility and advantages of a convection oven due to their architecture. Smoker-grills with wood pellets is safe and easy to work.

In the 1990s, wood pellet smoker-grills were first launched by a small business named Traeger Grills in Oregon.

Only after Traeger's initial patent expired did the business expand by leaps and bounds. More and more people have been introduced to the amazing, mouth-watering food from a wood pellet smoker-grill, but only two firms created wood pellet smoker-grills as recently as 2008: Traeger and its competitor MAK, both located in Oregon. Currently, a wide variety of retailers from small BBQ stores, grocery stores, produce stores, hardware stores, huge box stores, online outlets, and direct from the retailer hold more than twenty brands of incredible wood pellet smoker-grill makers.

In the present era, it is a must in every household that loves to have a barbeque meal at weekends.

This book is a guide that provides us with information regarding the wood pellet smoker grill and provides the recipes for starting up with grilling.

We hope that all your queries are clear with regards to wood Pellet Smoker Grill cooking.

Thank you and good luck!

The Ultimate Electric Smoker Cookbook

25+ Recipes and 13 Tricks to Smoke Just Everything

By

Chef Carlo Leone

Table of Contents

Introduction

Barbeque is a huge part of American cuisine and culture. Smoked meats are a favorite among the entire country. Barbeque becomes a must in summers when families get together on long summer weekends, spending quality time together. Nowadays, this has become nearly impossible because of the tough work-life balance and people's desire to grab an easy bite. No one has the time and energy to set up the conventional-style barbeque. Some people might still be up for doing all the hard work, but most of the population would welcome a quick and easy way to enjoy the smoked flavors of barbequed meat.

Technology has made this difficult feat possible. Electric Smokers are a great appliance that makes our job simple. There was a time when you had to spend the whole day in front of the Smoker to prepare a good smoked steak. With the electric Smoker, you can enjoy the authentic flavor of barbeque with little effort. What the electric Smoker does is that it uses the same conventional method for cooking, but you do not have to do all the hard work manually; the electric Smoker does it for you. All you must do is prepare the meat, set up the electric Smoker, pour in some water in the water tray, throw in some wood chips, turn up the heat according to your needs and set the timer.

Meanwhile, you go about your business, run your errands, have a chat with your friends, and your yummy food is being prepared all on its own. You do not need to worry about temperature control or about managing the charcoal. The electric Smoker fits best with the modern way of life. Another huge advantage of electric smokers, apart from them being super easy to operate, is that they are easy to clean. They are just like little closets which have removable racks. You can remove every part, clean it, and place it back. Also, because the temperature and the smoke can be regulated and controlled, the result is perfect most of the time. The chances for mishaps are rare, unlike the traditional style, where things can get tricky quite often.

If you want to enjoy a delicious barbeque with the least effort, you should read on about this amazing appliance, making you a pro at family barbeques in no time. Enjoy reading!

485

Chapter 1: What is an Electric Smoker?

In this chapter, the basic introduction and working of the electric Smoker will be discussed. Before understanding the Electric Smoker, we must first understand the meaning of the cooking method that the Electric Smoker uses.

This technique is known as 'Smoking,' and it is a type of process related to barbeque.

1.1. What is Smoking?

Smoking is a more specialized and extreme type of barbecuing. You will be using the smoke from different types of aromatic wood chips or wood chunks in smoking. You may use wood chips of cherry, apple, hickory, mesquite, and many others. These impart their unique flavor and smoky aroma to the meat being smoked.

The process of smoking takes longer than barbecuing. The temperature is also lower than barbecue. The temperature is usually set between 125 to 175°F. The temperature is kept lower because if the temperature is turned up, then the meat's outer layer will be cooked and will not allow the smoke to reach throughout the meat and impart its rich aroma and taste.

Smoking is an advanced technique, and it required a much longer time for food preparation than grilling and normal barbeque. This method also requires a maximum amount of expertise to understand the texture of different types of meat and how they will be perfectly smoked.

1.2 The Electric Smoker

An electric smoker is a cooking appliance that is used outside. Smoking is an advanced type of variation of barbecue. The electric Smoker uses an electric source and heating rods to produce heat for cooking and smoking. The conventional way to smoke is to burn charcoal to produce the required heat, but the electric Smoker is easier to use and simple to operate. The whole process is cleaner as compared to the conventional style. The body of the electric Smoker is either made of stainless steel or cast iron.

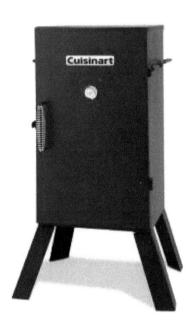

(An electric smoker)

There are numerous different types of electric smokers available in the market. You have an option to choose a smoker that is according to your requirements. Different models vary in their specific features, size, number of cooking racks present, temperature control features, number of cycles, preheat options, keep warm option, manual settings, automatic settings, digital displays, and control panels.

Sometimes variety can also overwhelm a buyer. To buy an electric smoker, it is recommended to first determine your requirements and then research the market too but the proper kind of Smoker for yourself. In the following pages, you will also find guidelines to help you decide whether you even need an electric smoker or not. Before that, we will briefly discuss the common features present in almost all electric smokers.

1.3 Working of an Electric Smoker

Normally, when you see an electric smoker, it looks like a cabinet; it is quite efficient in smoking the meat with relatively few components. The basic heating function is that the electric rods heat the entire cooking chamber, and the heated air is spread throughout the chamber. This causes the meat to cook by convection. There are six basic components of the electric Smoker:

- Cooking Chamber
- Woodchip tray
- Electric Heating rods or other heating elements
- Racks or grills to place the meat.
- Water Pan

1.3.1 Cooking Chamber

Like the gas smokers and the charcoal smokers, the electric smokers also have a vertical alignment. The space designated for cooking is at the top. The electric heating rods are placed at the bottom of the cooking chamber. Above the heating, rods are the grills, wood chips drawer and the water pan.

1.3.2 Electric Heating Rods:

The electric rods are placed at the base of the electric Smoker. They are the main source of heat for cooking. Some models of the electric Smoker have one heating rod, and some have more than one rods. This depends on the shape and size of the electric Smoker.

1.3.3   Wood Chip Tray

This is a specific space or tray provided above the electric rods to place the wood chips or wood chunks within the heating chamber. When the woodchips burn slowly, they cause smoke, which spreads within the cooking chamber and surrounds the meat. This smoke gives the meat a smoky and rich flavor. The woodchip tray is sometimes called the firebox as well.

Different types of hardwood are available to put in the electric Smoker. You can use various wood chips and chunks of mesquite, oak, alder, apple, cherry, maple, and hickory.

1.3.4   Water Pan

This is like a slightly deep pan or tray, fixed like a rack in the electric Smoker. Before starting the Smoker, this tray is filled with cold water. The main function is that when the heating rods are turned on, this cold water keeps the temperature from rising quickly inside the heating chamber. The other function is that steam is created when the water is heated up to a boiling point, which helps cook the meat. The steam helps the convection cooking process.

1.3.5   Grills or Racks

Above the water, the tray has placed the racks or grills. These are made of stainless steel. The food is placed on these for cooking. You can put the meat directly on the grill, or you can use heatproof skillets or barbecue utensils.

1.3.6   Vents and Dampers

the vents are usually placed at the top part of the electric Smoker. When the Smoker's temperature gets too high, the vents are opened to release some hot air and bring the temperature down.

The dampers are there for exactly the opposite reason. They are placed at the bottom part of the electric Smoker. When you open the dampers, oxygen enters the cooking chamber. The flames of the woodchips feed on this oxygen and increase the temperature inside the chamber.

Chapter 2. Why buy an Electric Smoker?

If you are someone who loves barbecue and the rich flavor of smoked meat, you might have thought about investing in an electric smoker. Even though you think about it, you are not quite sure whether you should invest in an electric smoker or not. You cannot deny that it is an expensive appliance and if you only occasionally barbecue, this appliance is not for you. Having said that, if you enjoy preparing delicious barbecue now and then, you might want to consider the electric Smoker. Using an electric smoker is easier than the conventional barbeque method, and it is much easier to clean. If you enjoy the smoky aroma and taste in each bite of meat, you might want to ditch the conventional method and adopt electric smoking. This is perfect for that tender, aromatic, and rich smoke flavor. However, you must be warned against the prejudice that surrounds electric smokers. The die-heart conventional barbecue community may argue that the electric Smoker does not give off the meat's authentic smoky flavor. You may agree or not to this argument but investing in an electric smoker would be your best bet if you are new to smoking.

In this chapter, we will discuss the top five reasons to buy an electric smoker. The five arguments in favor of the electric Smoker are:

- Perfect choice for beginners
- The cost
- The easy usage
- You can set it up where conventional barbeque grills might not be allowed.
- The option to cold smoke

2.1. Perfect Choice for Beginners

Investing in an electric smoker is a safe choice for beginners. Smoking is a slightly tricky technique. If you go by the conventional way, it might take you longer to learn and maybe you might give up early on. With the electric Smoker, you can operate it with ease. The temperature and length of cooking can be regulated, and the best part is that the results are almost always perfect. Getting perfect results in cooking is a huge plus because it further motivates you.

Using the electric Smoker, you can learn and become familiar with the basic method and technique involved. Once you have learned the basics, you can either move on to the more conventional style or even decide to stick to the electric Smoker.

2.2. The Cost

If you survey the market, you will find that electric smokers are cheaper than their conventional counterparts. When you look closely, the amount of food they can cook in one session is quite commendable. Another reason the electric Smoker might feel more appealing is that it needs only a one-time setup. After the initial setup, no maintenance is required. Cleaning is easy. To operate is easy. So, in the long run, this seems to be a better investment.

2.3. The Easy Usage

If you see the conventional system of smoking and barbecue, you have a lot to manage. You must control the optimum temperature, need the expertise to light the charcoal, maintain airflow to keep a smooth temperature and manage any temperature spikes or accidents during the entire procedure. In short, you will be on your toes the whole time. Now, flip the situation to the electric Smoker. You prepare your food items, place them on the grills, fill in the water tray, put them in the woodchips, and turn on the heating rods. You can even set the time. It is as easy as this. In case you are hosting a few people over, you will have plenty of time to set up the area and interact with your guests.

2.4. Can Carry the Electric Smoker Anywhere with Power Supply

The appliance comes in handy in two situations. Many states have a fire ban in summers, meaning you cannot set up a charcoal grill or do any cooking outside. There is a fear of forest fires due to the dry summer air. You can take out your electric Smoker and enjoy proper smoked food with friends and family in such a situation.

Another situation where the electric Smoker comes in handy is in small houses and apartments where space is an issue. In apartments, there is a prohibition on barbequing and smoke. You can easily set up your electric Smoker on your balcony and enjoy your favorite food in this situation.

2.5. The Option to Cold Smoke

Sometimes you want to cold smoke some food items like cheese and bacon. It is not easily possible on conventional smokers. It would help if you bought the cold smoke attachments with an electric smoker, generally available easily with all-electric smoker models. This attachment can be used to prepare a variety of preparations like meatloaves, deserts, dried meat, and fish sausages.

Chapter 3. Proper Usage of the Electric Smoker

After you have purchased the Electric Smoker, comes to the process of setting it up. Most electric smokers are easy to install and setup. It is best to read the manual to understand the working of the specific model.

This chapter will discuss step-by-step how we should prepare our food items and the correct method and sequence to smoke our desired food product.

3.1. Preparation of Meat

The meat preparation will be done the same way you would do for conventional barbecue and smoking as usual. Some people follow their family recipes passed down through generations. Some people prefer a marinade kept overnight; some perform a dry rub to season and prepare the meat. It is entirely up to you how you want to season the meat you want to prepare. The electric Smoker can smoke every kind of meat, so do not be shy and prepare your favorite meat for smoking. Be sure that the electric Smoker will prepare the same flavor and texture you expect from the traditional style smoker will give.

3.2. Setting up the Electric Smoker

Few points should be kept in mind when setting up the electric Smoker. The first and most important is that this is an outdoor appliance. Please keep it in a properly ventilated space. It cannot be kept indoors. It must be set up outside. It should be set up on a flat and strong surface that can withstand high temperatures. Sometimes the appliance can heat-up up to high temperatures. Please keep it in an open space with room to move about so that the appliance is in no danger to be tripped over and become a hazard. Keep children away from the electric Smoker while operating and afterward until it cools down after one or two hours.

3.3. Read the Electric Smoker Manual

Different models of Electric Smokers have a different set of instructions. The basic working of thee the Electric Smokers is the same, but there is a slight difference in how each Smoker is operated. It would help if you had a complete understanding of how your appliance is turned on and off, how to regulate temperature, when is it safe to open the appliance, what temperatures are suitable for which meat, how much time it requires for specific meats. It will help if you read up about all such details to use your Electric Smoker to its fullest.

3.4. Seasoning the Electric Smoker

This is an important process. You only need to do this once when your electric Smoker is brand new. To get rid of any harmful chemicals left in the Smoker during manufacturing, this procedure is done. All manuals have detailed descriptions of the seasoning. You must follow the exact instructions of your Electric Smoker because they are model specific.

However, a common procedure followed for seasoning is that you apply any cooking oil on all the electric Smoker's inner surfaces such that the surfaces are completely coated. Now turn on the Electric Smoker and let it operate empty for 2 to 3 hours. Then let it cook, and then your appliance is ready for use.

3.5. Preparing the Cooking Chamber

First, make sure that the cooking chamber is clean. Fill the water tray with water. This must be done before turning on the heat. Fill in the wood chip tray with wood chips or woodchucks that you wish to use. Usually, the wood chip compartment should be filled if the meat will be smoked for 3 to 4 hours. Next, set up the temperature and time for smoking. Always remember that the heating chamber should be preheated. Do not put the meat in the cold chamber and turn on the heat afterward. It is always recommended to put the meat in a well-heated chamber. This is a pro tip for the best results.

3.6. Putting in the meat

First, let the cooking chamber reach a certain temperature, then place the meat on the grills. You will need to open the chamber, place the meat, and then close it. Take care of that you put in the meat swiftly so that less heat is lost from within the chamber during this action. Temperature and the correct amount of heat are essential for the meat to be prepared to perfection. It is also recommended not to open the chamber when the meat is being smoked. This might disrupt the smoking process and bring the temperature down. The same rule applies to smoking as the one that applies in baking. Optimum temperature is essential.

3.7. The Process of Smoking

This is a slow process. It usually takes three or more hours. Only fish takes a shorter while to smoke. Otherwise, all other meats take much longer. Always take care to replenish the woodchips during the smoking process.

The smoking process will be carried out on its own, so there will be no other precaution except for keeping an eye on the wood chips.

Another thing to look out for will be the water. This water serves as the steam that gives the meats the required moisture that does not let them dry out. If the water is dried up, the meat will also become dry and difficult to chew on. So, it is always important that there is enough moisture circulation in the heating chamber. Always keep an eye out for the water tray. It should not be dry.

3.8. Taking out the meat

Before taking out the meat from the heated chamber, always check if the meat is cooked properly. Every meat has an internal temperature that indicates its doneness. So before bringing the meat out, insert the thermometer to the thickest part of the meat can see that the optimum temperature has been achieved or not. If you think the meat is undercooked, keep it in the chamber for 20 more minutes and check again. If all seems well, take out the Smoker's rack and place it on the counter to let it rest and then slice your meat.

Serve the meat with traditional side dishes like coleslaw, corn on the cob or baked potatoes. With the electric Smoker, you do not need to worry about the meat not being cooked properly. With the temperature regulation, the chance for accidents is reduced significantly.

Chapter 4. Tips and Tricks to Smoke Anything

Knowing some tricks and hacks about appliances always helps in preparing perfect meals. The same is the case with an electric smoker. This chapter discusses a few tricks and tips to help you in preparing smoked meats and foods. Usually, we start learning with experience but learning from other's experiences can give you a head start. Here is a list of tried and tested tricks and tips for the usage of an Electric Smoker. These tips and tricks will help you along your journey with the electric Smoker. Read all the points carefully to get the best results.

4.1. Do not Over Smoke the Food

When you first buy an electric smoker, you might be tempted to use many strong aromatic woodchips. But the reality is that you do not need an overpowering smoke flavor to make the barbecue delicious; only a mild smoky flavor will do the job. It is also true for poultry that over-smoked chicken becomes bitter and inedible. So always be careful about the amount of smoke you want for your food. In the case of smoke, the less is more saying is true.

4.2. Smoke Chicken at High Temperature

Chicken is not one of those meat groups which need a lower temperature for a longer time to be perfectly cooked. The chicken cooks at a higher temperature. The rule of thumb is to take the temperature to 275°F and smoke the chicken for around one to two hours. To check the chicken for doneness, insert a probe inside the chicken thigh and see that the internal temperature is about 165°F. The proper cooking of chicken is important because undercooked chicken can cause harmful effects and infections to the body.

4.3. Do not Soak the Wood Chips

It is common practice to soak woodchips in water before use. What happens is that when we soak the wood chips and put them in the Smoker and the smoking starts, white smoke is created. We think that this white smoke gives a smoky, rich flavor to the meat, but it is not true. This white smoke is just steam that dilutes the smoke's flavor and interferes with the temperature inside the chamber.

What you should do is that use the wood chips directly. The smoke that will be created will be thin blue smoke, which is the type of smoke that imparts a rich aromatic flavor to the smoked dishes.

4.4. Season your Electric Smoker before Use

This point is more of a health concern rather than a tip or trick. Seasoning is the process performed before cooking anything in the Smoker. This is usually done to eliminate all factory residue, chemicals, and dust from inside the cavity that has been left over from the manufacturing plant.

This process also has a good effect on subsequent smoking as well. After the seasoning, a black layer of smoke is formed on the electric Smoker's inner surfaces. So, after seasoning, whatever you will smoke, the black coating will impart the smoky flavor.

4.5. Preheat the Cooking Chamber

Always preheat the cooking chamber. Turn on the electric heat rods before putting in the meat and wait till the optimum temperature is reached; only then should you put in the meat. This will ensure that the meat will neither remain undercooked or overcooked.

4.6. Put Poultry in Oven to Finish

Most of the electric smokers have a maximum temperature of 275°F. This temperature is enough to cook poultry to perfection, but the desired crispy skins cannot be achieved at this temperature. So, if you want crispy skins, take out the chicken from the Smoker and place it in the oven at around 300∘F for 10 minutes. You will have yummy crispy skins.

4.7. Cover the Racks and Grills with Aluminum Foil

This tip is more for cleanliness than the taste of the smoked good. It would help if you covered all your racks and trays with aluminum foil. This will protect the racks and grills, and whenever the aluminum gets dirty, it can be replaced with a fresh layer of aluminum foil.

4.8. Do not use the Wood Chip Tray

In the electric Smoker, you fill the wood tray with woodchips. Often, people have experienced that they must refill the wood chip tray repeatedly, and it can be a bit inconvenient. Rather than wood chips, you can use a pellet smoker. A pellet smoker is a separately available tube that gives off thin blue smoke, which gives the aroma and amazing flavor to the smoked meats.

4.9. Leave the Vent Open

It is a good idea to keep the vent of the Electric Smoker completely open. This is to prevent the accumulation of creosote. Creosote is a substance in smoke that gives a smoky flavor to the foods. This substance is good to impart a smoky flavor to the dish, but a high quantity of this substance can accumulate over the meat and gives off a bitter flavor.

4.10. Control the Temperature Swings

The temperature swings are phenomena that are seen in all heating appliances using heating rods. What happens is that if you set the temperature of the appliance at 220∘F, the rod, when it reaches this temperature, will turn off; however, the temperature still keeps rising and is risen to about 240∘F and then starts coming back, it gets lower and lower about 210∘F, and then the rods turn on again, and it takes a while to get to 220∘F. you need to learn to manage this situation by keeping the temperature selection about 10∘F lower than the desired temperature. This way, the temperature swings will be controlled.

4.11. Invest in a Good Thermometer

In smoking, you can often be confused if the meat is done or not. Sometimes you can be fooled but the appliance's internal thermostat. But the doneness of meat is determined by the internal temperature of the meat. So, to check the internal temperature of the meat, you should have a separate thermometer. Such thermometers are commonly known as probes. You can insert the probe into the thickest part of the meat and determine the internal temperature. We must understand that the thermostat of the electric Smoker and the meat's internal temperature are different, and the doneness of the meat depends on the meat's internal temperature. Different meats have the different internal temperature that determines that they are fully cooked. Some meats are done at lower internal temperatures, such as fish and seafood. Some meats require high temperatures, like beef and lamb. Understanding this is especially important, and the first step towards this understanding is investing in a good thermometer.

4.12. Keep the Meat Overnight Before Smoking

To achieve the meat's full flavors, it is always a good idea to keep the meat overnight. It does not matter if you decide to marinate, dry rub, or brine the meat; leaving it in the refrigerator overnight will cause the flavors to fully absorb in the meat, and the meat will also become tender before smoking. The meat will be cooked even if you decide not to let it stay overnight, but the results might not be as good as the meat that has been kept overnight. In smoking and barbecue, patience plays an important role. The more patient you are, the better your food will cook and taste.

4.13. Do not Hurry.

Smoking is a long process. It takes time for meats to properly smoke. Whenever you decide to smoke meat, always keep in mind that you must have the patience to let the meat cook completely. Sometimes the temptation to check on our dishes can be harmful to the recipe. When you open the electric smoker door, the temperature is disrupted, and the recipe might be affected. Even opening the door for one or two minutes can even have such an effect. So, you must be patient while the Smoker is working. This is an amazing appliance, and you should trust it to work its wonder. All you must do is sit back and relax.

Chapter 5. Ultimate Electric Smoker Recipes

In this chapter, you will find easy-to-follow recipes that you can make in your Electric Smoker. You must follow all recipes exactly according to the instructions for the best results.

5.1. Beef BBQ Brisket

This is an easy recipe for BBQ brisket that you will prepare in your Electric Smoker. Be assured that you will enjoy the original BBQ flavor. The meat will have a beautiful texture on the outside and will be tender inside. Just follow the instructions carefully, and you are in for a treat. They this recipe and you will not be disappointed.

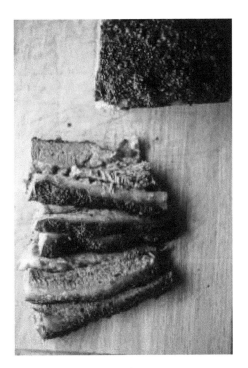

- Course: Dinner

- Cuisine: American BBQ

- Total Time: 8 hours 50 minutes

- Preparation Time: 30 minutes

- Cooking Time: 8 hours

- Rest Time: 20 minutes

- Serving Size: 2 servings

- Nutritional Value Per Serving

  - Calories: 564 calories

  - Carbohydrates: 0 g

  - Protein: 77.3 g

  - Fats: 27.4 g

Equipment Used:

- Electric Smoker

Ingredients:

1. BBQ rub (store-bought) 5 tbsp.
2. Beef Brisket ½ kg.

Instructions:

- Preheat the electric Smoker at 225∘F.

- Then prepare the beef brisket. Wash the meat and pat it dry.

- Trim all the excess fat from the brisket, leaving only one-fourth of an inch of fat on the meat.

- Next, remove the excess skin from the underside of the meat cut.

- Now, apply the BBQ rub on the beef on both sides generously.

- Put the brisket in the Electric Smoker and insert the probe in the thickest part of the beef.

- Smoke the beef until the temperature has reached 160◦F. This usually takes six hours. It might take longer, so you must see when the temperature reaches a certain point.

- At this stage, please take out the brisket very carefully and wrap it tightly in aluminum foil.

- Place it back into the Smoker and wait until the brisket's temperature reaches 190◦F. This usually takes additional 2 hours. The time might be a bit more depending on the brisket.

- When the beef is at 190◦F, take it out of the Smoker.

- Let it rest for 20 to 30 minutes.

- Then unwrap the brisket and slice it.

- Enjoy the delicious BBQ brisket.

5.2.   Smoked Salmon

The best thing about this recipe is that it is easy to make and quick to prepare. Minimum ingredients are used to achieve perfection with this smoked salmon. Try this recipe, and you will be in for a mouthwatering treat.

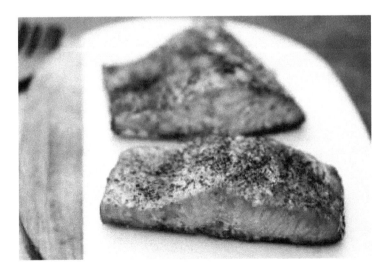

- Course: Lunch
- Cuisine: American

- Total Time: 2 hours 10 minutes

- Preparation Time: 10 minutes

- Cooking Time: 1 hour

- Rest: 20 minutes

- Serving Size: 3 servings

- Nutritional Value Per Serving

    - Calories: 454 calories

    - Carbohydrates: 0 g

    - Protein: 57.5 g

    - Fats: 24.2 g

Equipment Used:

- Electric Smoker

Ingredients:

1. Fresh Salmon 1 kg.

2. Brown Sugar 2 tbsp

3. Dried Dill 1 tsp

4. Pepper 1 tsp

5. Salt 1tsp

Instructions:

- Wash and pat dry the fish carefully. You must be careful with raw fish meat because it is delicate and can break.

- Mix the salt, pepper, sugar, and dill in a bowl.

- Rub this sugar mixture on the top side of the fish.

- Put it in the refrigerator for one hour. This will allow the fish to dry brine.

- Preheat the Electric Smoker at 250°F.

- Place a probe into the thickest part of the meat.

- Let it smoke until the meat reaches 145°F. It takes about 45 minutes to one hour.

- The dish can be served at room temperature or even cold.

- For this specific dish, you can use pecan, cherry, or oak wood for a subtle flavor.

5.3. Smoked Chicken

Chicken is one of the most widely popular food throughout the world. This recipe gives smoked chicken a spicy and flavorful twist. The brown sugar used in the rub gives it a caramelized look and texture and adds richness to the taste. Try this recipe out and you will not be disappointed.

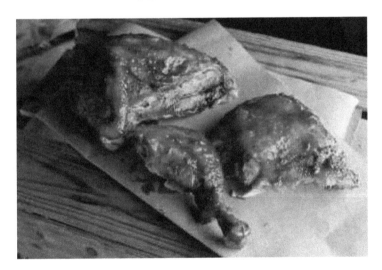

- Course: Dinner

- Cuisine: American BBQ

- Total Time: 5 hours

- Preparation Time: 30 minutes

- Cooking Time: 4 hours

- Rest Time: 30 minutes

- Serving Size: 4 servings
- Nutritional Value Per Serving
  - Calories: 240 calories
  - Carbohydrates: 0 g
  - Protein: 21 g
  - Fats: 17 g

Equipment Used:

- Electric Smoker

Ingredients:

1. Medium sized whole chicken with skin
2. Thyme 1 tbsp
3. Cayenne Pepper 2 tbsp
4. Garlic Powder 1 tbsp
5. Chili Powder 2 tbsp
6. Salt 1 tbsp
7. Sugar 2 tbsp
8. Onion Powder 1 tbsp
9. Black Pepper 2 tbsp
10. Olive Oil 3 tbsp

Instructions:

- Arrange the woodchips in the electric smoker tray. You can use peach, apple, or cherry woodchips. Then turn on the electric Smoker to preheat at 225°F.

- In a medium-sized mixing bowl, mix the thyme, cayenne pepper, garlic powder, chili powder, salt, sugar, onion powder, and black pepper. This will make the perfect rub for the chicken.

- First, rub the whole chicken with olive oil. All sides and inside the hollow cavity of chicken as well.

- After that, apply the prepared rub on the chicken generously. Rub it on the entire surface of the chicken.

- Put the skin over the breast of the chicken and apply the rub under the skin as well.

- Put the prepared chicken in the electric Smoker and insert a probe in the thigh.

- Check the chicken after every hour and take it out when the meat's internal temperature reaches 164∘F. The whole process takes about 4 hours.

- Served the smoked chicken warm.

5.4.   Smoked Corn on the Cob

Corn on the cob is a crowd's favorite side dish. It is popular among kids and adults alike. These complement all sorts of meats in a barbecue and give us that much-needed light and sweet flavors in the middle of a high protein barbecue. Try this easy recipe, and you will not regret preparing some smoked corn on the cob.

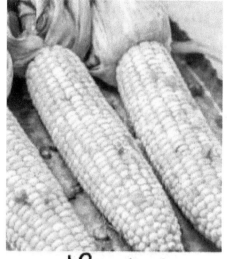

Smoked
CORN ON THE COB

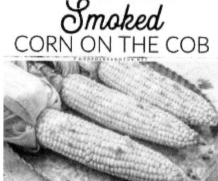

- Course: Side Dish

- Cuisine: American

- Total Time: 5 hours 10 minutes

- Preparation Time: 4 hours

- Cooking Time: 1 hour

- Rest Time: 10 minutes

- Serving Size: 6 servings

- Nutritional Value Per Serving

  - Calories: 142 calories

  - Carbohydrates: 16.6 g

  - Protein: 2.7 g

- Fats: 8.6 g

Equipment Used:

- Electric Smoker

Ingredients:

1. Ear corn with husks 6 pieces
2. Brown sugar 2 tbsp
3. Salt ½ tsp
4. Garlic powder ½ tsp
5. Melted butter ¼ cup.
6. Onion powder 1 tsp
7. Sliced green onion 3 pieces.

Instructions:

- Take a large roasting pot and fill it half with room temperature water.
- Pull the husks of all the corn cobs and remove the silks. Let the husks remain attached to the cob but just pulled back.
- Soak the corn cobs in the water and if needed, fill the pot with more water to completely immerse the cobs into water.
- Soak for 4 hours.
- After that remove, the cobs from the pot and place them on paper towels and let them dry.
- Preheat the electric Smoker at 225∘F. Place the woodchips inside the electric Smoker.
- In a mixing bowl, mix the butter, sugar, salt, onion powder, and garlic powder to make a rub for the corn on the cob.

- With the help of a brush, apply the rub generously to the corn cobs.

- Pull the husks back on the corn cobs. Place them in the electric Smoker.

- Leave for 60 minutes and then take them out.

- Let them rest for 10 minutes, and then serve them as a delicious side dish.

5.5. Grilled Chicken Thighs with Asparagus

This delicious chicken recipe is perfect for enjoying on the weekend. It is easy to make and takes only 2 hours to prepare. The juicy chicken with the light smokiness is a success with kids and adults alike. This dish will be a crowd favorite. Try out this recipe and enjoy it with friends and family.

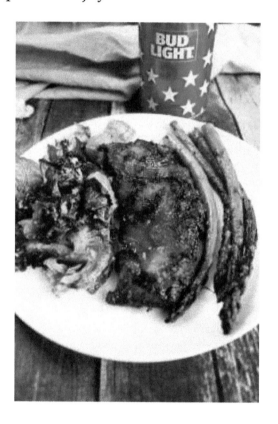

- Course: Lunch

- Cuisine: American

- Total Time: 5 hours

- Preparation Time: 3 hours

- Cooking Time: 2 hours

- Rest Time: 10 minutes

- Serving Size: 3 servings

- Nutritional Value Per Serving

    - Calories: 482 calories

    - Carbohydrates: 58.8 g

    - Protein: 58.5 g

    - Fats: 19.3 g

Equipment Used:

- Electric Smoker

Ingredients:

For Chicken:

1. Chicken thighs 3 to 4 pieces

2. Store-bought BBQ rub 5 tbsp.

3. Water as required.

4. Sugar 1 tsp

5. Salt 1 tsp

6. ¼ cup apple cider vinegar

For Asparagus

1. Asparagus 1 bunch

2. Red pepper flakes 1 tsp

3. Balsamic Vinegar ¼ cup

4. Pepper 1 tsp

5. Salt 1 tsp

Equipment Used:

- Electric Smoker

Instructions:

- Prepare to brine the chicken thighs. Put the chicken in a large zip lock bag, then add Vinegar, salt, and sugar.

- Then, fill the bag with water such that the chicken pieces are completely soaked. Put it in the refrigerator for 2 to 3 hours.

- The brining process will ensure that the chicken does not dry out while in the electric Smoker.

- Similarly, prepare a marinade for the asparagus bunch as well. Please put it in a large zip lock bag. Add the balsamic vinegar, salt pepper, pepper flakes and water to soak the asparagus. Please leave it in the refrigerator for 3 hours.

- Prepare a small BBQ spray bottle having one part vinegar, two parts water and 1 tsp sugar. Mix it properly. This will be used to spray on the chicken while it is being smoked.

- Take the chicken out of the refrigerator after 2 hours and wash and dry the pieces.

- Apply the BBQ rub generously on the chicken pieces.

- Preheat the electric Smoker at 225∘F for 15 minutes. Put the apple woodchips in the wood tray.

- Place the chicken thighs in the electric Smoker.

- Spray with the BBQ spray bottle after every 20 to 30 minutes. This will prevent the chicken from drying.

- Smoke the chicken for about two hours.

- Take the chicken out of the Smoker and let it rest for 10 minutes.

- Meanwhile, please take out the asparagus and spread it on a paper towel and pat dry.

- Put the asparagus in the electric Smoker and leave for 10 minutes, and then take it out.

- Serve the chicken with a side of asparagus.

- This is a good pairing to serve, and the asparagus complements the smoked chicken beautifully.

5.6. Smoked Turkey Breast

Turkey has often been bland and boring meat. This recipe gives the turkey a tasty and spicy twist. The BBQ sauce mixed with hot sauce and honey gives the smoked turkey a rich flavor and an amazing texture. Try out this mouthwatering and delicious recipe and enjoy the aromatic and tender turkey meat. This recipe never disappoints.

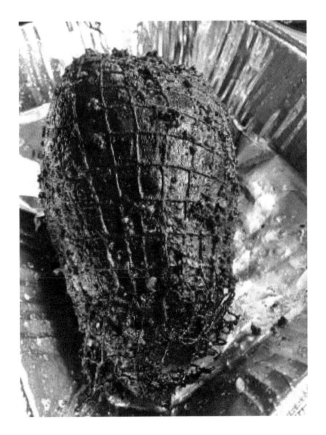

- Course: Lunch

- Cuisine: American

- Total Time: 3 hours 20 minutes

- Preparation Time: 5 minutes

- Cooking Time: 3 hours

- Resting Time: 10 minutes

- Serving Size: 3 to 4 servings

- Nutritional Value Per Serving

  - Calories: 380 calories

  - Carbohydrates: 16.5 g

  - Protein: 28.2 g

  - Fats: 20.8 g

Equipment Used:

- Electric Smoker

Ingredients:

1. Turkey breast 1 piece

2. Store-bought BBQ rub 4 tbsp.

3. Olive oil 3 tbsp.

4. Butter 100 g

5. Hot Tabasco sauce 2 tsp

6. Honey 1tsp

Instructions:

- First, preheat the electric Smoker at 250°F for at least 15 minutes.

- Put in the mesquite woodchips in the Smoker.

- Next, prepare the turkey meat. Cover the whole meat with a layer of olive oil. Rub the oil generously.

- Then apply the BBQ rub on the whole meat piece. Rub the mixture generously so that the whole turkey breast is covered with the BBQ rub.

- In a heatproof cup, prepare the basting mixture for the turkey. Add the butter, cut into small cubes to the cup. Put in the honey, hot sauce and ¼ teaspoon BBQ rub.

- Put the turkey and the cup in the electric Smoker and let it remain closed for approximately 45 minutes. Put a probe in the turkey meat at the thickest part of the meat.

- When you open the electric Smoker after 45 minutes, you will see that the basting mixture is prepared and is steaming.

- Pour the basting mixture about 2 tbsp on the meat and let it smoke.

- Repeat the procedure with the basting mixture after every 20 minutes.

- When the internal temperature of meat is near 170∘F, raise the electric Smoker's heat to 270∘F for the last 10 minutes.

- Take out the meat when the internal temperature reaches 170∘F.

- Let the meat rest for 15 minutes and then slice it.

- Serve this mouthwatering and delicious meal to your friends and family.

5.7.   Smoked Potatoes

Baked potatoes are an all-time favorite side dish. They go well with all meats, especially chicken. They can be served as it is or with a rich sour cream. This is an easy and useful recipe to smoke potatoes perfectly. This recipe is simple and easy to prepare and goes well with almost anything. You can even make this and have it on its own. It is great comfort food. Try it out and you will not be disappointed.

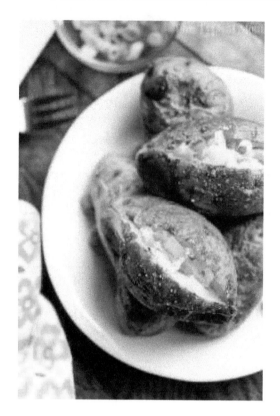

- Course: Side Dish

- Cuisine: American

- Total Time: 2 hours 20 minutes

- Preparation Time: 10 minutes

- Cooking Time: 2 hours

- Rest Time: 10 minutes

- Serving Size: 4 servings

- Nutritional Value Per Serving

  - Calories: 119 calories

  - Carbohydrates: 10 g

  - Protein: 1.8 g

  - Fats: 8.5 g

Equipment Used:

- Electric Smoker

Ingredients:

1. Medium sized potatoes 4 pieces
2. Olive oil ¼ cup
3. Granular Salt ¾ cup

Instructions:

- Preheat the electric Smoker at 275°F. Put in the wood chips of your choice. Preheat for at least 15 minutes.

- Wash the potatoes and dry them on a paper towel.

- Poke each potato with a fork 5 or six times at different places on the potato surface. This will prevent the potato from exploding when it is exposed to a high temperature in the electric Smoker.

- Pour the oil in an open cup and coat each potato with a thin layer of oil.

- Next, pour the salt into a shallow dish. Coat the potatoes with this salt.

- Place the potatoes in the electric Smoker and wait for approximately 2 hours.

- After 2 hours, check the potatoes for doneness. The potatoes should be cooked and soft.

- Take the potatoes out and let them rest for 10 minutes.

- Slit the potatoes from the entrance and fill them with American-style chili if you want to serve as a main dish.

- Another serving idea is to slit the center and fill it with sour cream and top it with sliced green onions. This makes a perfect side dish.

5.8. Smoked Burgers

Burgers are a staple food in American cuisine. These smoked beef burgers have a smoky flavor and are perfect for a quiet weekend lunch with the family. The burgers do not have a sauce but are still delicious and mouthwatering. The best part about this recipe is that it is easy to make, and it takes less time for preparation and cooking. Try this recipe and enjoy it with friends and family.

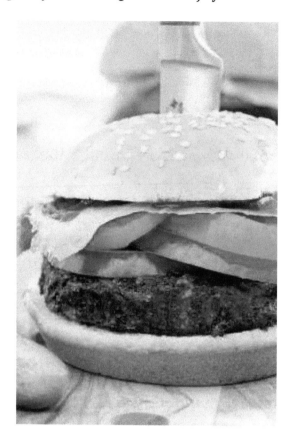

- Course: Lunch

- Cuisine: American

- Total Time: 1 hour 20 minutes

- Preparation Time: 10 minutes

- Cooking Time: 1 hour

- Rest Time: 10 minutes

- Serving Size: 6 servings

- Nutritional Value Per Serving

  - Calories: 160 calories

  - Carbohydrates: 1 g

  - Protein: 11 g

- Fats: 11 g

Equipment Used:

- Electric Smoker

Ingredients:

1. Pre-prepared beef burger patties 6 pieces
2. Salt 2 tbsp
3. Garlic Powder ½ tbsp
4. Pepper 1 tbsp
5. Dehydrated onion ½ tbsp

Instructions:

- Make sure that the burger patties are at room temperature.
- In a mixing bowl, add the salt, pepper, garlic powder, and dehydrated onion. Mix these ingredients well such that a rub is formed.
- Apply this rub on the burger patties. Cover both sides of the burger patty with the rub.
- Preheat the electric Smoker at 275∘F for 15 minutes. Add the woodchips to the electric Smoker.
- Next, place the burger patties in the Electric Smoker.
- If you want your burger to be medium-well done, smoke for 45 minutes and if you want it to be well done, smoke for 60 minutes. This depends entirely on your preference.
- Once the patties are cooked, take them out of the Smoker and let them rest for 10 minutes.

- Next, prepare the buns and put them in the burger patties. These can be served as it is or some raw vegetables and sauce can be added.

5.9. Smoked Chicken Drumsticks

This is a recipe for mouthwatering and flavorful drumsticks. The flavors are sweet and spicy. This recipe is prepared in 2 ½ hours, and you can enjoy these tasty drumsticks with BBQ sauce. Do try this recipe; this is a hit among kids and adults alike.

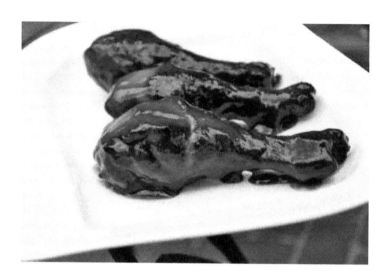

- Course: Dinner
- Cuisine: American
- Total Time: 3 hours
- Preparation Time: 15 minutes
- Cooking Time: 2 hours 30 minutes
- Serving Size: 6 persons
- Nutritional Value Per Serving
    - Calories: 180 calories
    - Carbohydrates: 8 g
    - Protein: 17 g
    - Fats: 8 g

Equipment Used:

- Electric Smoker

Ingredients:

1. Chicken Drumsticks 1.5 kg.
2. Store-bought Steak Rub ½ cup.
3. Cayenne Pepper 1 tsp
4. BBQ sauce ½ cup
5. Tabasco sauce 5 tbsp

Instructions:

- Wash and pat dry the drumsticks.
- Do not remove the skins from the chicken drumsticks.
- Rub the drumsticks with the store-bought steak rub and the cayenne pepper. Keep the drumsticks in the refrigerator for 2 hours.
- After a while, prepare the Electric Smoker.
- Put in the apple woodchips for a mild smoky flavor.
- Fill in the water tray with cold water.
- Turn on the electric Smoker at 250∘F to preheat.
- In the meanwhile, arrange the drumsticks in a stainless-steel wings rack.
- Put in the drumsticks in the Smoker and leave for 2 hours.
- At the end of 2 hours, check the internal temperature of drumsticks. The drumsticks are ready when the thermometer shows 160∘F as the internal temperature of the meat.
- Take out the drumsticks and let them rest for 5 minutes.
- Meanwhile, mix the BBQ sauce and tabasco sauce in a bowl.
- Dip all the drumsticks in the sauce one by one and arrange them on a platter.

- Serve hot.

5.10. Smoked Mac and Cheese

Mac and cheese as comfortable as comfort foods get. It serves as a great side dish with your barbeque. It is conventionally made in an oven, but you can also use a smoker to prepare this dish to give an extra smoky richness.

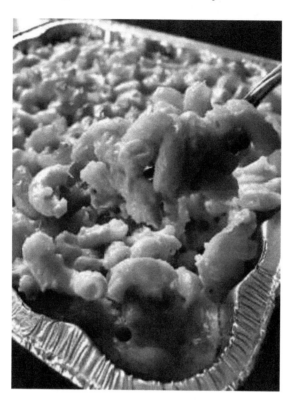

- Course: Side Dish

- Cuisine: American

- Total Time: 2 hours 30 minutes

- Preparation Time: 30 minutes

- Cooking Time: 2 hours

- Serving Size: 4 servings

- Nutritional Value Per Serving

  - Calories: 380 calories

  - Carbohydrates: 50 g

- Protein: 8 g
- Fats: 4 g

Equipment Used:

Electric Smoker

Ingredients:

1. Elbow Macaroni 1 packet, about ½ kg
2. Milk 3 cups
3. Flour ¼ cup
4. Cheese of your choice (grated) 500 g.
5. Cream cheese 250 g
6. Butter ¼ cup
7. Salt to taste
8. Pepper to taste

Instructions:

- First, boil 12 cups of water in a medium cooking pot. When the water comes to a boil, add the elbow macaroni, and let it boil for 8 to 10 minutes. When the macaroni is boiled, remove all the water, and put the macaroni aside.
- Next, you will prepare the cheese sauce.
- In a medium-sized pan, put in the butter in melt it over the flame. After the butter is melted, add the flour, and mix it. Cook for about two minutes till the flour starts to brown.
- Next, add the milk and cook for five minutes with constant stirring or whisking to not form lumps. Let the milk thicken. When the milk starts to thicken, take the saucepan off the flame, and add cream cheese.
- Mix the cream cheese and make a smooth mixture.

- In a heat-resistant bowl, add the cheese. Pour this mixture over the cheese and mix well.

- At this point, prepare the electric Smoker and put it to preheat at 225∘F.

- Now take an aluminum tray and spread the cooked macaroni in its base.

- Pour the cream and cheese mixture over the macaroni such that it is fully immersed in the mixture.

- Put the aluminum tray in the Smoker for two hours.

- Take out the dish after two hours. The upper layer will come out crusty with cheesy and gooey richness beneath.

- Enjoy your mac and cheese separately or with barbequed chicken or meat.

5.11. BBQ Smoked Ribs

If you are someone who enjoys the ribs on the bone, this recipe is just for you. You will enjoy the rich smokiness of the ribs flavored with mild herbs served with BBQ sauce. Preparing BBQ ribs might be a bit tricky if you go the conventional way, but the ribs prepared in the electric Smoker save you all the hassle, giving you the same flavor.

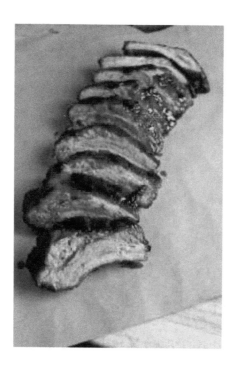

- Course: Dinner

- Cuisine: American

- Total Time: 4 hours 30 minutes

- Preparation Time: 30 minutes

- Cooking Time: 4 hours

- Rest Time: 15 minutes

- Serving Size: 4 servings

- Nutritional Value Per Serving

  - Calories: 302 calories

  - Carbohydrates: 0 g

  - Protein: 22 g

  - Fats: 23 g

Equipment Used:

- Electric Smoker

Ingredients:

1. One cut of ribs 1.5 kg

2. Black pepper 1 tsp

3. Paprika 1 tsp

4. Garlic Powder 2 tsp

5. Brown Sugar ¼ cup

6. Salt 1 tsp

7. BBQ sauce ¼ cup

Instructions:

- Prepare the ribs. Trim the extra fat and cut the ribs to easily fit on the Electric Smoker grills.

- Next, prepare the rub for the ribs. In a bowl, mix the pepper, paprika, salt, garlic powder, brown sugar, and salt.

- Rub this mixture on the ribs generously such that all parts of the ribs are rubbed with the herbs.

- Put the ribs in a large zip lock bag and put them in the refrigerator overnight.

- The next day, prepare the electric Smoker with applewood chips. Fill the water tray and turn on the Smoker at 225°F.

- Let the Smoker preheat for 20 minutes.

- Bring out the ribs and arrange them in the smoker racks.

- Place them in the Smoker and let them smoke for 2 hours.

- After 2 hours, take them out, wrap them in aluminum foil, and put them back in the Electric Smoker.

- Let them smoke for a further two hours.

- Take the ribs out and let them rest for 15 minutes.

- After that, unwrap the ribs and serve.

5.12. Smoked Beef Jerky

Commercially prepared beef jerky is commonly available in the market. But there is nothing as flavorful and delicious as homemade beef jerky. In this recipe, we will learn how to prepare beef jerky from scratch.

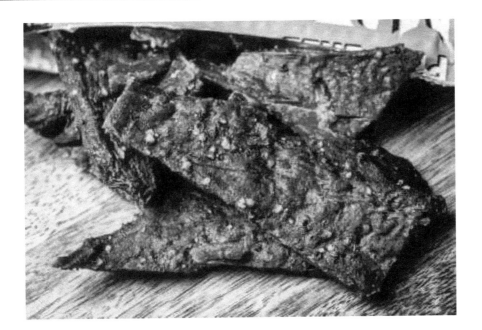

- Course: Snack

- Cuisine: American

- Total Time: 5 hours

- Preparation Time: 30 minutes

- Cooking Time: 3 hours

- Resting Time: 1 hour

- Serving Size: 5 servings

- Nutritional Value Per Serving

  - Calories: 240 calories

  - Carbohydrates: 1 g

  - Protein: 50 g

  - Fats: 4 g

Equipment Used:

- Electric Smoker

Ingredients:

1. Round beef steak 1.5 kg

2. Honey ¼ cup

3. Soy sauce ¼ cup

4. Worcestershire sauce ¼ cup

5. Brown sugar ¼ cup

6. Garlic Powder 2 tsp

7. Red pepper flakes 1 tbsp

8. Salt 1 tsp

9. Onion Powder 2 tsp

Instructions:

- First, prepare the beef by trimming the extra fat and skin from the meat.

- Next, cut the meat into ¼ inch slices. Make sure that the slices are evenly cut.

- Set the meat aside.

- In a medium-size saucepan, add the honey, soy sauce, Worcestershire sauce, pepper, salt, garlic powder, onion powder, and sugar. Simmer it over the flame until a uniform mixture is formed.

- Let the mixture reach room temperature. Apply the mixture generously on the beef slices and put them in a zip lock bag.

- Pour the remaining sauce into the zip lock bag. Let it in the refrigerator overnight.

- The next day, prepare the electric Smoker with wood chips and water. Turn on the heat at 175° F and preheat for 10 minutes.

- Meanwhile, take out the beef slices and set them on a tray and let them reach room temperature.

- After that, arrange them in an aluminum tray and put them in the Smoker.

- Let the beef smoke for 3 hours.

- Take it out after three hours and rest for about 2 to 3 hours until it becomes dry.

- You can consume it as a snack and store it in an airtight container for up to 2 weeks.

5.13. Striped Bass Recipe

This is a delicious recipe having a mouthwatering flavor. Smoking the fish gives a much better flavor than just grilling. The smokiness makes this dish worth enjoying on a warm summer day. You can have it with a rich tartar sauce, or a little lime juice drizzled on it. If you try this recipe, you are in for a treat.

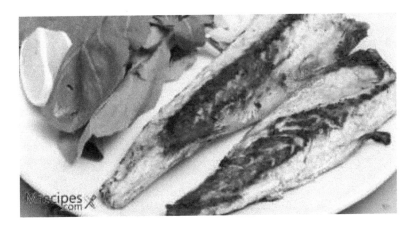

- Course: Lunch

- Cuisine: American

- Total Time: 3 hours

- Preparation Time: 45 minutes

- Cooking Time: 2 hours

- Serving Size: 6 servings

- Nutritional Value Per Serving

  - Calories: 154 calories

  - Carbohydrates: 0 g

  - Protein: 4 g

- Fats: 28 g

Equipment Used:

- Electric Smoker

Ingredients:

1. Striped Bass Fillets 1 kg
2. Brown Sugar ¼ cup
3. Water 4 cups
4. Salt ¼ cup
5. Bay leaves 2 leaves.
6. Black pepper 2 tsp
7. Lemon 5 to 6 slices
8. Dry wine ½ cup for brine ½ cup for Smoker
9. Olive oil 3 tsp

Instructions:

- Clean and wash the fish fillets.
- Heat the four cups of water and dissolve salt and sugar in them. Let it come to room temperature.
- When it is at room temperature add, bay leaves, pepper, wine, and lemon slices.
- Put in the fish fillets inside this brine such that they are completely soaked.
- Cover them and leave them overnight.
- The next day prepares the Electric Smoker. Put the alder woodchips in the tray. Fill the water tray half with water and half with white wine.
- Turn on the burner at 180∘F.

- Bring out the fish fillets and take them out of the brine and wash them with cold water. Ste them on the counter on a tray lined with paper towels. Let them dry and come to room temperature.

- Meanwhile, coat the smoker grills with olive oil.

- When the fish fillets have reached room temperature, set them on the grills and smoke for two hours.

- The doneness is checked by inserting a thermometer; the internal temperature should be 145◦F.

- Please take out the fish and let it rest for 10 minutes before serving.

5.14. Smoked Cajun Shrimp

Shrimps are a crowd favorite seafood. They are easy to make, and preparation also takes a few minutes. Either you are using fresh shrimps or frozen ones, this recipe works best for both. The only thing is that for frozen shrimps, you will have to defrost them first. This recipe is easy and simple to follow and seldom goes wrong. You will thank us when you have tried this one.

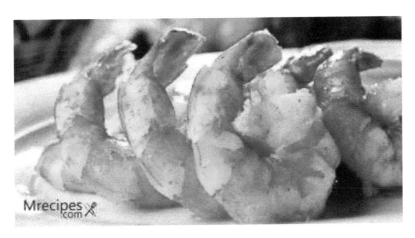

- Course: Appetizer

- Cuisine: American

- Total Time: 1 hour

- Preparation Time: 20 minutes

- Cooking Time: 30 minutes

- Serving Size: 6 servings

- Nutritional Value Per Serving

  - Calories: 92 calories

  - Carbohydrates: 2.2.g

  - Protein: 4.6 g

  - Fats: 7.6 g

Equipment Used:

- Electric Smoker

Ingredients:

1. Jumbo Shrimps 1 kg

2. Salt ¼ cup

3. Dried thyme 2 tbsp

4. Paprika 3 tbsp

5. Cayenne Pepper 2 tsp

6. Onion Powder 2 tbsp

7. Black Pepper 3 tbsp

8. Garlic Powder 2 tbsp

9. Olive Oil 3 tbsp

10. Lemon Juice ¼ cup

11. Fresh Parsley 1 bunch chopped.

Instructions:

- Prepare the shrimps. Take out the shells and devein them. Wash and pat them dry.

- In a bowl prepare the dry rum. Add salt, sugar, cayenne pepper, paprika, garlic powder, thyme, and onion powder. Mix this carefully.

- Next, prepare an aluminum tray by greasing it with olive oil.

- Place the shrimps on the tray in a single layer.

- Apply the dry rum to the shrimps generously.

- Start the electric Smoker at 225∘F. Put in the wood chips and water.

- Let it preheat for 20 minutes.

- Meanwhile, pour lemon juice over the shrimps.

- Put the shrimps in the oven for thirty minutes, moving them after every ten minutes.

- Please take out the shrimps after 30 minutes or as soon as they start turning pink.

- This dish can be served warmed or even at room temperature.

5.15. Smoked Scallops

Scallops are juicy and delicious, either grilled or cooked. In this recipe, we have smoked the scallops to give them a rich smokiness. The scallops can be enjoyed with a side of a fresh green salad. This is the ultimate healthy dish to eat for lunch. Do try it out for a different and mouthwatering experience. You will not be disappointed.

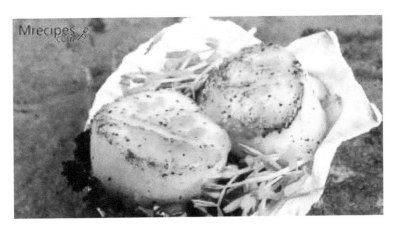

- Course: Appetizer

- Cuisine: American

- Total Time: 50 minutes

- Preparation Time: 5 minutes

- Cooking Time: 30 to 40 minutes

- Serving Size: 5 servings

- Nutritional Value Per Serving

    - Calories: 105 calories

    - Carbohydrates: 5 g

    - Protein: 8.7 g

    - Fats: 5.3. g

Equipment used:

- Electric Smoker

Ingredients:

1. Sea Scallops 1 kg

2. Olive oil 3 tbsp

3. Salt 1 tsp

4. Garlic 2 cloves minced.

5. Pepper 1 tsp

Instructions:

- Wash the scallops under cold running water and dry them on a paper towel.

- In a bowl, mix the oil, salt, pepper, and lemon juice.

- Apply the mixture to the scallops.

- Turn on the electric Smoker and prepare it with water and add the wood chips.

- Let it preheat for 10 minutes at 225∘F.

- Meanwhile, lightly grease an aluminum pan and place the scallops on it such that the scallops do not touch each other.

- Put the scallops in the Smoker and smoke for 20 to 30 minutes.

- Check the internal temperature of the scallops.

- Take them out when the temperature reaches 145∘F.

- Let the scallops rest for 10 minutes and then serve with a fresh green salad and a vinaigrette.

Smoked Curried Almonds

Almonds are an extremely healthy source of good fats. One enjoys munching them around. This recipe tries a twist on the good old roasted almonds. Let us make snack time fun with these delicious smoked curried almonds. You can keep them for as long as a month and keep enjoying a fistful every day. Heath and taste go hand in hand with this yummy snack.

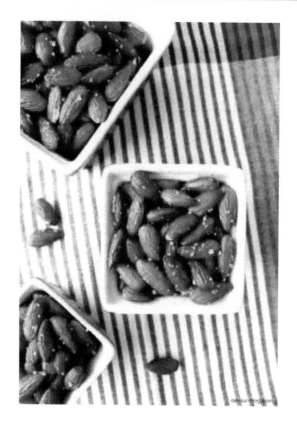

- Course: Snack

- Cuisine: American

- Total Time: 1 hour 5 minutes

- Preparation Time:5 minutes

- Cooking Time: 1 to 2 hours

- Serving Size: 6 servings

- Nutritional Value Per Serving

  - Calories: 170 calories

  - Carbohydrates: 5 g

  - Protein: 6 g

  - Fats: 15 g

Equipment Used:

- Electric Smoker

Ingredients:

1. Raw Almonds with skins ½ kg
2. Butter 2 tbsp
3. Curry powder 2 tbsp
4. Raw Sugar 2 tbsp
5. 2 tbsp
6. Salt 1 tsp
7. Cayenne Pepper 1 tsp

Instructions:

- Preheat the electric Smoker at 225°F. Fill the water tray half with water and put in the pecan wood chips.
- In a large bowl, mix the butter, salt, sugar, cayenne pepper and curry powder.
- Toss all the almonds in this mixture.
- Prepare an aluminum tray, spread the almonds in the tray as a layer and put it in the Smoker.
- Leave the almonds for one hour and take them out.
- Delicious, curried almonds are ready.
- Let them rest to reach room temperature and enjoy this rich flavorful snack.
- These can be stored in an airtight container for up to 3 months.

Smoked Apples with Maple Syrup

If you have a sweet tooth and enjoy fruity desserts, this one is just for you. The naturally citrus flavor of apples is balanced perfectly with the sweetness of maple syrup and raisins. Do try out this recipe; you will not regret it.

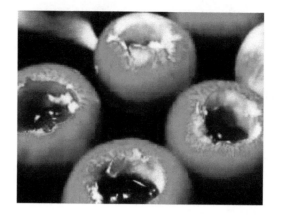

- Course: Dessert

- Cuisine: American

- Total Time: 2 hours

- Preparation Time: 30 minutes

- Cooking Time: 1 hour 30 minutes

- Serving Size: 6 servings

- Nutritional Value Per Serving

  - Calories: 224 calories

  - Carbohydrates: 47 g

  - Protein: 1 g

  - Fats: 5 g

Equipment Used:

- Electric Smoker

Ingredients:

1. Apples 6 pieces

2. Maple Syrup ½ cup

3. Raisins ½ cup

4. Cold Butter ¼ cup cut in small cubes.

Instructions:

- Prepare the electric Smoker with water and pecan woodchips. Turn it on at 250°F.

- Take the apples, wash them, and pat dry. Core the apples such that their outer shape is maintained, and a small cavity is formed inside. The apple should still be able to stand without support.

- Fill the lower part of each apple with a small number of raisins, followed by some butter and then the maple syrup.

- Grease an aluminum tray and arrange the apples in the tray.

- Put the apples in the electric Smoker and let them smoke for 1 hour 30 minutes.

- Take them out and let them rest for 10 minutes.

- Serve warm with vanilla ice cream.

Smoked Bean Sprouts

Bean sprouts are a great option for a side dish. They can be served with barbecued chicken and are a great source of vitamins and fiber. These are an excellent option for a side dish because they are easy to make and are prepared quickly.

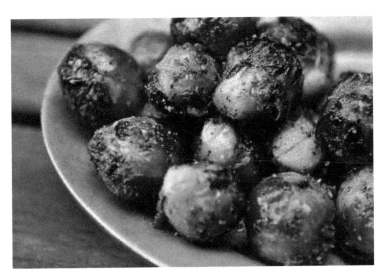

- Course: Side Dish

- Cuisine: American

- Total Time: 1 hour 30 minutes
- Preparation Time: 15 minutes
- Cooking Time: 1 hour
- Serving Size: 6 servings
- Nutritional Value Per Serving
    - Calories: 45 calories
    - Carbohydrates: 8 g
    - Protein: 3 g
    - Fats: 0 g

Equipment Used:

- Electric Smoker

Ingredients:

1. Brussel Sprouts ½ kg
2. Olive Oil 3 tsp
3. Salt 1tsp
4. Pepper ½ tsp

Instructions:

- Wash the Brussel sprouts with cold water and dry them out in a colander.
- Remove the base of the Brussel sprouts and the dried-out parts.
- In a bowl, mix the olive oil, salt, and pepper.
- Apply the mixture to the sprouts and put them in a single layer in an aluminum tray.
- Turn on the electric Smoker at 225∘F. Prepare with water and wood chips.
- Let the Smoker preheat for 10 to 15 minutes and then put in the sprouts.

- Let them smoke for 60 minutes.

- Take them out and serve as a side dish with barbeque chicken.

Smoked Cauliflower

Cauliflower is super healthy food. It is a rich source of vitamin C and dietary fiber. It contains eighty percent of the recommended amount of Vitamin C required for a day. It fills up your stomach and is slowly digested, thus keeping the stomach filled for a long while.

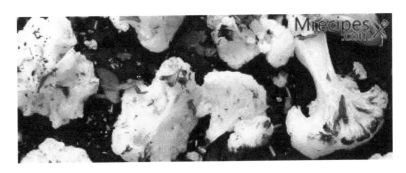

- Course: Side Dish

- Cuisine: American

- Total Time: 2 hours

- Preparation Time: 5 minutes

- Cooking Time: 2 hours

- Serving Size: 6 servings

- Nutritional Value Per Serving

  - Calories: 129 calories

  - Carbohydrates: 8 g

  - Protein: 3 g

  - Fats: 11 g

Equipment Used:

- Electric Smoker

Ingredients:

1. Cauliflower head 1 big
2. Salt 1 tsp
3. Olive Oil 3 tsp
4. Pepper 1 tsp
5. Balsamic Vinegar 3 tbsp

Instructions:

- Preheat the electric Smoker at 225∘F. Fill the water tray and the woodchip tray accordingly.
- Cut the cauliflower head into small florets and wash them with cold water.
- In a bowl, mix the olive oil, balsamic vinegar, salt, and pepper.
- Toss the cauliflower florets in the bowl.
- In an aluminum tray, layer the cauliflower florets and put them in the Smoker.
- Smoke for 2 hours, turning the florets once midway.
- Take out after two hours and serve as a side dish.

5.20. Smoked Cherry Tomatoes

Smoked cherry tomatoes are not a dish in themselves but can form a base for other dishes like salads and pasta. This recipe is included here because smoked cherry tomatoes add flavor and richness to the foods they are mixed with. To add a rich smoky flavor to pasta, you can add cherry tomatoes. Adding smoked cherry tomatoes to a salad hive is the required kick to the otherwise boring salad. Smoked cherry tomatoes are uses as a side dish in Middle Eastern food commonly.

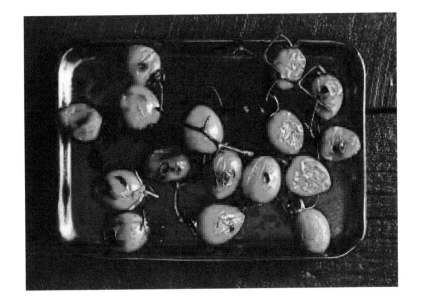

- Course: Side Dish

- Cuisine: American

- Total Time: 1 hour 5 minutes

- Preparation Time: 5 minutes

- Cooking Time: 1 hour

- Serving Size: 4 servings

- Nutritional Value Per Serving

  - Calories: 25 calories

  - Carbohydrates: 3.6 g

  - Protein: 1.1 g

  - Fats: 0.5 g

Equipment Used:

- Electric Smoker

Ingredients:

1. Cherry Tomatoes 300g

Instructions:

- Preheat the electric Smoker to 225∘F. Fill half of the water tray of the Smoker and fill in the wood chips.

- Wash the cherry tomatoes with cold water and spread them on a paper towel.

- Arrange the cherry tomatoes in the aluminum tray and put them in the Smoker.

- Leave the tomatoes for 60 minutes and then take them out.

- You will observe that the cherry tomatoes have burst open, and the juices are oozing out.

- Do not waste the juices; these juices also give off a smokey and delicious taste to salads and pasta.

5.21. Sweet and Spicy Chicken Wings

Chicken wings are another crowd favorite. This recipe used a lot of spices and cut the overpowering spicy flavor; sugar is used. The sugar gives a sweet taste and a crispy finish with its caramelization. This is a perfect dish if you are planning to host a barbecue party.

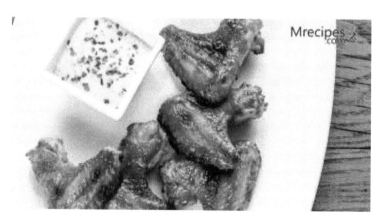

- Course: Lunch

- Cuisine: American

- Total Time: 1 hour 50 minutes

- Preparation Time:20 minutes

- Cooking Time: 1 hour 30 minutes

- Serving Size: 4 servings

- Nutritional Value Per Serving

  - Calories: 356 calories

  - Carbohydrates: 23.9 g

  - Protein: 15.6 g

  - Fats: 22.7 g

Equipment Used:

- Electric Smoker

Ingredients:

1. Chicken wings 2.5 kg

2. Salt 2 tsp

3. Pepper 1 tsp

4. Onion Powder 1 tsp

5. Garlic Powder 1tsp

6. Paprika ¼ cup

7. Cayenne Pepper 1 tsp

8. Brown Sugar ½ cup

Instructions:

- Wash the chicken wings with cold water and trim them.

- If you wish, you can break the wings in half or keep them full. Depends on your preference.

- Next, mix the paprika, salt, pepper, onion powder, garlic powder, sugar, and cayenne pepper in a big mixing bowl.

- Toss the chicken wings into this spice rub. Use your hands to coat the chicken wings with the spice rub.

- Turn on the electric Smoker at 250∘F. Put water in the water tray and fill the wood chip tray with wood chips.

- Let the Smoker preheat for 15 minutes.

- Meanwhile, take out the grill from the Smoker and arrange the wings on the grill.

- Put in the wings in the Smoker and smoke for 2 hours. Check the internal temperature of the chicken should be 165∘F.

- Take out the chicken wings and serve them hot.

5.22. Herbal Chicken Wings

This is a delicious recipe of chicken wings that has a strong flavor of herbs and spices. This recipe is inspired by French cuisine. Make this recipe to enjoy the Parisian feel in the comfort of your own house.

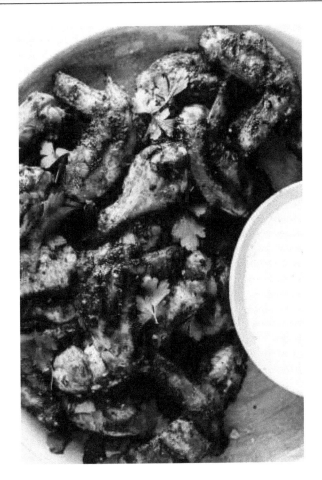

- Course: Lunch

- Cuisine: American

- Total Time: 3 hours 20 minutes

- Preparation Time: 10 minutes

- Cooking Time:

- Serving Size: 4 servings

- Nutritional Value Per Serving

  - Calories: 220 calories

  - Carbohydrates: 0 g

  - Protein: 18 g

  - Fats: 16 g

Equipment Used:

- Electric Smoker

Ingredients:

1. Chicken Wings 2.5 kg
2. Olive oil ½ cup
3. Garlic 2 cloves minced.
4. Rosemary Leaves 2 tbsp
5. Fresh basil leaves 2 tbsp.
6. Lemon Juice 2 tbsp
7. Salt 1 ½ tsp
8. Pepper 1tsp
9. Oregano 2 tbsp

Instructions:

- Prepare the chicken wings by trimming them. Wash the wings under cold running water.
- It is your choice to break the wings into half or use them as it is.
- In a large mixing bowl, add all ingredients and herbs and make a smooth mixture.
- Save half and toss the chicken wings in the other half.
- Use your hands to toss the wings in the mixture so that it is evenly applied.
- Preheat the electric Smoker at 250°F and prepare it with water and wood chips.
- Arrange the wings on the smoker racks and smoke them for two hours.
- The doneness is determined by achieving a 165°F temperature internally.
- Take out the wings and serve them hot.

5.23. Smoked Redfish

In this fish, we are using a dry brine technique. This is an easy and quick recipe; however, it requires the fish to marinate overnight. If you are planning to call guests over, you can prepare the fish fillets in advance.

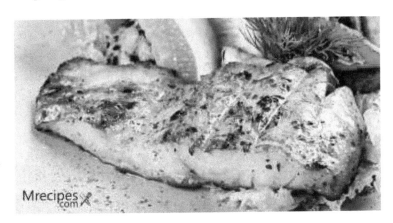

- Course: Lunch

- Cuisine: American

- Total Time: 2 hours 10 minutes

- Preparation Time: 10 minutes

- Cooking Time: 2 hours

- Serving Size: 6 servings

- Nutritional Value Per Serving

  - Calories: 160 calories

  - Carbohydrates: 2 g

  - Protein: 18 g

  - Fats: 4 g

Equipment Used:

- Electric Smoker

Ingredients:

1. 2 redfish fillets with skin 600g
2. Salt half cup
3. Black pepper 1tsp
4. Lemon Zest 1 tsp
5. Garlic powder 1tsp
6. Lemon 2or 4 slices

Instructions:

- Wash the fish fillets with cold running water.
- Next, prepare a rub by mixing all the ingredients and spices.
- Apply the rub on the fish fillets generously. Wrap the fish fillets in cling film and refrigerate them overnight.
- The next day take out the fish fillets and bring them to room temperature.
- Prepare the electric Smoker with wood chips and water. Turn it on at 170∘F.
- When the fillets are at room temperature, wash them and pat them dry.
- Put them in the Smoker for two hours.
- After two hours, check the internal temperature. It should be 140∘F.
- Let the fillets rest for 30 minutes before serving.

5.24. Smoked Dory

This fish is easy to cook and quickly prepared. We will use the dry rub method to prepare the dory fish fillets. This turns out to be a delicious recipe and is a crowd favorite.

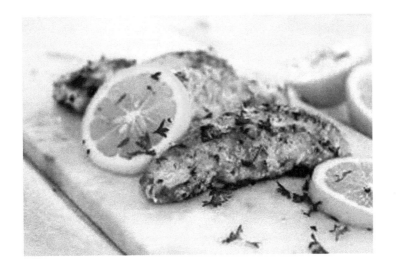

- Course: Dinner

- Cuisine: American

- Total Time: 1 hour 15 minutes

- Preparation Time: 15 minutes

- Cooking Time: 1 hour

- Serving Size: 4 servings

- Nutritional Value Per Serving

    - Calories: 175 calories

    - Carbohydrates: 2 g

    - Protein: 22 g

    - Fats: 8 g

Equipment Used:

- Electric Smoker

Ingredients:

1. 4 fillets of dory fish 800g

2. Onion Powder

3. Salt half cup

4. Black pepper 2tsp

5. Ginger powder 1 tsp

6. Garlic powder 1tsp

7. Coriander for garnish

8. Lemon slices for garnish

Instructions:

- Wash the fish fillets with cold running water.

- Next, prepare a rub by mixing all the ingredients and spices.

- Apply the rub on the fish fillets generously. Wrap the fish fillets in cling film and refrigerate them overnight.

- The next day take out the fish fillets and bring them to room temperature.

- Prepare the electric Smoker with wood chips and water. Turn it on at 220◦F.

- When the fillets are at room temperature, wash them and pat them dry.

- Could you put them in the Smoker for two hours?

- After one hour, check the internal temperature. It should be 160◦F.

- Let the fillets rest for 30 minutes before serving.

- Garnish the fish fillets with coriander and lemon slices for serving.

5.25. Herbal Smoked Salmon

Salmon is one fish variety that is consumed very often among people. The reason for this is that it is an excellent source of protein, and it cooks easily. Smoked salmon is something that you can enjoy at family dinners and other gatherings. You can never go wrong with smoked salmon.

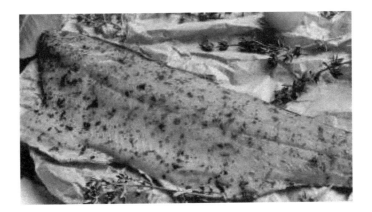

- Course: Dinner

- Cuisine: American

- Total Time: 4 hours 30 minutes

- Preparation Time: 30 minutes

- Cooking Time: 4 hours

- Serving Size: 4 servings

- Nutritional Value Per Serving

    - Calories: 210 calories

    - Carbohydrates: 0 g

    - Protein: 22.3. g

    - Fats: 12.3 g

Equipment Used:

- Electric Smoker

Ingredients:

1. Salmon fillets 750 g

2. Salt ¼ cup

3. Sugar ¼ cup

4. Water ½ cup

5. Black Pepper 2 tbsp

6. Lemon 2 slices

7. Fresh dill chopped 1 bunch.

Instructions:

- Prepare the marinade for the fish. In a flat dish, pour water, salt, sugar, and pepper. Mix them well.

- Soak the fish fillets in the marinade and cover them with dill and lemon slices.

- Wrap the fillets in cling wrap and refrigerate overnight.

- The next day, prepare the Electric Smoker. Put the wood chips and water in the water tray.

- Turn on the electric Smoker at 180∘F. Put the fish fillets on the grill and smoke for four hours.

- In this recipe, we are smoking the fish at a lower temperature for a longer time. If you have a time constraint, you can use a higher temperature for a shorter period.

- Check the doneness of the fish by inserting the thermometer. The internal temperature must be 130∘F.

- Take out the fish and let it rest for 30 minutes before serving.

5.26. Smoked Stuffed Mushroom

These stuffed mushrooms can be served by themselves and can be served as a side dish as well. Try this recipe, and you will not be disappointed.

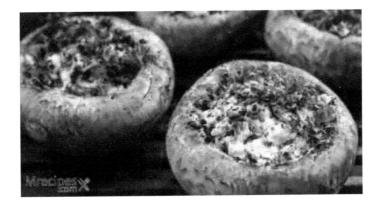

- Course: Side Dish

- Cuisine: American

- Total Time: 1 hour 15 minutes

- Preparation Time: 20 minutes

- Cooking Time: 55 minutes

- Serving Size: 6 servings

- Nutritional Value Per Serving

    - Calories: 320 calories

    - Carbohydrates: 22 g

    - Protein: 8 g

    - Fats: 7 g

Equipment Used:

- Electric Smoker

Ingredients:

1. Button Mushrooms with stem 24 mushroom

2. Onion 1 minced

3. Garlic 2 cloves minced.

4. Salt ½ tsp

5. Black Pepper 1 tsp

6. Breadcrumbs ¾ cup

7. Parmesan cheese ¾ cup

8. Olive Oil 1/3 cup

9. Parsley ¼ cup

Instructions:

- Preheat the electric Smoker at 250°F. Put the wood chips in the tray and water in the water tray.

- In a saucepan, put in some olive oil and sauté the onion and garlic in it.

- In another mixing bowl, mix the breadcrumbs, cheese and salt and black pepper.

- Cut the stems of the mushrooms and chop them. Add the chopped stems to the saucepan with the onion and garlic and cook for one minute.

- Set an aluminum tray and set the mushroom heads up-side-down in a layer.

- Mix the onion, garlic, and mushrooms into the cheese mixture.

- Put a spoonful of mixture on the mushroom heads.

- Put the mushrooms in the Smoker and smoke for 45 minutes.

- Take out the mushrooms and let them rest for 20 minutes before serving.

5.27. Smoked Chicken Breast

This is a simple recipe and can never go wrong. Easy to make and delicious to taste. You can prepare this overnight and smoke it the next day. Family and friends will enjoy it alike.

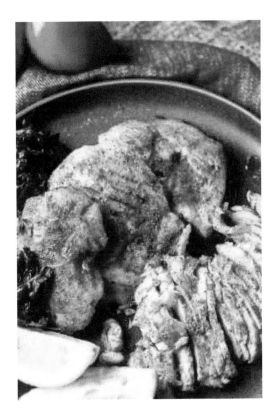

- Course: Dinner

- Cuisine: American

- Total Time: 5 hours

- Preparation Time: 20 minutes

- Cooking Time: 4 hours 30 minutes

- Serving Size: 4 servings

- Nutritional Value Per Serving

    - Calories: 280 calories

    - Carbohydrates: 2 g

    - Protein: 23 g

    - Fats: 4 g

Equipment Used:

- Electric Smoker

Ingredients:

1. 4 chicken breast pieces 1 kg
2. Black pepper 2 tsp
3. Salt 2 tsp
4. Lemon Juice 4 tbsp
5. Paprika 2 tbsp

Instructions:

- Wash the chicken breast pieces. It is your choice to remove the skin or keep it.
- Pat the chicken dry.
- In a flat dish, mix the salt, pepper, paprika and lemon juice.
- Apply the mixture generously on the chicken and wrap the pieces with cling wrap and leave it in the refrigerator overnight.
- The next day, prepare the electric Smoker with the wood chips and water. Preheat the Smoker at 180°F.
- Bring the chicken fillets at room temperature and wash them under cold running water.
- Pat the chicken dries with paper towels and arrange them on the racks of the Smoker.
- Smoke the chicken for about 4 hours and 30 minutes.
- Check the temperature of the chicken. It will be done when the internal temperature reaches 165°F.
- Take out the chicken and let it rest for 30 minutes before serving.
- Serve with your choice of side dishes.

Conclusion

This book gives you a detailed overview of the usage and benefits of an Electric Smoker. An electric smoker is a brilliant appliance that has been created following present-day needs. In the busy lifestyle we lead today; no one has the time or energy to sit around a barbeque all day to prepare food. This appliance is a cookery solution keeping up with times. Reading the book will give you clear instructions and illustrations to guide you through understanding the appliance. The recipes shared are precise and straightforward. Tried and tested tips and tricks are shared for your convenience. The beginners and the regular Electric Smoker users will benefit from this book alike.

The recipes mentioned in this book are all tried and tested, and all have amazing results. The quantities mentioned will not disappoint you. Even the first-time user of the electric Smoker can create these recipes like a pro. But patience is the key. Most of the recipes take longer than five hours, and the temptation to check on your dishes may ruin the dish. Checking on your dish repeatedly means that you will open the smoker time and again, which will cause the temperature to fluctuate and might cause the recipe to produce unsuccessful results.

Using an electric smoker is a wonderful experience, but sometimes it feels a bit overwhelming. Without guidance, you might feel lost. This book will help you in this situation. Read this book and become a pro at using the electric Smoker.

9 781802 2457